Laboratory and Diagnostic Tests with Nursing Implications

Laboratory and Diagnostic Tests with Nursing Implications

Joyce LeFever Kee, MSN, RN

Associate Professor
Coordinator, Undergraduate Field of Study
College of Nursing
University of Delaware
Newark, Delaware

With the assistance of

Helen Liang Tang, BS, MT (ASCP), CLS

Assistant Professor
Medical Technology
School of Life and Health Sciences
University of Delaware
Newark, Delaware
(Reviewer [Part I] and Contributor)

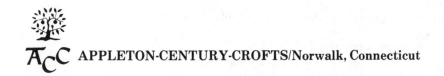 APPLETON-CENTURY-CROFTS/Norwalk, Connecticut

83 84 85 86 87/10 9 8 7 6 5 4 3 2

Prentice-Hall International, Inc., London
Prentice-Hall of Australia, Pty. Ltd., Sydney
Prentice-Hall of India Private Limited, New Delhi
Prentice-Hall of Japan, Inc., Tokyo
Prentice-Hall of Southeast Asia (Pte.) Ltd., Singapore
Whitehall Books Ltd., Wellington, New Zealand

Library of Congress Cataloging in Publication Data
Kee, Joyce LeFever.
    Laboratory and diagnostic tests with nursing implications.

    Includes bibliographies and index.
    1. Nursing.   2. Diagnosis, Laboratory.   I. Tang, Helen L.
[DNLM: 1. Diagnosis, Laboratory—Nursing tests.
QY 4 K26L]
RT48.K43   1983   616.07'5   82-11353
ISBN 0-8385-5583-7

Cover and text design: Jean M. Sabato

PRINTED IN THE UNITED STATES OF AMERICA

This book
I dedicate in
loving memory of
Connie O'Neill
for her
inspiration and encouragement

Contents

Preface

The advances made in identifying health care needs through communication and assessment skills and technology have greatly increased in the last several decades. Nurses are active participants in identifying health needs and providing quality care. Nursing responsibilities are forever increasing. Nurses should understand laboratory and diagnostic tests and attend to their nursing implications—i.e., assessment, nursing judgment, teaching, and interaction.

For the past ten years I have been stating that nursing needs a book on laboratory/diagnostic tests that "spells out" nursing implications. Because of the increasing number of nursing functions, the nurse needs to identify quickly the responsibilities related to ordered laboratory/diagnostic tests. Today this is especially true, with the numerous tests being performed. This book, *Laboratory and Diagnostic Tests with Nursing Implications,* is designed to be a quick reference book for nurses and for other health professionals. The format is similar to that of a book by Govoni and Hayes, *Drugs and Nursing Implications,* with emphasis on nursing implications.

In this book there are nearly 200 current laboratory/diagnostic tests, and these are considered to be today's commonly performed tests. The book is divided into two parts. Part I covers laboratory tests and Part II covers diagnostic tests. The tests in both sections are arranged in alphabetic order so that tests can be rapidly located without the use of an index. However, there is an index for cross-reference.

Each test is arranged in seven subsections: the name(s) of the test, normal range/finding, description, clinical problems, procedure, factors affecting laboratory or diagnostic results, and nursing implications with rationale. Following the name(s) and initials for each test there may be names of other closely associated tests. *Normal range/finding* values are given for children and adults. The *description,* brief and concise, focuses on background data, general purpose, and pertinent information related to the test. *Clinical problems* include disease entities, drugs, and foods that cause or are associated with abnormal tests results. *The procedure* is explained with a rationale for the test and gives pertinent steps which the nurse and other health professionals can follow. *Factors affecting laboratory or diagnostic results* alert the nurse to the important factors that could cause an abnormal test result. The last subsection for each test, and the most valuable part, concerns the *nursing implications with rationale.* For the *laboratory tests,* nursing implications are listed for decreased and for elevated abnormal results. For most of the *diagnostic tests,* nursing implications are given as "pre-test" and "post-test."

The introduction chapter, "The Importance of Specimen Collection and Handling," by Helen L. Tang, Assistant Professor at the University of Delaware, describes pertinent general information that nurses need to know in the collection of specimens. It would be helpful to nurses (students and graduates) if they read the chapter first. Professor Tang gives many suggestions and answers to questions nurses frequently ask or should ask.

This test is appropriate for students in various types of nursing programs—i.e., graduate students in Master of Nursing programs and students in baccalaureate, diploma, associate degree, and practical nursing programs. This book should be most valuable to the RN and LPN in hospital settings (ICU, Emergency Room, and general floors), clinics, and in independent nursing practice.

The list of references used in Part I follows the last laboratory test and the list for Part II follows the last diagnostic test. The numbers which appear at the end of the *Description* section for each test are reference numbers. Also included is a bibliography of all the references used in Parts I and II. There are three appendices: "Abbreviations of Measurements Used for Normal Values," "Abbreviations for Laboratory and Diagnostic Tests," and "Laboratory Test Values for Adults and Children." The detailed index should be most helpful for locating the page of a test when the test name is different than the alphabetic listing used here.

Acknowledgments

My sincere thanks and deepest appreciation go to the following people: Helen L. Tang, Assistant Professor, Medical Technology in the School of Life and Health Sciences, University of Delaware, Newark, Delaware, contributor and a reviewer (reviewing all the laboratory tests) for Part I of this book; Susan Keri Jonas, MD, gastroenterologist, for reviewing the GI diagnostic tests; Josephine M. Piccone, PhD, nuclear physicist, for reviewing all the nuclear tests: John D. Miller, RT, Chief Technologist, V.A. Medical Center, for reviewing the radiologic tests; Geraldine M. Oldham, RCPT, Senior Cardiopulmonary Technologist, V.A. Medical Center, for reviewing the pulmonary function tests; Diane L. Wharry, EEG technician, V.A. Medical Center, for reviewing the electroencephalography test; Sheila Wentling, Special Technician, CAT department, Wilmington Medical Center, Wilmington, Delaware, for detailed information on CT scans; and Ann Dowling, supervisor, Pulmonary Function Laboratory, Wilmington Medical Center, for detailed information on pulmonary function tests. I also wish to extend my sincere appreciation to four outstanding medical technicians who reviewed my long list of laboratory tests and gave me feedback on tests that were obsolete, replaced by other tests, seldom or never ordered, named inaccurately, or had not been but should be included. The four are Peggy Sue Brandi, Chief Technologist, V.A. Medical Center; Nancy Bristol, Laboratory Manager, Crozer–Chester Medical Center, Chester, Pennsylvania; Rose Hilger, Laboratory Manager, Professional Clinical Laboratory, Wilmington, Delaware; and Helen L. Tang, Assistant Professor, Medical Technology, University of Delaware.

For secretarial assistance, I wish to extend my sincere thanks to Maureen Brady for typing the major part of the book on the word processor, Katherine E. Kee for typing the beginning of the manuscript, and Betty Armstrong for her help with the typing as needed. My sincere appreciation also goes to John F. Allison, Executive Editor, Appleton-Century-Crofts, for his helpful suggestions and support, and to Dean Edith Anderson, College of Nursing, University of Delaware, for her support. And last but not least, to my dear husband, Ed, an avid sailor, my love and appreciation for his support.

Laboratory and Diagnostic Tests with Nursing Implications

THE IMPORTANCE OF SPECIMEN COLLECTION AND HANDLING

Helen Liang Tang

Laboratory results are used to assist the physician in the diagnosis, prognosis, and monitoring of the patient in the course of treatment. Presently, there are more than 6,000,000 clinical laboratory tests performed each year in the United States, at an annual rate of $20,000,000.[21] The increase in volume can be attributed to new scientific knowledge and the development of automated technology.

On one hand, this progress has led to the improvement of the selectivity, accuracy, sensitivity, and precision of laboratory measurements.[19] On the other hand, the combination of analytic methods and automated instruments makes each laboratory a unique department. Such uniqueness often causes confusion for the physicians who order the tests and for the nurses who must transfer the orders to the laboratory and must frequently be responsible for the collection, handling and delivery of the analytic specimens. For this reason, the medical team should establish some form of cooperative plan, educational program, or manual to facilitate communication among themselves so that the goal of quality health care can be met. Such a goal has provided the impetus for writing this book.

The purpose of this first chapter is to assist nurses and professionals in better understanding the responsibilities of a medical laboratory and to emphasize the reasons that patient preparation, specimen collection, handling, preservation, and transport are important. Any one of these activities can be a limiting factor in the accuracy and reliability of the final result. Hence the duties mentioned above must be considered to be as crucial as the analysis itself. As the sources of error are eliminated, we can better serve the patient.

To assist nurses in selecting the appropriate requisition form, in contacting the proper section of a laboratory for inquiries, and in delivering a specimen promptly, it would be beneficial to first explain the general divisions and duties of a clinical laboratory.

THE PATHOLOGY LABORATORY AND ITS SECTIONS

Pathology is the study of the nature and cause of disease which involves changes in structure and function. The roles of a pathologist are to:[23]

1. Provide supervision in the medical laboratory.
2. Evaluate laboratory results.

1

3. Identify disease.
4. Evaluate treatment.
5. Ascertain the cause of death by means of autopsies.
6. Advance medicine through research.

The pathology laboratory in a modern hospital is usually divided into two major branches (anatomic and clinical) from which sections have evolved. Such divisions are necessary to simplify management, to concentrate the skills of specialists in one area, to reduce the duplication of equipment, and to conserve space.[24] The subdivision is primarily based on the material to be examined and the methods employed in the analyses.[13]

The two major branches and their subdivisions are as follows.[23,40]

Anatomic Pathology

This is the field of pathology that deals with structural changes. The changes may be apparent through the study of tissues with the naked eye (gross examination) or with the aid of a microscope (microscopic examination.)

Histology. Histologic technicians prepare the frozen sections and surgical and autopsy tissues by slicing them to less than paper thickness, mounting them on slides, and finally staining them with special dyes. The slides are then examined, evaluated, and interpreted by a pathologist.[23]

Cytology. Instead of tissue sections, single cells are investigated in the cytology department. The cytotechnologists are trained to do the preliminary screening by recognizing the minute abnormalities in color, size, and shape of cell substances—for example, the familiar "Pap smear." Any suspicious smears are checked by a pathologist.[40]

Clinical Pathology

This is the field of pathology that applies to the solution of clinical problems, and especially the use of laboratory methods in clinical diagnosis. In addition to the pathologist, the laboratory is staffed with technicians (associate degree), medical technologists (baccalaureate degree), and scientists with specialization (master's or doctorate degree). As a team, they perform a wide variety of tests for the prevention, diagnosis, and treatment of disease.

There are six major sections in a clinical pathology laboratory, as follows.

Blood Bank (Immunohematology).[40] The responsibilities of a blood bank is to obtain, preserve, and select properly matched blood for transfusion. The sources of blood may be donors who come directly to a blood bank in the hospital or donors from a local or regional blood donor center. The blood is typed and screening tests are performed to ascertain its qualification as "donor blood."

A patient requiring blood is typed and his blood is cross-matched with the donor's blood. Likewise, transfusion of special blood components—such as packed red blood cells, plasma, leukocytes, platelets, and antihemophilic globulins—also require specialized handling and cross-matching.

If the blood of a patient (recipient) is found to be incompatible with that of a donor, the blood bank must identify the incompatible factor(s) or antibodies. This necessitates further cross-matching(s) until the compatible blood is found. These processing procedures are time-consuming and require patience, professional skills, expert judgment, and *absolute* accuracy in technique and record keeping.

Whenever a transfusion is requested, it is essential that the laboratory be notified immediately, in view of the possible incompatibility problem. The search for compatible blood for a problem recipient may extend beyond a local or regional area. Time can be a critical factor in the life-or-death situation of an acute bleeder with an incompatibility problem.

Clinical Chemistry. The chemistry section performs analyses on whole blood, serum, plasma, urine, and other biologic specimens such as the cerebrospinal fluid, amniocentesis fluid, pleural fluid, peritoneal fluid, and feces. A majority of the chemical determinations are quantitative.

The number of inorganic and organic tests is constantly being expanded. Many older methods are being modified or replaced by new ones with better precision and accuracy. There may be several analytic methods available for a single constituent (plasma glucose can be quantified by at least six different methods). Furthermore, the same chemical method may be analyzed using several types of equipment. (It is not unusual to find three different instruments in a chemistry laboratory for quantifying glucose, all using the same "enzymatic" principle—one to be part of the admission profile, another for STAT work, and a third, manual or single-method analyzer that may be more economical.)

From the foregoing discussion, it is no wonder that the amount of information on policy, procedures, and reference values in the chemisty section can be overwhelming. It should be the responsibility of the laboratorians to inform and educate the nonlaboratory medical staff whenever new or modified tests or protocols are implemented.

The major groups of determinations performed in a clinical chemistry laboratory include:

1. Trace metals—lead, antimony, zinc.
2. Electrolytes—sodium, potassium, chloride, CO_2.
3. pH and blood gases.
4. Minerals—calcium, magnesium, copper, iron.
5. Carbohydrates—glucose, xylose.
6. Lipids—fatty acids, triglycerides, cholesterol.
7. Proteins and amino acids.
8. Electrophoresis and immunoelectrophoresis.
9. Radioimmunoassays.
10. Enzymes.
11. Hormones.

12. Therapeutic drug monitoring.
13. Toxicology—drug abuse.
14. Organ profiles—liver, cardiac, pancreas, kidney.
15. Vitamins.

Some of the chemical determinations are performed manually (by hand), while many others are done by automated equipment. The time required for a clinical result to reach a patient's floor will vary. It is a common practice that when an abnormal value is found, a repeat of the analysis may be indicated just to "double check" the abnormality. This type of precautionary action could result in a delay of the patient's report.

Hematology.[40] Hematologists are responsible for the quantification of cellular components, including the red and white blood cells and platelets. Enumeration of these cellular elements is done electronically. However, many manual methods are still employed, such as the differentiation of cells in the peripheral blood or bone marrow, the erythrocyte sedimentation rate test, and numerous special tests.

Coagulation (hemostasis) studies for the diagnosis and treatment of blood clotting problems are generally an integral part of the hematology section. Some of the common tests are prothrombin time, partial thromboplastin time, fibrinogen level, bleeding time, and factor assays.

In addition to patients with primary hematologic or coagulation problems, patients with secondary problems also require frequent blood test monitoring. The latter group includes those who are on chemotherapy for cancer treatment and cardiac patients who are on anticoagulant therapy. Hence it is not surprising that nursing staff members and their patients have many close contacts with hematology technologists.

Clinical Microbiology.[40] In the microbiology department, a technologist works with a variety of biologic specimens—blood, urine, feces, sputum, cerebrospinal fluid, drainage, transudate, exudates, nail, skin, tissue, and swabs from the throat, wounds, etc. Smears and cultures are essential for the identification of bacteria, funguses, or molds that may be the causative agents of infections. Once a pathogen is identified, the microbiologist also assists the physician in selecting the best chemotherapeutic substance by employing various susceptibility testing techniques.

Microbiologic methods require more time than the methods of other laboratory sections—sometimes hours, days, or even weeks, depending on the characteristic growth pattern of the microbial organism.

Clinical parasitology, the study of disease-producing parasites, is usually incorporated into the functions of the microbiology department. Stool specimens are commonly utilized to search for ova, cysts, and adult parasites. However, other specimens may also be used in parasitic studies—e.g., a blood smear for malaria and urine for trichomonas.

Serology.[11] In conjunction with microbiologic studies, which are designed to detect the disease-causing agent directly, serologic tests are used to detect the causative agent indirectly. At times, it is not possible to isolate the pathogenic organism, as in the subacute or chronic stage of infection.

When a pathogenic microbe (antigen) invades the human body, it stimulates the production of antibodies which can be detected in the serum. The antibodies are specific to the infecting organism.

The serologic techniques include diagnostic tests for syphilis, hepatitis, rheumatoid arthritis, infectious mononucleosis, rheumatic fever, and typhoid fever.

Urinalysis. The smallest but nonetheless an important section of the clinical laboratory deals with the chemical and microscopic study of urine. The components in a routine urine sample must be analyzed within 1 hour after collection. A fresh specimen is valuable in the diagnosis and management of kidney disease, diabetes, liver dysfunction, transfusion reaction, drug toxicity, and genetic disorders in newborns or infants.

With the use of a microscope, some miscellaneous procedures are also performed in the urinalysis section—namely cell counts on cerebrospinal fluid and other aspirate fluids and semen analysis.

REFERENCE VALUES[7,18,41]

To guide physicians in identifying the diseased individual (as separate from the "normals") and to monitor his course of treatment, the clinical laboratory is confronted with the need to establish a list of normal values. Ideally, specimens from every individual in a given population must be analyzed. In practice, this is not possible; hence only a group of apparently healthy individuals are selected, frequently the blood donors. The constituent or analyte* of interest is measured.

Generally, the "normal values" for an analyte are established to include an interval of values that represents 95 percent of a reference sample of apparently healthy subjects. It should be emphasized that these "apparently healthy" individuals are merely assumed to be normal due to the lack of any obvious signs of illness. Normal values may include measurements of both apparently healthy and possibly asymptomatic sick individuals. Due to the ambiguity in defining "normal," Grasbeck recommended in 1969 that the term "reference values" be used to replace the term "normal values."[16]

In the interpretation of a patient's laboratory result, the physician does not allow his evaluation to be restricted by the boundaries of the reference values. Usually, he compares the patient's present value for a given analyte with the patient's previous values (his reference values). Furthermore, a combination of tests may be requested to supplement the diagnosis, along with the patient's clinical findings.[41]

Analyte is another name for a constituent, substance or component.

One of the problems frequently encountered in health care is that medical personnel (and laymen) place a heavy judgment on a single test result, based on the reference values alone. This may lead to erroneous conclusions, for there are numerous factors that could influence a laboratory result other than the patient's clinical status. It is essential that medical professionals understand and be aware of these variables and attempt to eliminate or minimize them so that meaningful interpretation may be achieved.

Recent studies conducted by researchers Statland at al. indicated that numerous factors can bring about variations in the laboratory results.[32] In the following sections, some of the pronounced variables and examples will be discussed. Emphasis will be on blood tests, since they comprised the majority of the diagnostic procedures.

PATIENT CONSIDERATIONS

A value that appears on a laboratory report is assumed to represent the biologic problem for which the test was requested. This is to say that the "specimen represents the patient." Does it? To answer this, one must take into consideration the following variables.[32]

Preparation of the Patient[5]
Most clinical tests do not require extensive patient preparation. However, this should not be seen as a general rule. In fact, this is all the more reason to pay strict attention to those few tests that do. One must be knowledgeable as to why standardization is necessary.

Patient Identification[5,38]
This is simple, and obviously vital—it is the *most important* aspect of any collection. True identification of the patient and correct labeling of the specimen are equally crucial. If possible, let the patient tell you his own name. Then confirm the identification by a second method—e.g., a wrist band. Imagine the serious consequences of giving a pint of blood to the wrong recipient, or obtaining a tube of blood from the wrong patient for an intended cross-matching.

Physical Activity[33]
A laboratory should provide set guidelines for the patient, physician, and nurses in reference to the extent of muscular activities allowed before a specimen is collected. In general, it is advisable that a specimen be collected after a period of basal state. For hospital patients, this is no great concern, since "bed rest" is the norm.

Outpatients could be a problem. The effects of exercise were studied by Statland et al.[33] They reported that after 20 minutes of strenuous exercise by a group of healthy persons, the results of nine serum analyses showed significant changes. For example, serum potassium was decreased by 8 percent, while alanine aminotransferase (ALT or GPT) was increased by 41 percent. Exercise will also cause an increase in other muscle enzymes, namely creatine kinase (CK or CPK), aldolase, and lactate dehydrogenase (LDH).

Patient Posture[5,31,36]

When a specimen drawn from an individual who has been in a recumbent or supine position is compared to one drawn from a recently standing or ambulatory individual, differences in values are obtained in certain analytes. These differences can be attributed to the shift of body fluid from the vascular to the interstitial (tissue) compartment upon standing. This is to say that the vascular compartment is more diluted when one is lying down, due to the increase of water content, than when one is standing. Substances that are most affected by posture are proteins (enzyme, albumin, globulins) and protein-bound substances (triglyceride, cholesterol, calcium, iron).[5]

For example, in a healthy person, the enzyme alanine aminotransferase (ALT) can increase 14 percent in going from a supine to an erect position.[36] To avoid this type of measurement variability, a patient should be advised to avoid prolonged standing prior to a scheduled venipuncture. It takes 20 to 30 minutes for the fluids in the vascular and tissue compartments to establish an equilibrium after a shift in posture.

Diet[5,10,31,33]

Most laboratory tests do not require any special diet or restrictions in diet. On the other hand, there are a number of tests that require very specific guidelines. The patient should be instructed carefully, both verbally and in writing, to be sure he understands the directions. Otherwise, the interpretation of his test results may be meaningless. For example, when a patient is scheduled for a glucose tolerance test, his diet should contain 1.75 g/kg day of carbohydrates for 3 days prior to the test.[5] This is especially significant when a physician attempts to interpret the values of a borderline diabetic.

In certain tests, the patient may be required to avoid a certain drug or food. One of the screenings tests for carcinoid tumor is the urinary 5-hydroxy indole acetic acid (5HIAA) determination. A diet rich in bananas, pineapples, tomatoes, walnuts, or avocados will produce an elevation in 5HIAA levels. All of these foods contain serotonin, which can be metabolized to 5HIAA. To prevent a false positive diagnosis, the patient should be on a restricted diet for 3 to 4 days prior to the urine collection. On the other hand, the patient may give a false negative result if he is taking phenothiazine drugs.[10]

Fasting[5,25,31]

Only a few laboratory tests require that blood be drawn in the fasting state (fasting for 12 to 14 hours before the test). The important tests are worth remembering.

1. Serum glucose, triglycerides, and potassium are elevated after a meal.
2. A diet extremely high in protein will cause a slight elevation in serum and urine urea, urate, and ammonia.

3. A highly unsaturated diet will result in an increase in serum cholesterol.
4. Serum inorganic phosphorus is decreased after a meal.

The above analytes are influenced directly by the diet. There are numerous tests that can be affected due to the high chylomicron (turbidity of the serum due to lipids in the diet). The lactescent serum will interfere with the analytic procedure (an in vitro variable) and frequently result in false positive or negative results. For this reason, blood collection is best carried out at least 4 to 6 hours after a meal.

Furthermore, the established "reference values" are generally derived from fasting specimens. For ideal comparisons, the patient's specimen should be obtained under the same conditions experienced by the reference group.

Drug Interference[5,31,33]

With the increased usage of prophylactic, therapeutic, and adjuvant agents in the present society, it is important for physicians, nurses, and technologists to be aware of the possible effects of these medications on test results. Close communication is essential in dealing with these particular interferences.

A drug may have physiologic (in vivo) effects on an analyte. For example, the pharmacologic effects of oral contraceptives will cause an increased value in the following tests: iron, transferrin, tryglycerides, ceruloplasmin, thyro-binding globulin, and many more.

Some drugs may have toxic effects on the liver and kidney, causing elevation in the results of the organ function tests. Diagnosis and treatment of patients with a primary hepatic dysfunction or renal disease can be difficult and confusing in the presence of drug toxicity.

In addition to the above in vivo effects of drugs, many pharmacologic agents can produce in vitro interference in the testing procedures. These interferences can be attributed to either the parent (original) drug or its metabolites (products of the drug when degraded in the body). Blood, urine, and even other biologic specimens may be altered.

In this book, the author lists many of the frequently encountered drugs and indicates their effects (increase or decrease) on each laboratory test. When the patient is being given a drug that is known to alter the values for a given analyte, the attending physician should whenever possible be made aware of this so that he may discontinue the drug (or postpone its initiation) until the test is completed. If this protocol is not possible, it is essential that the drug(s) taken by a patient be noted on the laboratory requisition.

As the number of medications on the market continues to rise, the laboratory will find it increasingly difficult to avoid this problem. It was impossible to compress all known drug interferences within the limits of this book. For further information, the reader should refer to the comprehensive list of over 15,000 drugs compiled by Young et al., as well as their more than 2000 references on the subject.[43]

COLLECTION CONSIDERATIONS

In the foregoing section, the importance of patient standardization and its relationship to reference values were emphasized. The following section will concentrate on the collection and handling of specimens. The quality of the specimen correlates directly to the quality of care a patient receives.

Laboratory Requisition[3]

Each institution has a characteristic way of structuring and departmentalizing its laboratory. The subdivisions of a laboratory are often reflected in the requisition form. Nursing personnel should consult the laboratory procedure manual so that the proper tests are requested according to the organization's protocol.

Test requests written on an incorrect form may end up in a different section of a laboratory, which will result in a delay in having the request processed.

Generally, the following information should be on a requisition form:

1. Patient's full name: the middle name should be included to avoid confusion in the event that there is another person with the same first and last name.
2. Location: inpatient, room and unit; outpatient, address.
3. Patient's identification number: this second and specific identification can be very useful—for instance, in a blood bank.
4. Patient's age and sex: in evaluating laboratory results, the reference values may differ for age and sex; disease prevalence may be age- or sex-linked.
5. Name(s) of physician(s): name all of the physicians on the case; "panic values" should be called to the attention of the physician ordering the test; a physician may have some specific test guidelines for his patients.
6. Name of the test and the source: reference values may be different for the different biologic specimens (e.g., serum and CSF glucose); in microbiology, it is essential to know the source of a swab.
7. Possible diagnosis: essential for evaluating the laboratory results and selecting the appropriate methodology—e.g., the media selection in microbiology.
8. The date and time the test is to be done: some tests must be scheduled by the laboratory; blood transfusion may require ample advanced notice; patient preparation and diet regulations need to be considered.
9. Special notation: provide relevant information to assist the laboratory— e.g., medications taken; for hormone assay, the point in the menstrual cycle when the specimen was obtained; for microbiology, the patient's sensitivity to drugs.

Blood Collection

General Consideration. According to Page and Culver, a sample of blood is often "regarded as a 'biopsy specimen' of the most widely distributed, most representative, and most easily obtained 'tissue' in the body."[25] It is no wonder that blood samples are the biologic specimens most frequently analyzed in the evaluation of health and disease. In fact, every section of a laboratory uses blood for its analytic work.

The composition of blood is divided into two main parts: (1) the liquid component, plasma, which contains various proteins, carbohydrates, lipids, minerals, gases, and products of metabolism, and (2) the blood corpuscles, which are the individual cells enclosed in membranes and are classified as erythrocytes (red blood corpuscles), leukocytes (white blood corpuscles), and thrombocytes (platelets).[22]

When blood is circulating in the body it is a fluid. When withdrawn from the body, the blood will clot or coagulate. Once it is clotted, it appears to be solid, although the clot still contains the same amount of fluid distributed throughout the clot mass. This fluid in the clotted blood is known as serum. The chemical composition of plasma and serum are identical except for the fibrinogen. In the clotting process the fibrinogen, a soluble protein, is converted to a nonsoluble protein, fibrin. Hence the serum does not contain any fibrinogen, but the plasma does.

Many laboratory tests are performed using the blood serum after the blood clots. As a general rule, the clotted blood after separated from the serum is useless (one exception is that the Lupus Erythematosus (L.E.) preparation and blood bank use both the serum and the clot.

If whole blood in liquid form or plasma is required, an anticoagulant must be added to the blood to prevent coagulation. There are several types of anticoagulants and each serve some specific functions. The details will be covered in a subsequent section.

Too frequently, the terms serum and plasma are used interchangeably among medical personnel. Since the numerical values are identical (except for the presence or absence of fibrinogen) in both types of fluid, it has been acceptable to ignore the technical differences. However, to be technically correct, one must know whether a test is performed on the serum or plasma.

Approaching the Patient. No individual enjoys having his blood taken. A venipuncturist (phlebotomist)—physican, nurse, or technologist—must resort to his psychologic know-how in implementing a positive attitude even when the patient seems frightened, nervous, and hostile. A patient's anxiety will affect some of the laboratory results, such as the adrenal hormones, blood gases, lactate, and nonesterified fatty acids.

Collection Sites. The reference values of certain analytes may differ for blood obtained from veins, arteries, or capillaries. For meaningful interpretation of results, the site of collection should be stated on the laboratory report.

Arterial collection is generally performed by a physician. Except for the blood gas studies, very few requests are made for arterial blood. The potential hazards are greater in obtaining blood from an artery than in obtaining blood from other vessels due to the higher pressure.

Venipuncture has been the method of choice in blood collection. It is assumed that any medical personnel performing venipuncture should be trained properly. The reader will also find the recent guidelines published by the National Committee for Clinical Laboratory Standards (NCCLS) to be extremely informative.[38]*

Capillary blood collection has primarily been the responsibility of the laboratories. This may change in the future in view of the advancements made in the automated instruments. Many of the recent micromethods require smaller specimens. Therefore, capillary blood is assuming a new and important role.

Thomas A. Blumenfield, M.D. of Babies Hospital in New York City has indicated that skin puncture is a procedure of choice in obtaining blood from infants and children less than 2 years old.[3] There is less hazard involved in skin puncture than in venipuncture, provided correct technique is carried out. Venipuncture could increase the risk of lowering the total blood volume in pediatric patients. Probing a vein too deeply may result in cardiac arrest, uncontrolled bleeding, damage to the surrounding tissue, or even infection.

On the other hand, skin puncture techniques are extremely important and should require just as much training, taking of precautions, and practice as venipuncture. The procedure should never be performed by untrained personnel. The following points are extremely crucial for the accuracy of the test and the safety of the patient[27]:

1. Locating the proper zone of the blood vessels on the finger, toe, or heel.
2. Warming the area to assure arterialized blood flow and to avoid tissue fluid contamination.
3. Cleansing the site thoroughly to avoid infection.
4. Avoiding contamination of the specimen with antiseptics.
5. Puncturing the skin to the proper depth to avoid damage to the tissue or bone.
6. Selecting and handling the specimen collection apparatus appropriately.

Intravenous Infusions.[5,36] One must try to avoid collecting a specimen from a patient's intravenous (IV) arm. If this is not possible, request that the IV be turned off 3 to 5 minutes before obtaining the blood. Notation must be made on the laboratory report to indicate that a specimen was drawn from an IV limb.

Tourniquet Application.[31,36,38] In recent years, there has been greater emphasis on the proper techniques of specimen collection as a result of many research data. The reliability of laboratory results is influenced not only by the analytic technique, but also by the way a specimen is collected, how it is handled after the collection, and the time interval between collection and analysis.

One of the very first and important steps is the proper application of a tourniquet. Too frequently, a tourniquet is left on an arm longer than is necessary, which can result in erroneous results. A tourniquet should never be left on for

---

*NCCLS Publications may be obtained from the National Committee for Clinical Laboratory Standards, 711 E. Lancaster Avenue, Villanova, PA 19085.

longer than 1 minute. The stasis caused by the tourniquet application produces a shift of plasma fluid into the interstitial fluid. Variability as a result of the fluid shift was discussed earlier under "Patient Posture." Statland's group found in their study of healthy individuals that a 3 minute tourniquet application, in comparison to the 1 minute, causes an increase of 5 to 10 percent in protein or protein-bound substances—total protein, total lipids, cholesterol, iron, bilirubin, and aspartate aminotransferase.[36]

It should be pointed out that some tests are extremely "pressure sensitive," and in these tests the tourniquet should be released once the vein is located. These tests include blood pH and blood gases and lactate level.

Tourniquets are potential germ carriers. They should be cleansed with antiseptic after each use.

Collection Apparatus.[5] Along with the technological advancements in the laboratory, many changes and improvements have occurred within the past 5 years in the collection, preservation, and handling of blood specimens. Phlebotomy is not merely an art of "hitting a vein" and filling a tube with blood. A venipuncturist should look upon his technique as a critical beginning step in the total analytic procedure. A laboratory result should reflect the exactness of the physiologic state when a specimen is drawn from the patient. If any change takes place in a specimen between the time of collection and the time of analysis, the changes may invalidate the test result.

The objective for improving or modifying some of the collection apparatus— needles, holders, stoppers, tubes, preservatives, anticoagulants, separators, labels—is aimed at stabilizing and/or preventing contamination of the natural analyte. The more a medical professional understands the laboratory procedure, the procurement, and the apparatus, the less the need for a repeat collection. Unlike a hospital manual, this book includes descriptions of many of the common laboratory procedures so that the nurse and other readers will have a greater appreciation as to *why* a certain specimen requires special handling.

Within the last decade, there has been a wide acceptance of "one-step" blood collection with evacuated tubes. In addition to the standardized collection technique in venipuncture,[38] NCCLS has developed guidelines and standards for the collection tubes.[29] Some of these guidelines will be presented, along with background, usage, and key points.

Manufacturers. As of this writing, there are three major companies that produce a variety of collection apparatuses. It is recommended that the venipuncturist use parts all from the same manufacturer, as the parts may not be interchangeable—e.g., the needle and the holder.

MANUFACTURER	TRADE NAME	PRODUCTS
Becton–Dickinson Company (BD)	Vacutainer Brand	Needle, holder, tube
Terumo Medical Corporation	Venoject	Needle, holder, tube
Sherwood Medical Industries	Monoject	Needle, holder, tube

Needles.[38] The most commonly used needles are 20, 21, and 22 gauge. The large gauge number (22) indicates a small needle, and the small gauge number (20) indicates a large needle. Some needles are for single tube collection while others are for multiple tubes. The designation will be on the container of a needle.

For pediatric or geriatric use, or for individuals with small or difficult veins, a syringe with a small needle or a butterfly needle with attached tubing will be more successful in obtaining blood.

Holders for the Evacuated Tubes and Needles.[38] Be sure to select the proper holder for the correct diameter collection tube.

Evacuated Tubes with Color-coded Stoppers.[38] The rubber stoppers are color-coded to indicate the presence (or absence) of different types of additives in the tube. As recommended by NCCLS, the manufacturers also use a common coding system to label each tube for the additive(s) it contains. As new and more specific tubes are produced, one would expect to find a larger variety of colored stoppers, and some even bear multicolored coding.

Although it is helpful to remember the colors and codings for the common tests, it is even more beneficial, and important, to understand why a test requires a particular tube. For instance, when one is confronted with an urgent situation (such as in the emergency room, operating room, or intensive care unit), judgment, instead of memory, is crucial in deciding on the correct tube(s).

ADDITIVES. An *additive* is any substance, either solid or liquid, that is added to a specimen collection container. The two common classes are preservative and anticoagulant.

A *preservative* is a substance that prevents chemical or physical changes in the natural component in the biologic specimen.

An *anticoagulant* is a substance that inhibits clot formation or coagulation. The calcium ion is one of the chemicals required for the coagulation process. The majority of the anticoagulants (citrates, EDTA, oxalates) prevents coagulation by forming a complex molecule with calcium. When calcium is "tied up," blood will not clot. Another important anticoagulant is heparin, which inhibits clotting by preventing the transformation of prothrombin, an inactive enzyme, to thrombin, an active enzyme.

THE RELATIONSHIP OF TYPES OF BLOOD, TESTS, AND COLLECTION TUBES. The three types of blood samples used for laboratory determinations are whole blood, serum, and plasma. Whole blood, collected in an anticoagulated tube, is mainly used for hematologic tests, such as the complete blood count (CBC), or chemical tests whenever a chemical constituent is located within a cell—e.g., glucose-6-phosphodehydrogenase (G6PDH), an enzyme within the erythrocytes. When blood is collected in a plain tube (no additives), it will clot. This semisolid material can *not* be used for hematologic work even though it is whole blood. Clotted whole blood may be used in a blood bank and for typing and cross-matching.

Serum is the liquid component obtained from a clotted or defibrinated blood. Plasma is the liquid component obtained from nonclotted blood due to the addition of an anticoagulating agent in the container. As mentioned previously, serum and plasma are the same except that plasma contains fibrinogen and serum does not.

The advantages of using plasma over serum are:

1. When an analysis must be performed quickly, an anticoagulated tube of blood needs no waiting time for it to clot. An analysis may begin as soon as the blood and plasma are separated by centrifugation. A plain tube of blood, without additives, takes 45 to 60 minutes for a firm clot to be formed.
2. When the concentrations of an analyte differ appreciably in comparing erythrocytes and plasma, it is essential to separate these two components expeditiously by centrifugation to avoid diffusion. Remember: a test result should represent the in vivo condition.

The advantages of using serum over plasma are:

1. Hemolysis is less likely to occur after the blood has clotted completely.
2. When an additive is incorporated into a tube of blood, such a "foreign substance" may cause interference in an analysis and sacrifice the accuracy of the result.
3. Anticoagulated tubes are more costly to produce and have a shorter shelf life.
4. Greater precautions must be exercised with anticoagulated tubes, such as filling the tube to the maximum blood volume because the ratio of blood to anticoagulant is critical to the analysis. A proper amount of mixing of the tube contents is essential. Undermixing may result in clot formation, while overmixing may produce hemolysis.

Unfortunately, there is no single tube that could be used for the many functions of a laboratory. If one is faced with a crucial decision of limiting the selection to three choices, it is the author's opinion that the following combination would be sufficient to accommodate 95 percent of the common tests: a red-top tube (15 ml), a lavender-top tube (7 ml), and a green-top tube (10 ml).

The interior of the collection tubes can be either sterile or nonsterile. Such information is indicated on the label. Nonsterile tubes may be a source of infection, especially when backflow occurs during the venipuncture procedure. To prevent backflow, make sure the venipuncture arm or site is in a downward position and the collection tube is below the level of the needle.[38]

Description of Commonly Used Collection Tubes. A brief outline is given on the individual collection tube. The information provided is intended to serve as a general guideline only. The list of tests included under the usage section is by no means a comprehensive one. They are mentioned for illustrative purposes. Due to the differences in methodology, it is advisable that nursing staff members also consult their institutional procedure manuals.

SERUM TUBES.[29,37,38] When a tube contains no anticoagulant, the blood entering the container will clot within 1 hour. When a tube contains only a preservative that has no anticoagulant effect (e.g., iodoacetate), the blood will also clot. There are two types of serum tubes, both with red color-coded stoppers. One contains no separator, while the other one does.

1. Red-top tube (without separator).
   a. Additive: none.
   b. Code: not applicable (NA).
   c. Usage.
      (1) Blood bank:
         (a) Typing and cross-matching antibodies.
         (b) Identification.
      (2) Chemistry
         (a) Admission profile.
         (b) Inorganic substances.
         (c) Proteins and enzymes.
         (d) Lipid studies.
         (e) Electrophoresis: proteins, lipids.
         (f) Hormones.
         (g) Drug monitoring.
         (h) Radioimmunoassay (RIA).
         (i) Special organ profiles: cardiac, liver, kidney, pancreas.
      (3) Serology: all immunologic tests.
   d. Precautions.
      (1) Blood needs no mixing or inversion since there are no additives in the tube.
      (2) Agitation may produce hemolysis.
2. Red-top tube (with separator).
   a. Additive: none.
   b. Code: NA.
   c. Contents of the tube.
      (1) A gel material will be found on the bottom of the tube. This serves as a barrier that separates the coagulum and serum layer after the process of coagulation and centrifugation.
      (2) Silicon is coated onto the interior wall of the tube to accelerate the clotting process (usually 15 to 30 minutes).
      (3) A special synthetic polymeric stopper is used which minimizes red cell adherence so that the tube can be centrifuged with the stopper on. This feature prevents sample evaporation and aerosol formation during the centrifugation process.
   d. Usage: serology, immunology, and chemistry as discussed under "Red-top tube (without separator)" above.
   e. Precautions.
      (1) *Do not* use the tube for a blood bank because of the possible interference of the gel. False interpretations in typing and cross-matching may result.

(2) The filled tube should be inverted gently five times. Further inversion may cause alterations in sample integrity.

f. Note:

(1) The cost of the separator tube is approximately 50 percent greater than that of the regular red-top tube without separator.

(2) One should be familiar with the brand names of these tubes:

		TUBE CONTENTS		
		Gel	Clot Activator	Cell Repellent Stopper
MANUFACTURER	**TRADE NAME**			
Becton–Dickinson Co. (BD)	Sterile Serum* Separator (SST)	X	X	X
Becton–Dickinson Co. (BD)	Clot Activator Tube (CAT)		X	X
Sherwood Medical Ind.	COVAC	X	X	X
Terumo Medical Corp.	Autosep	X	X	X

PLASMA TUBES.[29,37,38] There are several types of anticoagulant tubes, and each serve specific functions. Some tubes contain a single anticoagulant, while others may contain a preservative and an anticoagulant. These additives may be either a dry powder, a dried solution, or clear solution.

1. Lavender-top tube.
   a. Additives.
      (1) Sodium ethylenediamine tetraacetate (EDTA), dry powder: code N_2E.
      (2) Potassium EDTA, clear solution: code K_3E.
   b. Usage.
      (1) Hematology: complete blood count (erythrocyte and leukocyte counts, differential, hemoglobin, hematocrit, indices), sedimentation rate, platelet count, hemoglobin electrophoresis.
      (2) Immunohematology/blood bank: blood grouping and typing.
      (3) Chemistry: some special tests when plasma, instead of serum, is needed.
   c. Precaution: sodium EDTA, a powder, requires thorough but gentle mixing. This anticoagulant is not as soluble as the liquid potassium EDTA.
   d. Comment.
      (1) EDTA salt is superior in preserving the cellular integrity of both the red and white blood cells in comparison to other anticoagulants.
      (2) EDTA prevents clotting by chelating or binding with the calcium in blood.
      (3) The Microtainer (BD) containing EDTA is used for capillary collection.

*BD also produces a capillary tube for skin puncture (Microtainer).

2. Green-top tube.
   a. Addtives.
      (1) Lithium heparin, dry powder: code LIH.
      (2) Sodium heparin, dried solution: code NAH.
      (3) Ammonium heparin: code NA.
      (4) Sodium heparin with glass beads: code NA.
   b. Usage: chemistry—pH, blood gases, electrolytes, hormones, amino acids, chromosome karyotype, drug level, G6PD, lupus erythematosus (LE) preparation, etc.
   c. Precaution.
      (1) Heparinized blood should not be used for making differential smears in hematology due to the unusual staining property of the cells.
      (2) Heparin salts exist in three forms, as indicated above. A test will be invalidated if the analyte in question is also found as a component of the anticoagulant. For example, a lithium test should *not* be done with the plasma collected in a green-top tube that contains the anticoagulant lithium heparin. But if a green-top tube contains sodium or ammonium heparin, it would be acceptable for lithium analysis.
      (3) For the LE test, blood should be collected *only* in a green-top tube with glass beads. This special tube contains less heparin than the other green-top tubes. The LE factor is inhibited if the heparin concentration is greater than 75 USP units.[4]
   d. Comment.
      (1) Since heparin is a natural psychologic substance found in the blood, it causes the least amount of chemical interference in comparison to other anticoagulants.
      (2) Heparin tubes may be used for many chemical tests (like the serum tubes). However, the laboratory prefers the serum tubes because they are more economical.

3. Blue-top tubes.
   a. Additive.
      (1) Trisodium citrate (0.105 M or 0.129 M): 1:9 ratio, code NC9.
      (2) Trisodium citrate (0.105 M or 0.129 M): 1:4 ratio, code NC4.
   b. Usage.
      (1) Coagulation studies: prothrombin, fibrinogen, factor assays, partial thromboplastin time (PTT).
      (2) Chemistry: plasma hemoglobin.
   c. Precaution.
      (1) For coagulation studies, the tube must be filled to the maximal level; otherwise the inaccurate ratio of blood to anticoagulant will invalidate the test.
      (2) Tissue fluid contamination will cause erroneous results. Ideally, the specimen should be collected without a tourniquet. Furthermore, to avoid tissue fluid contamination, the second tube should be used for coagulation.
   d. Comment: the coagulation process is activated when the blood comes in contact with a wettable surface in the tube. This may result in a falsely low

prothrombin time. Recently, a special nonwettable coagulation tube (BD) was marketed to eliminate this problem.

4. Gray-top tubes.
   a. Additives: may be any of the following five combinations.
      (1) Potassium oxalate/sodium fluoride: code NFX.
      (2) Potassium oxalate.
      (3) Sodium fluoride.
      (4) Sodium fluoride/thymol.
      (5) Iodoacetate/lithium salt.
   b. Usage: mainly for glucose determinations.
   c. Precaution: gray-top tubes may contain various types of additives. All bear the objective of preserving the integrity of the glucose concentration, as in the vivo state. Being a nutrient, glucose is utilized for energy by all cells (erythrocytes, leukocytes, and even bacteria).
      (1) Sodium fluoride is a mild anticoagulant and serves as an excellent preservative by preventing glycolysis (breakdown of glucose).
      (2) Thymol is a microbial inhibitor (prevents bacterial growth).
      (3) Iodoacetate is another glycolytic inhibitor. This preservative can also be used for BUN determinations.
      (4) Potassium oxalate is an anticoagulant.
      (5) In combination, sodium fluoride and potassium oxalate will inhibit glycolysis and allow the blood to be centrifuged immediately. Separation of plasma from the cellular components lessens the chance of the glucose being metabolized.
      (6) Gray-top tubes containing a glycolytic inhibitor (sodium fluoride) should not be used for any enzymatic determinations because the inhibitory effort is directed at the enzyme reactions.
      (7) Red- and green-top tubes may also be used for glucose if the test can be done STAT, but the reliability of the value is still best with the gray-top tubes.

Special Tubes.[37] Some evacuated tubes are restricted for highly specialized testings. They are made to provide better reliability and are frequently much more expensive.

1. Black-top tube.
   a. Additives.
      (1) Sodium oxalate.
      (2) Sodium citrate.
      (3) Sodium heparin.
   b. Usage.
      (1) Coagulation studies (prothrombin test of Quick).
      (2) Sedimentation rate (Wintrobe method).
   c. Comment: black-top tubes are less popular than the blue-top ones for coagulation work. The latter have a wider application for the new coagulation methods.

2. Yellow-top tube.
   a. Additive: a modified Alserver's solution containing dextrose, sodium chloride, and sodium citrate.
   b. Usage: blood bank only.
   c. Comment: the additives preserve the integrity of the many components in the blood. Hence this tube has a longer shelf life than a regular red-top tube for cross-matching.
3. Brown-top tube.
   a. Additive: sodium heparin.
   b. Usage: lead determination only.
   c. Comment.
      (1) This is one of the most expensive tubes manufactured.
      (2) Lead is a ubiquitous chemical in many additives, even the glass itself, and hence can be a source of contamination.
      (3) Unlike the sodium heparin in a regular green-top tube, the chemical in the brown-top tube is highly purified and the lead content is eliminated.
4. Royal blue-top tube.
   a. Additives.
      (1) None (serum).
      (2) Sodium heparin (plasma).
      (3) EDTA.
   b. Usage: zinc, lead, antimony, cadmium, and other trace metals.
   c. Precaution: hemolysis should be avoided, for it will falsely increase the zinc level.
   b. Comment: the royal blue-top tube could be used for either serum or plasma (comments for the brown-top tube also apply here).

Antiseptic Agents.[2,29,39] The commonly used antiseptics are:
1. 70 percent isopropyl alcohol.
2. Povidone–iodine swab (for skin puncture and blood culture).
3. 0.5 percent chlorhexidine gluconate in 70 percent isopropyl alcohol.

The antiseptic agents should be totally removed using plain sterilized gauze or cotton balls before the insertion of a needle. Alcohol antiseptics *should not* be used for blood alcohol level testing. Povidone–iodine *should* be used, but with caution, for it may cause contamination to some chemistry tests—e.g., potassium, phosphate, and uric acid.

Waste Disposal.[29] Clearly labeled containers should be provided to collect the used needles and other wastes. Prompt disposal of these will prevent their reuse or accidental injury. Ideally, a needle cutter should be available for such precautionary purposes.

Specimen Labeling.[38] Once the specimen has been drawn, the tube should be labeled immediately in ink or indelible pencil. The required information on the tube may vary with different institutions. In general, the following must be included.

1. Patient's full name.
2. Floor location (in hospital); address (outpatient)
3. Patient's identification number.
4. Physician's name.
5. Time and date of collection.
6. Initials of venipuncturist.

Note the following.
1. Blood bank specimens must be labeled according to the guidelines set by the American Association of Blood Banks (AABB). It is recommended that the nursing staff consult the laboratory to determine how this can be handled. Positive identification of the blood recipient is of the utmost importance.
2. The laboratory will not accept unlabeled specimens; nor will it accept verbal identification.
3. A specimen should accompany the requisition form.
4. If there are any discrepancies between the requisition and the labeled specimen, a laboratory may refuse to accept the specimen. This practice is important in order to avoid potential medical–legal problems.

Checking the Patient.[38] Before leaving the patient after a venipuncture procedure, check to make sure that bleeding has stopped. If bleeding persists, apply pressure on an adhesive or gauze bandage over the punctured site. When bleeding lasts longer than 5 minutes, a physician should be notified. Special care should also be considered for semiconscious or comatose patients. Hematoma can be hazardous to the patient and can also make subsequent venipuncture more difficult for the patient and the phlebotomist. Specimens collected from a hematoma area may give inaccurate results.

Speciman Handling and Transport.[5,25,38] Many of the blood constituents undergo rapid changes after they leave the body. Specimens must be sent quickly to the laboratory and not left in the patient's room or the nursing station.

In addition to the effects of preservatives in a collecting tube on slowing down deteriorations, chilling the tube by submerging it in ice and water will further preserve the integrity of the analytes. Some of the tests that require this type of special handling include prothrombin time, activated partial prothrombin time (APTT), coagulation factor assays, hormone assays (gastrin cortisol, renin, pressoramines), ketones, lactate, pH, and blood gases.[38]

When the specimen reaches the laboratory, make sure a laboratorian is notified. The time when a specimen arrives in the laboratory is recorded on the requisition form. Every specimen should be handled with the attitude that the patient's life depends on it. There may not be a chance for repeating a specimen collection, as with surgical specimens and special aspirates (CSF, amniocentesis fluid).

Precautions should also be exercised to protect oneself and others from potential pathogen substances. If an infectious disease (hepatitis) is suspected or known, precautionary labels should be attached to the requisition form and the specimen so that proper handling and isolation techniques can be enforced.

Preventing Hemolysis.[22,38] Hemolyzed blood is the major reason for repeating a blood collection, because a hemolyzed sample is unsatisfactory for many chemical tests. Repeat of a venipuncture not only causes unnecessary discomfort to the patient, it results in time and reagent wastes and delay in the initiation of treatment. The following steps will help prevent hemolysis when performing a venipuncture.

1. Be sure the venipuncture site is dry.
2. Avoid using too small a needle.
3. If a syringe is used, (a) make sure the needle has a tight fit to avoid frothing, (b) avoid pulling the plunger back too forcefully, and (c) transfer the blood by first removing the needle from the barrel and then slowly forcing the blood to the side of the glass tube.
4. Avoid drawing blood from a hematoma.
5. Do not agitate a specimen. Mix anticoagulated specimens gently by inversion.

The following steps will help to prevent hemolysis during specimen delivery.

1. Do not hold the specimen too long. Avoid warming the specimen.
2. Do not permit the specimen to freeze.
3. If possible, do not transport specimens in pneumatic tubes.

Microbiologic Specimens

General Considerations. If reliable results are to be obtained from isolating pathogens (disease producing organisms), it is essential that the physician, nurse, and microbiologist work in a cooperative and communicative environment. This is usually accomplished through consultation and the laboratory's provision of a procedure manual. Attention to the details in collecting and transporting the microbiologic specimen is of paramount importance.

The main challenge for a microbiologist is to differentiate the pathogens from the indigenous (normal or commensal) flora. The success or failure of a diagnostic procedure is often dependent on the quality of the specimen. There are several parameters to be consider: the time of collection, the quantity of the specimen, the collection apparatus, and the preservation and delivery of the specimen. All of these factors will facilitate the accuracy and speed of detecting the significant pathogens, reporting the findings, and initiating treatment.

Time of Collection.[11,14] The optimal period for successful isolation of the pathogen is related to the pathogenesis of the disease. For this reason, the patient's clinical history can be extremely useful. Frequently, one is more likely to isolate the causative agent during the acute stage or early onset of the disease. For example, the pathogen responsible for typhoid can be isolated in the blood culture during the first 10 days of the disease but is less likely to be found a week later.[11]

Whenever possible, the specimen should be collected, before the therapeutic agents have been administered. A microbial culture may show no pathogens after an antimicrobial drug has been given. If a specimen is collected under this condition, the microbiology laboratory should be notified so that an attempt can be made to neutralize the effects in the culturing process—e.g., by adding penicillinase to counteract the effect of penicillin.[14]

Collection Techniques.[11,14,39] Normally, the skin, nasopharynx, mouth, lower part of the ileum, cecum, and colon have an abundance of indigenous flora. On the other hand, the blood and cerebrospinal fluid (CSF) are sterile, and microbial flora are not usually found in the muscle, bone, lower bronchi, kidneys, urinary tract, liver, or other vital organs due to efficient defensive mechanisms.[11]

In vivo, the commensal bacteria have a defensive role in denying the pathogens an opportunity to colonize under normal conditions. However, such normal commensalism between man and the indigenous flora may be altered by a person's resistance or the use of immunosuppressive drugs.[11]

The competition for survival between the indigenous flora and pathogens also exists in vitro. When collecting a specimen for the isolation of a pathogen, it is essential to avoid or minimize the contamination of the indigenous flora. When a specimen is contaminated with a large amount of normal flora, it is not only time-consuming to isolate and identify these flora, but accuracy may be sacrificed in the interpretation of the result. Furthermore, this may lead to inappropriate recommendation of an antimicrobial drug.[39]

Some general guidelines are essential in resolving the contamination problem:

1. For collection in which skin contact (wound) is involved, cleanse the area with a disinfectant thoroughly with enough friction to completely void the normal flora before obtaining the culture by swab or syringe. Povidone— iodine and 70 percent alcohol are acceptable antiseptics.
2. A biologic specimen from an internal area may be collected by bypassing the location of normal flora. A throat swab should not touch the tongue, cheeks, or lips.[14]
3. In the collection of a biologic fluid when aspirates are involved (such as blood, exudates, and CSF), be sure the skin and all of the collection apparatus are sterile before the aspiration takes place.[39]
4. Urine collection for microbial culture requires special precautions. The distal urethra and perineum are contaminated with normal flora. The contamination can be eliminated or minimized by first cleansing the tip of the penis, the labia fold, or the vulva with at least two washings of detergents followed by sterile water rinses. The first part of the voiding will flush out the urethra. This urine is discarded. The subsequent midstream

urine is used. Since urine is a rich medium for bacterial growth, it is absolutely essential that the specimen be delivered to the laboratory immediately. If this is impossible, the specimen must be stored in the refrigerator. However, any specimen stored longer than 1 hour is not worth processing for bacterial growth. Even with the above precautions, it is impossible to eliminate all of the normal flora. The microbiologist interprets the disease-causing agent by counting the colonies; the predominant and high-concentration ones are used to determine the drug therapy regimen. Hence it is very important that the collection and transport procedures be followed strictly.[14]

5. Sputum cultures require the cooperation of the patient and proper instructions from the nurses. Saliva is definitely unsatisfactory. It may contain indigenous flora which will obscure the true infecting agent. Any unsatisfactory specimen will be discarded by the microbiologist because it would be costly to process and would provide misleading information.[14]

6. A stool specimen should be collected in a wide-mouth plastic or waxy container. The specimen must be processed within 2 hours after collection; otherwise a preservative must be added to the specimen. When a fecal specimen is unobtainable, a rectal swab is satisfactory. However, if the infection involves the small intestine, isolation of the pathogen may not be reliable.[11]

7. Besides preventing contamination with patient's indigenous flora, it is also essential that external contamination be eliminated. All collection containers should be sterile, so that the original flora will not multiply or decrease in growth.[14]

8. The above general guidelines are by no means comprehensive. Nurses should also consult the laboratory procedure manual for the specifics of their own institution.

Quantity of the Specimen.[14] The amount of specimen needed for isolation and identification of the pathogenic bacteria varies. An amount ranging from 1 to 3 biologic aspirates, such as cerebrospinal, synovial, pleural, or peritoneal fluid. Blood cultures require two to three 10 ml specimens of venous blood taken over a 24 hour period. Other scanty material from the eye, throat, nasopharynx, genitals, or a wound may be submitted on a swab moistened with broth. In general, the greater the amount of specimen, the more complete the microbial examination.

Specimen Labeling.[26] All specimens should be clearly labeled with the following information.

1. Patient's full name.
2. Floor location (in hospital); address (outpatient).
3. Patient's identification number.
4. Physician's name.

5. Time and date of collection.
6. Nature of specimen and site of collection (e.g., swab: wound on left leg). The specimen should be accompanied by a requisition form. There should be no discrepancies between the information provided on the label and that on the requisition slip. See "Requisition Form" above.

Specimen Transport[14]

1. Check the specimen container to be sure there is no leakage. The outer surface of the container should not be soiled by the contents. If it is, disinfect it accordingly. All specimens should be handled with caution to avoid contamination of the nursing staff, the ward clerk, other patients, and laboratory personnel.
2. Prompt delivery of the specimen is essential to preserve the viability of the pathogens and minimize the overgrowth of the commensal organisms.
3. When delay is absolutely unavoidable, the nurse should contact the laboratory for special instructions. Some general guidelines are as follows.
   a. The Culturette,* a disposable sterile plastic tube containing a swab and moistening broth, will provide sufficient moisture for storage for up to 72 hours at room temperature.
   b. A variety of transport media are available to preserve the viability of the microorganism when there is a delay between collection and culturing. A fresh supply is kept by the laboratory.
   c. Anaerobes will not tolerate atmospheric oxygen. These microbes are extremely fragile. Special anaerobic collection devices (gassed out) are required to preserve these pathogens.
4. Some microbes, such as the meningococcus in the cerebrospinal fluid, are very sensitive and fragile at low temperatures. CSF should not be refrigerated. These microbes require immediate culturing. Delay in transporting the CSF to the laboratory is absolutely intolerable.[20]

Urine Specimens

General Considerations.[22] Urine is the most easily obtainable specimen, and the urine assay is one of the simplest assays to perform. The examination of urine provides a great deal of information if the specimen has been collected properly and carefully.

There are four types of specimens, each of which is related to a specific function:

1. The sterile specimen for microbiologic examination, discussed under "Microbiologic Specimens" above.
2. The first morning specimen for routine urinalysis and pregnancy tests.

---

*Becton–Dickinson Co.

3. The random specimen for qualitative determinations—this can be collected any time.
4. Timed or 24 hour specimens for chemical quantification or clearance tests.

Routine Urinalysis.[8] Routine urinalysis is part of the physical examination and an integral part of the admission laboratory work. The preferred specimen is the first morning sample, since it is more concentrated. A sample that is diluted due to increased fluid intake will tend to dissolve some of the cellular components—e.g., red blood cells, pus, and casts.

After a specimen is collected, it should be sent to the laboratory as soon as possible. If delay is unavoidable, refrigeration of the specimen for up to 1 hour is permissible. Further delay may result in the deterioration of certain components due to the normal flora present. Bacterial contamination will cause increased alkalinity (higher pH) due to the breakdown of the urea to ammonia. A decrease in glucose, ketones, bilirubin, and urobilinogen and the deterioration of cellular components are also attributed to the microbial attack. Hence a specimen must be analyzed immediately to ensure reliability of the results.

Vaginal contamination, mucoid discharge, and bleeding will produce false positive results, such as epithelial cells and red blood cells.

Chemical or Qualitative Tests.[8,22] A random specimen, collected anytime, is used for qualitative or semiqualitative determinations. There are usually no restrictions in fluid or food intake. Examples of these assays include calcium, hemoglobin precursors (phorphobilinogen or porphyrins), hemoglobin metabolites (urobilinogen or bilirubin), and some toxic substances such as salicylates.

The pregnancy test, another screening test, should be performed with urine with high specific gravity. Usually the first morning specimen is ideal.

Twenty-four Hour Specimens or Timed Specimens.[8] A timed specimen is utilized for chemical quantitative determinations, including the various kidney function clearance tests. Many substances (e.g., protein, glucose, electrolytes, and hormones) are excreted in a variable concentration during a 24 hour period. A more meaningful comparison can be made between a 24 hour collection and a reference value for the same time interval than with a random specimen.

For proper evaluation of an analyte in a 24 hour sample, it is essential that a complete and accurate collection be made. Patients should be given written instructions for the collection of timed specimens. For example, for a 24 hour collection, the patient is instructed to empty his bladder completely at 8:00 A.M.; this specimen is discarded. All the subsequent specimens, including a final one obtained at 8:00 A.M. the next morning, are collected in a large container.

A preservative, usually an antimicrobial agent, is added into the collection container. The type of preservative depends on the analyte and the methodology employed. All specimens should be refrigerated during the collection period. Specimens should be brought to the laboratory promptly after the collection is completed.

In addition to the general information provided on the label and the requisition slip (see previous sections on specimen labeling), the collection period or interval should be included—e.g., "collection: March 20, 1983, 8:00 A.M. to March 21, 1983, 8:00 A.M."

The total volume and the timed collection interval are factors used in calculating the 24 hour urinary excretion of the analyte. Hence it is of great importance that specimens are recorded accurately and reflect the data for the actual collection.

Fecal Specimens[14,30]

General Considerations. A fecal specimen may be utilized for microbiological studies, parasitic examinations, and chemical determinations. Each type of analysis requires specific guidelines in the collection and handling of the specimens. A preservative required for one test may be inappropriate for any other tests.

Microbiologic Studies. See "Microbiologic Specimens."

Parasitic Examinations[14]

Patient Considerations. Due to the excess crystalline material found in a stool specimen after the use of barium sulfate for radiologic studies, a patient should schedule his parasitic studies for performance prior to the x-ray procedure. The exogenous debris may obscure the parasites.

Intestinal protozoa may not be detected after certain medications are given, such as tetracycline, mineral oil, insoluble antidiarrheal preparations, and bismuth compounds.

Specimen Collection and Transport. Stool for oval, parasite, and cyst examinations should be collected in a clean, wide-mouth container with a tight-fitting lid. The specimen should not be mixed with urine since this may result in destruction of the motile organisms.

For successful isolation of the infective agents, multiple specimens (three to six) are recommended, depending on the type of parasites. A physician may suggest that a specimen be collected after a cathartic, such as a Fleet Phospho-Soda, has been given.

The specimen should be delivered to the laboratory immediately after collection as some organisms require examination within 30 minutes after passage. If delay is unavoidable, the specimen should be divided into three parts.

1. *Unpreserved stool* is used for detecting occult blood and for determining the specimen type, such as liquid, soft, or formed. Knowledge of the consistency of the specimen will assist the parasitologist in searching for a specific developmental stage of the infective protozoon.
2. *Polyvinyl alcohol* (PVA), a fixation solution, is added to a second part. This will preserve the protozoan cysts and trophozoites for later examination. (A commercial kit or vial with PVA is available.)

3. *Ten percent formalin* is added to a third portion of the specimen. Tapeworm eggs, larvae, and protozoan cysts are preserved for a long period in this mixture. Note that the latter two specimens require thorough mixing of the feces and the fixatives.

The collection procedure for pinworms should be part of the laboratory manual.[14] Pinworm can be better diagnosed by using the clear cellophane tape technique than by using the anal swab. The pinworm eggs are deposited on the perianal area during the night by the adult female worm. Therefore, the specimen should be taken in the morning, before bathing.

Chemical Examination.[6] Occult (hidden) blood is the most common chemical determination of the feces. The test reagents are extremely sensitive; even a small trace of blood, such as iron or the myoglobin from red meats in the diet, may give a false positive result. A patient should be on a diet free from meat and fish for 2 days prior to the test.

Random stool specimens are used for several qualitative tests, such as tests for bile pigments and trypsin. No special patient preparation is required.

Twenty-four hour or 3 to 5 day stool collection is required for quantitaive fecal fat determination. The test is primarily used in the investigation of steatorrhea due to any of a variety of such etiologies, such as malabsorption or pancreatic dysfunction. The major concern in this test is the accurate and complete collection of the specimens over the stated period.

Precaution. All fecal specimens must be handled with extreme care, for they represent a potential source of infective material.

THE LABORATORY REPORT

Units of Measurement[12,17]
Just as we are making the transition from our day-to-day conventional units of measurement (inch, pound, quart, Fahrenheit) to the metric system (meter, gram, liter, Celsius), the clinical laboratories are in the process of leaving the metric units for the SI units.

The abbreviation *SI units* stands for the "International System of Units" (Le Système International des Unités). The World Health Organization recommended at the 30th World Health Assembly in 1977 that the medical and scientific community throughout the world adopt the SI unit.[17] The advantage of such conversion is that it will provide a common language among the international scientists so that communication related to measurements will have no ambiguity. Most clinical laboratories in Canada, Australia, and western Europe, as well as most of the American medical journals, are presently using the SI units.[12] The major disadvantage is that all medical staff members must become accustomed to a new set of numerical data, and there is a great potential for misinterpretation. To alleviate this serious problem, most likely both metric and SI units will be reported.

The International System has adopted a number of conventions and units of measurements. This information may be found in many medical reference books, encyclopedias, and dictionaries. Some of the common standardized usage of the SI bears mentioning.[12]

1. A half space, instead of a comma, is used to divide large numbers into groups of three (1 234 000 not 1,234,000).
2. No periods or plural forms are used to symbolize a unit (1 kg, not kg.; 100 kg, not 100 kgs).
3. The degree sign is omitted for temperature scales (25C not 25 °C).
4. The preferred spelling is litre, not liter; metre, not meter.
5. A laboratory report of measurements should include five parameters, including system, component, kind of quantity, value, and unit. For example:

SYSTEM	COMPONENT	KIND OF QUANTITY	VALUE	UNIT
Serum	Total calcium	Concentration	1.2	mmol/l
CSF	Cell	Count	$5 \times 10^6/$	L
Sweat	Chloride	Concentration	60	mmol/l
Blood	Prothrombin	Time	12	S
Urine	Glucose	Concentration	2	+

Types of Measurements[17]

There are three types of analytic measurements performed by a clinical laboratory—namely, qualitative, semiquantitative, and quantitative. In qualitative tests, the physician is interested in the presence or absence of a particular substance, component, material, or microorganism. The results of these tests are given as "yes" or "no," or "positive" or "negative." Examples are the identification of a microorganism, the presence or absence of a toxic chemical, the typing of a blood group, and the identification of an antigen or antibodies.

Semiquantitative tests are those tests that provide some degree of positiveness or negativeness. Frequently, they are estimations judged by visual observation. These tests are subject to human error and therefore may show discrepancies (imprecisions) upon repeated testing. The semiquantitative tests have at least three choices for an answer. Nurses may be familiar with the dipstick test in urinalysis. The urinary glucose may be estimated as negative, 1+, 2+, or 3+. Another way of reporting the results is negative, weakly positive, moderately positive, or strongly positive.

Quantitative tests are those tests that require greater precision (reproducibility) and accuracy. The *exact* measurement of an analyte is given. High quality of methodology and instrumentation and careful techniques must be employed to produce a numeric value. The value obtained represents a specific concentration of an analyte in the biologic specimen. Quantitative measurements entail a great deal of quality control for monitoring and evaluating the reliability of the results. Most hematologic and chemical determinations are of this category.

Interpreting the Laboratory Report

The Patient's Values Versus the Reference Values.[1,7,19,32,42] There are many factors one should take into consideration in evaluating and interpreting a patient's laboratory results intelligently. (The first two items were discussed previously under "Reference Values.")

1. The reference values do not necessarily represent normal individuals.
2. The conditions under which specimens are obtained from individuals in the reference group may be different.
3. There are intrapersonal differences. The concentration of some substances may vary within a day (diurnal variation), from day to day, or from month to month in an individual.
4. Environment may affect an analyte—for example, the lead level may be normally high among certain industrial workers.
5. There are interpersonal differences due to race, age, sex, body surface, nutritional status, ovarian status, emotional state, and geographic location.
6. Some reference values are derived with inadequate numbers of individuals.
7. Multiple methods exist for the determination of an analyte. In some cases, the different methods do not give the same values. This is especially true for the many enzyme analyses.
8. Reference values are established with "apparently healthy" individuals. A chronically ill, undernourished, or nonambulatory person may exhibit normal values that are not related to a specific pathology.

Because of these complex factors, reference values should be used only as an integral part of other clinical parameters in assessing a patient's laboratory report.

Panic Values.[9,28] There are many occasions when a patient's test results fall outside of the reference values. A decision must be made as to whether the attending physician should be notified.

Each laboratory should have a list of the so-called panic, alarm, or critical decision values. When a patient's results appear on this list, the physician or charge nurse must be notified immediately. The "panic value" should be circled in red on the report sheet. Explicit guidelines should be made available to all members of the medical care team, outlining the reporting procedures and actions to be taken.

The panic value policy and list would be different for each institution. In general, the types of tests and intervals to be included are based upon the judgments of the pathology department, input from the medical staff, and recommendations from professional journals.

EXAMPLE: PANIC VALUES*

Chemistry	Less Than	Greater Than
Glucose	40 mg/dl	500 mg/dl
Calcium	7 mg/dl	14 mg/dl
Sodium	120 mEq/L	160 mEq/L
Potassium	2.5 mEq/L	6.5 mEq/L
CO_2	10 mEq/L	40 mEq/L
Lithium	—	1.5 mEq/L
BUN	—	75 mg/dl
Digoxin	0.8 ng/ml	1.6 ng/ml
Blood gases		
pH	7.25	7.55
PO_2	55 mmHg	—
PCO_2	20 mmHg	60 mmHg
Hematology		
PT	—	15 sec above control
PTT	—	20 sec above control
Hematocrit	15%	—
Hemoglobin	6.0 g/dl	—
WBC	2000/μl	—
Platelets	30,000/μl	—

Urinalysis
  Grossly bloody
  >50 WBC/1pf and numerous bacteria
Microbiology
  Blood
  CSF } Positive smear and culture
  AFB
  Parasites: Positive

Reliability of Measurements[1,7,31,32]

In performing any analytic measurements, regardless of how carefully they are done, there is a certain amount of errors or variations. An analytic procedure starts with the preparation of the patient; continues with the collection, handling, and transport of the specimen; and, in the laboratory, ends with the performance of the test and production of a report.

Errors may be of two types, random or systemic. Random error is considered to be due to chance, as with a hemolyzed specimen. The source(s) of error may not be completely identified or controlled. An error of this nature may cause a result to be either higher or lower than the true value (value without errors).

Systemic error is due to variation that is consistent or proportional throughout the analytic procedure. An incorrect test reagent (e.g., one that is too old) will affect all of the results that involved use of this bad reagent and may result in

---

*Average values taken from several hospitals and publications.

lowering of the values. The direction of error is consistent throughout. The sources of error are classified into three areas:

1. Variations due to preparation of the patient—exercise, posture, diet, drug interferences, etc.
2. Variations due to preparation of the specimens prior to the actual measurement—collection, labeling, handling, transport, and storage.
3. Variations due to performance of the analysis—sample identification; choice of methodology; quality of analytic equipment; the analysts' techniques; the physical environment of the laboratory; calculation, interpretation, and recording of results; and charting a report.

The emphasis of this chapter has been on eliminating sources of error in the firs two categories, which are more relevant to nurses' assignments.

The laboratory must concentrate on eliminating all possible sources of error and must be responsible for assuring the reliability of measurements. Such assurance in laboratory medicine is known as quality control, a program with goals of recognizing, minimizing (or eliminating), and controlling errors. Statistical methods are employed in evaluating the precision and accuracy of laboratory measurements.

Each quality control program is designed to accommodate the individual needs of a laboratory. Provision of the details is beyond the scope of this discussion. If a nurse is interested in this important area of health care, she should contact her laboratory.

It should be reassuring to know that before test results are reported to the physician, the laboratory must meet the established quality control guidelines.

The information provided in this chapter offers a means of achieving excellence and reliability in laboratory testing. Accurate and reliable results can only be obtained when the medical team members—the physician, the nurse, the technologist, and other supportive staff—begin with a common attitude that their performances will ultimately benefit the patient.

ACKNOWLEDGMENT

It is a pleasure to acknowledge my gratitude to Lorraine Holton for her expert secretarial assistance with this chapter.

REFERENCES

1. Annino, J.S., & Giese, R.W. *Clinical chemistry, principles and procedures* (4th ed.). Boston: Little, Brown, 1976, pp. 36–43.
2. *BD Lab Notes*, Rutherford, N.J.: Becton Dickinson & Co., 1977, *2*.
3. *BD Lab Notes*, Rutherford, N.J.: Becton Dickinson & Co., 1979, *7*.
4. *BD Lab Notes*, Rutherford, N.J.: Becton Dickinson & Co., 1980, *9*.
5. *BD Lab Notes*, Rutherford, N.J.: Becton Dickinson & Co., 1981, *11*.

6. Bauer, J.D., Ackermann, P.G., & Toro, G. *Clinical laboratory methods* (8th ed.). St. Louis: Mosby, 1974.

7. Bermes, E.W., Erviti, V., & Forman, D.T. Statistics, normal values and quality control. In N.W. Tiez, (Ed.), *Fundamentals of clinical chemistry* (2nd ed.). Philadelphia: Saunders, 1976, pp. 60–102.

8. Bradley, M., Schumann, G.B., & Ward, P.C.J. Examination of urine. In J.B. Henry, (Ed.), *Clinical diagnosis and management by laboratory methods* (16th ed.). Philadelphia: Saunders, 1979, vol. 1, pp. 559–634.

9. Chang, Y.W. Panic value reporting: How well does it work? *Medical Laboratory Observer*, 1981, *13*, 60.

10. Chattoraj, S. Endocrine function. In N.W. Tietz, (Ed.), *Fundamentals of clinical chemistry* (2nd ed.) Philadelphia: Saunders, 1976, pp. 818–20.

11. Collee, J.G., et al. Bacteria, fungi, and viruses. In R. Passmore, J.S. Robson, (Eds.), *A companion to medical studies.* London: Blackwell Scientific Publications, 1970, vol. 1, pp. 18.87–18.93.

12. Conn, R. Laboratory reference values of clinical importance. In B.F., Miller, C.B., Keane, (Eds.), *Encyclopedia and dictionary of medicine, nursing, and allied health* (2nd ed.). Philadelphia: Saunders, 1978, pp. 1132–48.

13. Davidsohn, I., & Carr, M.T.: *A curriculum for schools of medical technology* (5th ed.). Chicago: Registry Board of Medical Technologists of the American Society of Clinical Pathologists, 1964,pp. 5–8.

14. Finegold, S., Martin, W.J., & Scott, E.G. *Bailey and Scott's diagnostic microbiology* (5th ed.). St. Louis: Mosby, 1978.

15. Grannis, G.F., & Statland, B.E. Monitoring the quality of laboratory measurements. In J.B. Henry, (Ed.), *Clinical diagnosis and management by laboratory methods* (16th ed.). Philadelphia: Saunders, 1979, vol. 2, pp. 2049–68.

16. Grasbeck, R., & Saris, N.E. Establishment and use of normal values. *Scandinavian Journal of Clinical and Laboratory Investigation,* 1969, *24* (Suppl. *110*), 62.

17. Henry, J.B., & Lehmann, H.P. SI units. In J.B. Henry, (Ed.), *Clinical diagnosis and management by laboratory methods* (16th ed.). Philadelphia: Saunders, 1979, vol. 2, pp. 2083–85.

18. Hyde, T.A., Mellor, L.D., & Raphael, S.S. Quality control and statistical analysis. In S.S. Raphael, (Ed.), *Lynch's medical laboratory technology* (3rd ed.). Philadelphia: Saunders, 1976, vol. 1, pp. 42–72.

19. Kinney, M. *Mechanization, automation, and increased effectiveness of the clinical laboratory.* Washington, D.C.: DHEW, No. NIH-77-145, 1976, pp. 37–50.

20. Krieg, A. *Cerebrospinal fluids and other body fluids.* In J.B. Henry, (Ed.), *Clinical diagnosis and management by laboratory methods (16th ed.).* Philadelphia: Saunders, 1979, vol. 1, pp. 635–79.

21. Krieg, A., Gambino, R., & Galen, R.S. Why are clinical laboratory tests performed? When are they valid? *Journal of the American Medical Association,* 1975, *233, 76.*

22. McFate, R.P. *Introduction to the clinical laboratory* (3rd ed.). Chicago: Year Book Medical Publishers, HEW, 1972.

23. *What kind of career could I have in a medical laboratory?* National Committee for Careers in the Medical Laboratory, 1972.

24. Newell, J.E. *Laboratory management.* Boston: Little, Brown, 1972, pp. 15–74.

25. Page, L.B., & Daland, G.A. Collection of blood samples. In L.B. Page, P.J. Culver, (Eds.), *A syllabus of laboratory examinations in clinical diagnosis.* Cambridge, Mass.: Harvard University Press, 1962, pp. 21–26.

26. Raphael, S.S., Spencer, F., & Culling, C.F.A. Collection and examination of specimens for microbiological examination. In S.S. Ralphael, (Ed.), *Lynch's medical laboratory technology* (3rd ed.). Philadelphia: Saunders, 1976, vol. 1, pp. 657–78.

27. Schmidt, R.M., et al. *NCCLS document TSH-4: Collection of diagnostic blood specimens by skin puncture.* 1979.

28. Skendzel, L.P. How to judge the quality of laboratory testing. *Tech. Improve. Serv.* Chicago: American Society of Clinical Pathologists, 1976, *27,* 12.

29. Slockbower, J.M., et al. *NCCLS document ASH-1: Standard for evacuated tubes for blood specimen collection* (2nd Ed.), Villanova, PA: NCCLS, 1980.

30. Smith, J.W., & Gutierrez, Y. Medical parasitology. In J.B. Henry, (Ed.), *Clinical diagnosis and management by laboratory methods* (6th ed.). Philadelphia: Saunders, 1979, vol. 2 pp. 1731–1814.

31. Statland, B.E., & Winkel, P. Sources of variation in laboratory measurements. In J.B. Henry, (Ed.), *Clinical diagnosis and management by laboratory methods* (16th ed.). Philadelphia: Saunders, 1979, vol. 1, pp. 3–28.

32. Statland, B.E., Winkel, P., & Bokeland, H. Factors contributing to intra-individual variation of serum constituents, I: Within day variation of serum constituents in healthy subjects. *Clinical Chemistry,* 1973, *19,* 1374.

33. Statland, B.E., Winkel, P., & Bokelund, H. Factors contributing to intra-individual variation of serum constituents, II: Effects of exercise and diet on variation of serum constituents in healthy subjects. *Clinical Chemistry,* 1973, *19,* 1380.

34. Statland, B.E., Winkel, P., & Bokelund, H. Factors contributing to intra-individual variation of serum constituents, III: Use of randomized duplicate serum specimens to evaluate sources of analytical error. *Clinical Chemistry,* 1974, *20,* 1507.

35. Statland, B.E., Winkel, P., & Bokelund, H. Factors contributing to intra-individual variation of serum constituents, IV: Effects of posture and tourniquet application on variation of serum constituents in healthy subjects. *Clinical Chemistry,* 1974, *20,* 1513.

36. Statland, B.E., Winkel, P., & Bokelund, H. Factors contributing to intra-individual variation of serum constituents, V: Short term day-to-day and within-hour variation of serum constituents in healthy subjects. *Clinical Chemistry,* 1974, *20,* 1520.

37. *Scientific apparatus catalog 82/83.* Baltimore: VWR Scientific, 1982, pp. 208–18.

38. Van Assendelft, O.W. *NCCLS document ASH-3: Standard procedures for collection of diagnostic blood specimens by venipuncture,* Villanova, PA: NCCLS, 1980.

39. Washington II, J.A. Medical bacteriology. In J.B. Herny, (Ed.), *Clinical diagnosis and management by laboratory methods* (16th ed.). Philadelphia: Saunders, 1979, vol. 2, pp. 1574–1638.

40. Williams, M.R., & Lindberg, D.S. *An introduction to the profession of medical technology* (3rd ed.). Philadelphia: Lea and Febiger, 1979, pp. 38–41.

41. Winkle, P., & Statland, B.E. Reference values. In J.B. Henry, (Ed.), *Clinical diagnosis and management by laboratory methods* 16th ed.). Philadelphia: Saunders, 1979, vol. 1, pp. 22–52.

42. Winkle, P., Statland, B.E., & Bokelund, H. Effects of time of venipuncture on variation of serum constituents. *American Journal of Clinical Pathology,* 1975, *64,* 433.

43. Young, D.S., Pestaner, L.C., & Gibberman, V. Effects of drugs on clinical laboratory tests. *Clinical Chemistry,* 1975, volume 21 (5), ID-432D.

PART I
Laboratory Tests

A

ACETONE, KETONE BODIES (Serum or Plasma)

NORMAL RANGE
Adult: *Acetone:* 0.3–2.0 mg/dl; 51.6–344.0 μmol/liter (SI units). *Ketones:* 2–4 mg/dl.
Child: *Newborn to 1 week:* slightly higher than adult. *Over 1 week:* same as adult.

DESCRIPTION
Ketone bodies are composed of three compounds—acetone, acetoacetic (diacetic) acid, and betahydroxybutyric acid—which are products of fat metabolism and fatty acids. Ketone bodies result from uncontrolled diabetes mellitus and starvation due to increased fat catabolism instead of carbohydrate metabolism. In diabetic ketoacidosis, the serum acetone is > 50 mg/dl.

Ketones are small and excretable in the urine. However, the elevation is first in the plasma or serum, then in the urine. Serum acetone (as ketones) is useful in monitoring acidosis due to uncontrolled diabetes or starvation, since the serum level will decrease towards normal before the urine test (acetest) does.[9,11,30]

CLINICAL PROBLEMS
Elevated level *(↑ 2.0 mg/dl):* diabetic ketoacidosis, starvation/malnutrition, vomiting and diarrhea, heat stroke, exercise.

PROCEDURE
Collect 3 to 5 ml of venous blood in a red-top tube.
There is no food or drink restriction.

FACTORS AFFECTING LABORATORY RESULTS
Contamination can cause false positive results.

NURSING IMPLICATIONS WITH RATIONALE

Elevated level (↑ 2.0 mg/dl)

Relate elevated serum acetone levels to diabetes acidosis and starvation. Many of the diet programs call for high-protein and low-carbohydrate (CHO) diet. Daily CHO intake of less than 100 g can result in ketosis (excess ketone bodies) due to the substitution of fat metabolism for energy.

Explain to the patient the purpose of the test. Explanation could be brief, such as "to determine if there is any fatty acid accumulation in the blood from diabetes" or a similar response.

Obtain a history from the patient concerning his diet. If the patient is on a reducing diet, the elevated serum level (ketosis) could be due to a low-CHO diet.

Assess for signs and symptoms of diabetic ketoacidosis, such as rapid, vigorous breathing; restlessness; confusion; sweet-smelling breath; and a serum acetone level greater than 50 mg/dl.

Check the urine for ketone bodies. An acetest is usually performed and is positive.

ACID PHOSPHATASE (ACP) (Serum)
Prostatic Acid Phosphatase (PAP)

NORMAL RANGE
Adult: 0.1–2U/dl (Gutman), 0.5–2 U/dl (Bodansky), 0.1–5 U/dl (King–Armstrong), 0.1–0.8 U/dl (Bessey–Lowry), 0.0–0.8 U/L at 37°C (SI units).
Child: 6.4–15.2 U/L.

DESCRIPTION
The enzyme acid phosphatase is found in the prostate gland in high concentration. It is frequently referred to as PAP—prostatic acid phosphatase. There is another acid phosphatase that differs from PAP and is present in red blood cells (erythrocytes) and platelets. Various methods are used to distinguish between prostatic ACP and erythrocyte (RBC) ACP. Tartaric acid will inhibit prostatic ACP, and if the serum ACP level is still elevated, nonprostatic origin would be suspected.

An elevation of serum acid phosphatase above 5 Bodansky units can indicate carcinoma of the prostate gland. When prostatic cancer has metastasized beyond the capsule to the bone or elsewhere, the ACP will be markedly elevated. If prostatic cancer is confined to the capsule, the serum ACP will usually be normal. The use of radioimmunoassay for ACP is helpful when prostatitis or benign prostatic hypertrophy is suspected, for it shows a rise above the normal level—not, however, the high level that is seen in prostatic cancer. A markedly elevated alkaline phosphatase level may cause a false high serum acid phosphatase level.[8,11,14,27,30,36]

CLINICAL PROBLEMS
Decreased level: Down's syndrome. *Drug influence:* fluorides, oxalates, phosphates, alcohol.
Elevated level: carcinoma of the prostrate, multiple myeloma, Paget's disease, cancer of the breast and bone, sickle cell anemia, cirrhosis, chronic renal failure, hyperparathyroidism, benign prostatic hypertrophy, osteogenesis imperfecta, myocardial infarction. *Drug influence:* androgens in females, clofibrate (Atromid-S).

PROCEDURE
Collect 5 to 10 ml of venous blood in a red-top tube.
Hemolysis should be prevented and the specimen should be taken to the laboratory immediately. ACP is heat- and pH-sensitive. If the specimen is exposed to air and left at room temperature, there will be a decrease in activity after 1 hour.
There is no food or drink restriction.

FACTORS AFFECTING LABORATORY RESULTS
Hemolysis of the blood sample.
Drugs that decrease the serum ACP level (see *Drug Influence* above).
Blood specimen exposed to air and room temperature for longer than 1 hour.

NURSING IMPLICATIONS WITH RATIONALE

Decreased level
Know which drugs can cause a decreased serum acid phosphatase.

Elevated level
Recognize clinical problems associated with an elevated serum acid phosphatase level.
A high serum ACP level occurs with metastasized prostatic cancer.

Explain to the patient that the purpose of the test is to determine if there is an excess amount of this enzyme in the blood.

Inform the patient that he can eat and drink prior to the test. NPO is not necessary.

Indicate on the laboratory slip if the patient had a prostate examination 24 hours before the test. Prostatic massage or extensive palpation of the prostate can elevate the serum ACP.

Check the serum ACP following treatment for carcinoma of the prostate gland. With surgical intervention, the serum level should drop in 3 to 4 days; following estrogen therapy (when the treatment is successful), it should drop in 3 to 4 weeks. If serum ACP has not been ordered, a reminder or suggestion to the physician may be necessary.

Notify the laboratory before the serum acid phosphatase is drawn, so that immediate attention will be given to the specimen.

ALANINE AMINOTRANSFERASE (ALT) (Serum)
Serum Glutamic Pyruvic Transaminase (SGPT)

NORMAL RANGE
Adult: 5–35 U/ml (Frankel), 5–25 mU/ml (Wroblewski), 8–50 U/ml at 30°C (Karmen), 4–36 U/L at 37°C (SI units).
Child: similar to adult.

DESCRIPTION
ALT/SGPT is an enzyme found primarily in the liver cells and is effective in diagnosing hepatocellular destruction. Serum ALT levels can be higher than levels of its sister transferase (transaminase), AST/SGOT, in cases of acute hepatitis and liver damage from drugs and chemicals, with its serum levels reaching to 200 to 4000 U/L. ALT is used for differentiating between jaundice caused by liver disease and hemolytic jaundice. With jaundice, the serum ALT levels of liver origin can be higher than 300 units; from causes outside the liver, the levels can be less than 300 units.

ALT/SGPT levels are frequently compared with AST/SGOT levels for diagnostic purposes. ALT is increased more markedly than AST in liver necrosis and acute hepatitis, while AST is more markedly increased in myocardial necrosis (acute myocardial infarction, or MI), cirrhosis, cancer of the liver, chronic hepatitis, and liver congestion. ALT levels are normal or slightly elevated in myocardial necrosis. The ALT levels return more slowly to normal range than AST levels in liver conditions.[8,11,14,27,30,31,34,36]

CLINICAL PROBLEMS
Decreased level (↓ 4U/L [SI]): exercise. *Drug influence:* salicylates.

Elevated level (↑ 36U/L [SI]): Highest increase: acute (viral) hepatitis, necrosis of the liver (drug or chemical toxicity). Slight or moderate increase: cirrhosis, cancer of the liver, CHF, acute alcohol intoxication. *Drug influence:* Antibiotics: carbenicillin, clindamycin, erythromycin, gentamicin, lincomycin, mithramycin, spectinomycin, tetracycline. Narcotics: meperdine (Demerol), morphine, codeine. Antihypertensives: methyldopa, guanethidine. Other: digitalis preparations, indomethacin (Indocin), salicylates, rifampin, flurazepam (Dalmane), propranolol (Inderal), oral contraceptives (progestin–estrogen), lead.

PROCEDURE

Collect 5 to 10 ml of venous blood in a red-top tube.

Avoid hemolysis of blood specimen.

There is no food or drink restriction.

Drugs administered to the patient that can cause false positive levels should be listed on the laboratory slip along with the date last given.

FACTORS AFFECTING LABORATORY RESULTS

Hemolysis of the blood specimen.

Aspirin can cause a decrease or increase of serum ALT.

Drugs that increase the serum ALT level (see *Drug Influence* above).

NURSING IMPLICATIONS WITH RATIONALE

Elevated levels *(↑ 36U/L [SI units])*

Relate the patient's serum ALT/SGPT to clinical problems. A high serum elevation (> 2000 units) can be indicative of liver necrosis from toxic agents or from acute viral hepatitis.

Compare ALT and AST levels if both have been ordered. ALT is a better indicator of acute liver damage and will be at higher levels than AST in liver necrosis and acute hepatitis.

Explain to the patient that this test aids the physician in determining whether the liver is secreting more of this enzyme into the blood than it should. Further explanation may be needed.

Instruct the patient that he may eat and drink before blood is drawn.

Check for signs of jaundice. ALT levels rise several days before jaundice begins if it is related to liver damage. However, if jaundice is present and serum ALT levels are normal or slightly elevated, the liver may not be the cause of the jaundice.

ALCOHOL (Ethyl or Ethanol) (Serum or Plasma)

NORMAL RANGE

0.00 percent (normal)—no alcohol; < 0.05 percent or 50 mg/dl—no significant alcohol influence; 0.05 to 0.10 percent or 50 to 100 mg/dl—alcohol influence is present; 0.10 to 0.15 percent or 100 to 150 mg/dl—reaction time affected; > 0.15 percent or 150 mg/dl—indicative of alcohol intoxication; > 0.25 percent or 250 mg/dl—severe alcohol intoxication.

DESCRIPTION

Serum or plasma alcohol level is drawn on unconscious patients as requested by physician to determine whether alcohol intoxication is present. A person whose blood alcohol level is under 0.05 percent or 50 mg/dl is not legally considered to be under the influence of alcohol, according to the National Safety Council on Alcohol and Drugs.

Chronic use of alcohol has a number of metabolic and toxic effects on the body. Alcohol is toxic to the liver, and constant use can cause liver disease and malnutrition.

The test may also be requested to rule out metabolic disease or overdose due to other drugs when patient is unconscious.[8-11,27,30,31]

CLINICAL PROBLEMS
    Decreased level *(< 0.05 percent):* mild alcohol consumption.
    Elevated level *(> 0.15 percent):* moderate to severe alcohol intoxication; chronic alcohol consumption—cirrhosis of the liver, malnutrition, folic acid deficiency, red cell macrocytosis, leukopenia, acute pancreatitis, gastritis, hypoglycemia, hyperuricemia. *Drug influence:* alcohol and drug interaction—(1) increases the effects of sedatives, hypnotics, narcotics, and tranquilizers (especially chlordiazepoxide—Librium—and diazepam—Valium), depressing the CNS response, (2) antagonize the action of Coumadin and Dilantin.

PROCEDURE
    Collect 5 to 10 ml of venous blood in a green-, red-, or gray-top tube.
    Cleanse the venipuncture area with benzalkonium and then wipe the solution off with a sterile swab or sponge. *Do not use* alcohol or tincture to cleanse the area.
    Write on the specimen and laboratory slip the date and time the blood specimen was drawn. The signatures of the collector and a witness must be included on the tube.

FACTORS AFFECTING LABORATORY RESULTS
    Methyl alcohol (wood alcohol) and isopropyl alcohol (rubbing alcohol) can cause elevated serum alcohol levels and are very toxic.
    Cleansing the venipuncture site with alcohol or tincture can cause inaccurate results.
    Alcohol and drug interaction (see *Drug Influence* above).

NURSING IMPLICATIONS WITH RATIONALE

Elevated level (↑ 0.15 percent or 150 mg/dl)
Provide safety measures to prevent physical harm to the patient when the serum alcohol level is greatly increased. Side rails may be needed while the patient is sleeping off the effects of alcohol.
Recognize clinical problems which develop from chronic alcohol consumption.
Teach the patient not to consume alcoholic beverages when taking sedatives, hypnotics, narcotics, tranquilizers (Valium, Librium), anticonvulsants, (Dilantin), and anticoagulants (Coumadin). Alcohol and tranquilizers can depress respirations and can cause respiratory arrest.
Encourage the patient to attend AA meetings for chronic alcoholism.

ALDOLASE (ALD) (Serum)

NORMAL RANGE
    Adult: 3–8 U/dl (Sibley–Lehninger), 22–59 mU/L at 37°C (SI units).
    Infant: 12–24 U/dl (four times).
    Child: 6–16 U/dl (two times).

DESCRIPTION
    Aldolase is an enzyme present most abundantly in the skeletal and cardiac muscles. This enzyme monitors skeletal muscle diseases—i.e., muscular dystrophy, dermatomyositis, and trichinosis—but is not elevated in muscle disease of neural origin, such as multiple sclerosis, poliomyelitis, and myasthenia gravis.
    Serum aldolase is helpful in diagnosing early cases of Duchenne's muscular dystrophy before clinical symptoms appear. Progressive muscular dystrophy may cause elevated

serum aldolase levels 10 to 15 times greater than normal. In late stages of muscular dystrophy, the enzyme level may return to normal or below normal. Serum aldolase is not the most effective diagnostic test for myocardial infarction (MI), since there is only a slight rise. Following an acute MI, it peaks (two times normal) in 24 hours and returns to normal in 4 to 7 days.[9,11,34,36]

CLINICAL PROBLEMS

Decreased level *(↓ 3 U/dl):* late muscular dystrophy.

Elevated level *(↑ 8 U/dl):* early and progressive muscular dystrophy; trichinosis; der- dermatomyositis; acute myocardial infarction; acute hepatitis; cancer of gastroin- testinal (GI) tract, prostate, and liver; lymphosarcoma; leukemia. *Drug influence:* alcohol, cortisone, narcotics.

PROCEDURE

Collect 3 to 5 ml of venous blood in a red-top tube. Unhemolyzed serum must be used when measuring for aldolase.

There is no food or drink restriction.

FACTORS AFFECTING LABORATORY RESULTS

Hemolysis causes false positive results.

NURSING IMPLICATIONS WITH RATIONALE

Elevated level (↑ 8 U/dl [S-L], ↑ 59 mU/L at 37°C)

Recognize the purpose for monitoring aldolase levels. This is a useful test for diagnosing muscular disorders.

List any drugs the patient is receiving which can elevate the serum aldolase level on the laboratory slip.

Explain to the patient the reason for the aldolase blood test—e.g., to diagnose muscular problems.

Inform the patient that food and drink (with the exception of alcohol) are not restricted.

Check serum aldolase results and plan your nursing care according to symptoms present and psychologic needs.

ALDOSTERONE (Serum)

NORMAL RANGE

Adult: 1–9 ng/dl (supine position), radioimmunoassay method (RIA).

DESCRIPTION

Aldosterone is the most potent member of all mineralocorticoids produced by the adrenal cortex. Its major function is to regulate sodium, potassium, and water balance according to body needs. Aldosterone promotes sodium reabsorption from the distal tubules of the kidney and potassium and hydrogen excretion. With sodium reabsorp- tion, water is retained. Eighty to ninety percent of aldosterone is inactivated in the liver.

This hormone responds to various changes in the body. When there is a sodium loss and a water loss, aldosterone is secreted for re-establishing sodium and water balance. Other factors that influence aldosterone secretion are hyperkalemia (serum potassium excess) and an increased renin secretion (an enzyme produced by the kidney). Potassium excess causes an increase in aldosterone secretion; thus more sodium is reabsorbed from the kidney and potassium is excreted. Renin promotes aldosterone secretion, which causes more sodium and water to be retained and body fluid to be increased. Stress will increase aldosterone secretion. Hypernatremia (serum sodium excess) inhibits aldosterone secretion.

Serum aldosterone is not the most reliable test, since there can be fluctuations due to various influences. If the patient is in a lying-down position (supine), serum aldosterone will be lower than if he were in a sitting or standing position. A 24 hour urine test is considered more reliable than a random serum aldosterone collection. Also, the concentration of aldosterone in blood is low and difficult to measure. Several serum aldosterone levels may be requested.[14,17,19,27,31,36]

CLINICAL PROBLEMS

Decreased *(↓ 1 ng/dl—supine position):* overhydration with ↑ Na, severe hypernatremia (sodium excess), high-sodium diet, adrenal cortical hypofunction, diabetes mellitus, licorice ingestion (excessive), glucose—excess infusion.

Elevated *(↑ 9 ng/dl—supine position):* dehydration, hyponatremia (sodium deficit), low-sodium diet, essential hypertension, adrenal cortical hyperfunction, cancer of the adrenal gland, cirrhosis of the liver, emphysema, severe CHF. *Drug influence:* Diuretics (furosemide [Lasix] and others), hydralazine (Apresoline), Diazoxide (Hyperstat), nitroprusside.

PROCEDURE

Collect 5 ml of venous blood in a red-top tube. A green-top tube (heparinized) may also be used.

The patient should be in a supine position for at least 1 hour before the blood is drawn. Write the date and time on the specimen. Aldosterone levels exhibit circadian rhythm, with peak levels occurring in the A.M. and lower levels in the afternoon.

Food and drinks are not restricted, but excess salt and interfering substances (licorice) should not be consumed before the test. Normal salt intake is suggested.

FACTORS AFFECTING LABORATORY RESULTS

A high- or low-salt diet.

Prolonged use of potent diuretics.

Excessive licorice and glucose ingestion.

Sitting or standing position when blood is drawn.

NURSING IMPLICATIONS WITH RATIONALE

Decreased level (↓ 1 ng/dl—supine position)

Relate a decreased serum aldosterone level to hypernatremia, high salt intake, excessive licorice ingestion, and Addison's disease.

Mark on the specimen and laboratory slip the time the blood specimen was drawn. Aldosterone levels are frequently lower in the afternoon.

Elevated level (↑ 9 ng/dl—supine position)

Relate an elevated serum aldosterone level to hypovolemia (dehydration), low-sodium diet (< 2 g), excess use of diuretics, Cushing's disease, and stress.

Explain to the patient that the purpose of the test is to determine whether there is an excess aldosterone secretion in response to specific clinical problems, and that he must remain in the supine position for at least 1 hour before blood is drawn to prevent a false serum elevation.

Assess the patient for signs and symptoms of dehydration—i.e., poor skin turgor, dry mucous membrane, shock-like symptoms, and for hyponatremia when the serum aldosterone is elevated.

Compare the serum aldosterone and the 24 hour urine aldosterone results if both have been ordered.

Record vital signs on the patient. A rapid pulse and later a drop in blood pressure could be indicative of hypovolemia (fluid volume deficit).

ALDOSTERONE (Urine)

NORMAL RANGE

    Adult: 6–25 µg/24 hours.

DESCRIPTION

See the *Description* for *Aldosterone (Serum)*.

    Aldosterone causes sodium reabsorption and potassium excretion from the distal tubules of the kidney. Aldosterone secretion from the adrenal cortex influences sodium retention, fluid retention, fluid volume, and blood pressure.

    A 24 hour urine aldosterone has an advantage over serum aldosterone, since fluctuation levels can be eliminated. Both urine and serum aldosterone will be increased by hyponatremia, a low-salt diet, and hyperkalemia. Likewise, hypernatremia, a high-salt diet, and hypokalemia will decrease urine and serum aldosterone. A urine sodium test may be ordered for comparison purposes.[15,16,19,27,30,31]

CLINICAL PROBLEMS

    Decreased level *(↓ 6 µg/24 hours):* same as for serum aldosterone.

    Elevated level *(↑ 25 µg/24 hours):* tumors of the adrenal cortex or primary aldosteronism, same as for serum aldoesterone.

PROCEDURE

    Collect a 24 hour urine specimen in a large container with a preservative (usually 1 g boric acid tablet).

    Keep container on ice or refrigerate.

    Have the patient void or discard the urine before the test begins.

    Label the container with the exact date and time for the test (e.g., 4/9/83, 7:35 A.M. to 4/10/83, 7:35 A.M.).

FACTORS AFFECTING LABORATORY RESULTS

    Twenty-four hour urine container not refrigerated or iced.

    Failure to place all urine collected in a 24 hour period in the urine container.

    Toilet paper and feces in the urine.

NURSING IMPLICATIONS WITH RATIONALE

Explain to the patient why a 24 hour urine specimen collection is required. The purpose of this test is to determine if there is an excess or a decrease in aldosterone secretion.

Instruct the patient how to collect the 24 hour urine specimen. All urine should be
saved after the initial urine is discarded. The urine must be kept on ice or refrigerated. Toilet paper or feces should not be in the urine.

Answer the patient's questions concerning the test and the collection procedure.

Check at specified times to determine whether the urine collection is being properly
obtained.

ALKALINE PHOSPHATASE (ALP), With Isoenzyme (Serum)

NORMAL RANGE

Adult: 20–90 U/L at 30°C (SI units), 25–97 U/L at 37°C (SI units), 2–4 U/dl
(Bodansky), 4–13 U/dl (King–Armstrong), 0.8–2.3 U/dl (Bessy–Lowry).
Child: *Infant:* 40–300U/L. *Older child:* 60–270 U/L, 15–30 U/dl (King–Armstrong),
5–14 U/dl (Bodansky).

DESCRIPTION

Alkaline phosphatase is an enzyme produced mainly in the liver and bone; it is also
derived from the intestine, kidney, and the placenta. The ALP test is useful for determining liver and bone diseases. The liver excretes alkaline phosphatase into the bile,
and with obstructive biliary disease, either extrahepatic or intrahepatic, the serum
enzyme level is greatly increased. In cases of mild liver cell damage, the ALP level may
be only slightly elevated, but it could be markedly elevated in acute liver disease. Once
the acute phase is over, the serum level will promptly decrease, whereas the serum
bilirubin would still remain increased. For determining liver dysfunction, several
laboratory tests are performed—i.e., bilirubin, leucine aminopeptidase (LAP), 5′-
nucleotidase (5′-NT), and gamma-glutamyl transpeptidase (GGTP).

With bone disorders, the ALP level is increased because of abnormal osteoblastic
activity (bone cell production). In children, it is not abnormal to find high levels of
alkaline phosphatase during the prepuberty and puberty ages due to bone growth.

Isoenzymes of ALP are used to distinguish between liver and bone diseases. The heat
stability test is the most common method used to differentiate between the two, ALP[2]
of bone origin and ALP[1] of liver origin. ALP[2] of bone origin is inactivated by heat,
whereas liver ALP[1] is heat-stable. The placenta has the greatest heat stability. A heat
stability greater than 30 percent suggests liver origin, and a heat stability of less than
30 percent suggests bone origin.

Electrophoretic analysis of ALP is becoming available, and in the future, this method
should be a more effective means of identifying ALP isoenzymes.[8,11,14,27,30,34,36]

CLINICAL PROBLEMS

Decreased level *(↓ 25 SI U/L):* hypervitaminosis D, hypothyroidism, malnutrition,
scurvy (vitamin C deficit), hypophosphatasia, pernicious anemia, placental insufficiency. *Drug influence:* fluoride, oxalate, propanolol.
Elevated level *(↑ 97 SI U/L):* obstructive biliary disease (jaundice), cancer of the liver,
hepatocellular cirrhosis, hepatitis, hyperparathyroidism, leukemia, cancer of the bone
(breast and prostate), Paget's disease, osteitis deformans, healing fractures, multiple
myeloma, osteomalacia, late pregnancy, rheumatoid arthritis (active), GI ulcerative
disease. *Drug Influence:* intravenous (IV) albumin; antibiotics—erythromycin, lincomycin, oxacillin, penicillin; colchicine; methyldopa (Aldomet); allopurinol;
phenothiazine tranquilizers; indomethacin (Indocin); procainamide; oral contraceptives (some); tolbutamide; isoniazid (INH); PAS.

PROCEDURE
Collect 5 to 10 ml of venous blood in a red-top tube.
There are no restrictions on food and drink.
Drugs elevating the alkaline phosphatase levels may be held for 24 hours. The nurse should check with the physician before holding drugs, and the drugs taken should be listed on the laboratory slip.
State the age of the patient.

FACTORS AFFECTING LABORATORY RESULTS
Drugs which increase or decrease the serum alkaline phosphatase levels (see *Drug Influence* above).
Administered IV albumin can elevate the serum ALP to five to ten times its normal value.
Age of the patient—i.e., youth and aged cause a serum increase.
Late pregnancy to 3 weeks postpartum could cause a serum ALP elevation.

NURSING IMPLICATIONS WITH RATIONALE

Decreased level (↓ 20 U/L)
Recognize clinical problems that are related to a serum alkaline phosphatase deficit.

Elevated level (↑ 97 U/L)
Correlate the elevated serum alkaline phosphatase levels of patients to their clinical problems—i.e., liver and bone diseases.
Explain to the patient that the blood test is to determine liver function or disorders of the bone, or any other expected clinical problem.
Instruct the patient that he may eat or drink prior to the blood test.
Record on the laboratory slip whether the patient received IV albumin 5 days prior to the blood test.
Determine whether the age of the patient could be responsible for the elevated serum ALP. Rapid bone growth in children between the ages of 11 and 14 can cause a high alkaline phosphatase level. Older adults may have a slightly elevated serum ALP.
Recognize that pregnant women in the third trimester may have a slight to moderate serum ALP elevation.
Check the results of other ordered liver tests to determine the significance of the elevated serum alkaline phosphatase in liver diseases.
Assess for clinical signs and symptoms of liver disease and bone disease.

ALPHA-1-ANTITRYPSIN (α-1-AT) (Serum)
Alpha-1-trypsin Inhibitor

NORMAL RANGE
Adult: 159–400 mg/dl, 1.0–1.6 g/L.
Child: *Newborn:* slightly below range. *Infant:* similar to adult range.

DESCRIPTION
Antitrypsin or trypsin inhibitor is a protein produced by the liver. It inhibits specific proteolytic enzymes that are released in the lung by bacteria or by phagocytic cells. A deficiency of homozygous antitrypsin (heredity-linked) permits proteolytic enzymes to

damage lung tissue, thus cause emphysema. A low circulating α-1-AT level can also be associated with liver disease (rare) in children and young adults.

With inflammatory conditions, alpha-1-antitrypsin serum level can be markedly increased. Following the inflammatory insult that could result from a surgical wound, the serum α1-AT increases in 2 to 3 days and can remain elevated for 1 to 2 weeks. The serum level then returns to normal.[8,14,27,30,36]

CLINICAL PROBLEMS

Decreased level *(↓ 159 mg/dl):* pulmonary emphysema, chronic obstructive lung disease, (COLD), homozygous deficiency, cirrhosis (children—rare), severe liver damage.

Elevated level *(↑ 400 mg/dl):* acute and chronic inflammatory conditions, infections (selected), necrosis, late pregnancy, exercise (returns to normal in 1 day). *Drug influence:* oral contraceptives.

PROCEDURE

Collect 5 ml of venous blood in red-top tube.

Keep the patient NPO, except for water, for 8 hours before drawing blood.

Hold oral contraceptives for 24 hours before the test, with the physician's permission.

Any oral contraceptive taken should be listed on the laboratory slip.

FACTORS AFFECTING LABORATORY RESULTS

Oral contraceptives can increase the alpha-1-antitrypsin level.

Oral intake of food before the test can cause an inaccurate result, especially if the patient has an elevated serum cholesterol or serum triglycerides.

NURSING IMPLICATIONS WITH RATIONALE

Decreased level (↓ 159 mg/dl)

Recognize clinical problems that are associated with alpha-1-antitrypsin deficiency—e.g., emphysema.

Explain to the patient that the test is ordered to determine whether there is an antitrypsin (protein) deficiency which can cause a lung disorder (disease). A nonsmoker with an α-1-AT deficiency can have emphysema. Antitrypsin inhibits proteolytic enzymes in destroying lung tissue; with a lack of this protein, the alveoli are damaged.

Instruct the patient that he should have nothing by mouth except water for 8 hours before the blood test. NPO before blood test may vary among physicians.

List the name of the oral contraceptive the patient is taking on the laboratory slip and note the last time it was taken.

Teach the patient with an alpha-1-antitrypsin deficit to use preventive methods in protecting his lungs—i.e., avoid persons with upper respiratory infections (URI), seek medical care when having a respiratory infection.

Encourage the patient to stop smoking and to avoid areas having high air pollution. Air pollution can cause respiratory inflammation and promote COLD.

Elevated level (↑ 400 mg/dl)

Check the serum alpha-1-antitrypsin level 2 to 3 days after extensive surgery. Inflammation can markedly increase the serum level. A baseline serum level may be ordered before surgery for several reasons—e.g., for determining lung disease and the effects of surgery.

Report to the physician if the serum α-1-AT remains elevated 2 weeks after surgery.

Note that serum α-1-AT can be markedly elevated during late pregnancy.

AMMONIA (Plasma)

NORMAL RANGE
Adult: (depends on method used) 3.2–4.5 g/dl or 32–45 g/L (SI units), 11–35 μmol/L, 20–120 μg/dl (diffusion), 40–80 μg/dl (enzymatic method), 12–48 μg/dl (resin method).
Child: *Newborn:* 90–150 μg/dl, *Child:* 40–80 μg/dl.

DESCRIPTION
Ammonia is a by-product of protein metabolism and is formed from the bacterial action in the intestine and from metabolizing tissues. Most of the ammonia is absorbed into the portal circulation and goes to the liver, where it is converted to urea. The kidneys excrete urea.

With severe liver decompensation or when blood flow is altered to the liver, the plasma ammonia level remains elevated. A rising plasma ammonia level does not result from severe liver disease only, but from inadequate portal blood circulation to the liver, as well.

Plasma ammonia is best correlated with hepatic failure; however, it is not elevated in all patients with hepatocellular disorders. Other conditions that can interfere with liver functions—e.g., CHF, acidosis—may cause a temporary elevation of plasma ammonia.[8,9,11,27,30,36]

CLINICAL PROBLEMS
Decreased level *(↓ 32 g/L):* renal failure, malignant hypertension, essential hypertension. *Drug influence:* neomycin (Mycifradin), monoamino oxidase inhibitors, Benadryl, potassium salts, sodium salts, sodium salts, tetracycline (decreasing gut bacteria).

Elevated level *(↑ 45 g/L):* hepatic failure, hepatic encephalopathy or coma, portacaval tacaval anastomosis, erythroblastosis fetalis, cor pulmonale, congestive heart failure, pulmonary emphysema, high-protein diet with liver failure, exercise. *Drug influence:* antibiotics—tetracycline, polymyxin B, methicillin (Staphcillin); ammonia chloride; diuretics—thiazides (Hydrodiuril), furosemide (Lasix), ethacrynic acid (Edecrin); ion exchange resin; INH (isoniazid).

PROCEDURE
Collect 5 ml of venous blood in a green-top tube. The blood sample should be in a heparinized tube, delivered immediately in packed ice to the laboratory.

NPO is suggested for 8 hours prior to the collection of the blood specimen. Drinking water is permitted.

FACTORS AFFECTING LABORATORY RESULTS
Failure to place the blood sample on ice and analyze it immediately.
High- or low-protein diet.
Exercise might increase the plasma ammonia level.
Certain antiobiotics (neomycin and tetracycline) decrease the ammonia level.

NURSING IMPLICATIONS WITH RATIONALE

Decreased level (↓ 32 g/L)
Identify clinical problems and drugs which can decrease the plasma ammonia level.
Check the plasma ammonia levels in patients receiving antibiotics and receiving a low-protein diet. Antibiotics decrease bacteria (protein in nature), and low-protein diet decreases the protein consumption—thus less ammonia is being produced.

Elevated level (↑ 45 g/L)
Identify clinical problems and drugs which can increase the plasma ammonia level.
Notify the laboratory personnel when a plasma ammonia level is drawn so that it can
    be analyzed immediately to avoid false results.
List antibiotics on the laboratory slip. Certain antibiotics (such as neomycin and tetra-
    cycline) can decrease the ammonia level, causing a false result.
Explain to the patient why he may be NPO 8 hours before the test. Foods containing
    protein may cause a higher ammonia level.
Answer the patient's questions about the purpose of the test and how it is performed.
    The purpose would be to determine whether the liver is able to convert ammonia to
    urea for the kidney to excrete. Blood is drawn from a vein—in most cases, before
    breakfast.
Inform the patient that he may drink water before the blood sample is taken.
Observe for signs and symptoms of hepatic failure, especially when the plasma am-
    monia is elevated. There are many neurologic changes, such as behavioral and per-
    sonality changes, lethargy, confusion, flapping tremors of the extremities, twitch-
    ing, and later coma.
Recognize that exercise may be a cause of an elevated plasma ammonia level.
Know various treatments used in decreasing the plasma ammonia level. A few of these
    are: low-protein diet, antibiotics (such as neomycin) to destroy intestinal bacteria,
    enemas, cathartics (such as magnesium sulfate) to prevent ammonia formation, and
    sodium glutamate and L-arginine in IV dextrose solution to stimulate urea for-
    mation.

AMYLASE (Serum)

NORMAL RANGE
    Adult: 60–160 Somogyi U/dl, 111–296 U/L (SI units).
    Child: not usually done.

DESCRIPTION
    Amylase is an enzyme that is derived from the pancreas, the salivary gland, and the
    liver. Its function is to change starch to sugar. When there is an acute inflammation of
    the pancreas or salivary glands, serum amylase rises. In acute pancreatitis, serum
    amylase is increased to twice its normal level. Acute pancreatitis is frequently asso-
    ciated with inflammation, severe pain, and necrosis due to digestive enzymes (in-
    cluding amylase) escaping into the surrounding tissue.
    Increased serum amylase occurs following abdominal surgery involving the gall-
    bladder (stones or biliary duct) and stomach (partial gastrectomy). The serum level
    could be increased to two to five times its upper range (400 to 1000 units). Following
    abdominal surgery, some surgeons order a routine serum amylase for 2 days to deter-
    mine whether the pancreas had been injured.
    With acute pancreatitis, the serum amylase level begins to increase 2 to 6 hours after
    onset and reaches its peak between 20 and 30 hours. It may persist for 48 to 72 hours
    before returning to normal. The urine amylase level is helpful in determining the
    significance of a normal or slightly elevated serum amylase, especially when the
    patient has symptoms of pancreatitis.
    Amylase levels can also be obtained from abdominal fluid, ascitic fluid, pleural ef-
    fusion, and saliva.[8,9,11,27,30,31,36]

CLINICAL PROBLEMS

Decreased level *(↓ 60 Somogyi U/dl):* 5 percent dextrose in water IV, advanced chronic pancreatitis, acute and subacute necrosis of the liver, chronic alcoholism, toxic hepatitis, severe burns, severe thyrotoxicosis. *Drug influence:* glucose (5 percent D/W IV), citrates, fluorides, oxalates.

Increased level *(↑ 160 Somogyi U/dl):* acute pancreatitis, chronic pancreatitis (acute onset), partial gastrectomy, peptic ulcer perforation, obstruction of pancreatic duct, acute cholecystitis, cancer of the pancreas, diabetic acidosis, diabetes mellitus, acute alcoholic intoxication, mumps, renal failure, benign prostatic hypertrophy, burns, pregnancy. *Drug influence:* meperidine (Demerol), codeine, morphine, bethanechol (Urecholine), pentazocine (Talwin), ethyl alcohol (large amounts), ACTH, guanethidine, thiazide diuretics, salicylates, tetracycline.

PROCEDURE

Use a red-top tube and obtain 5 to 10 ml of venous blood. Food should be restricted for 1 to 2 hours before the blood sample is drawn. If the patient has eaten and received a narcotic near the same time, the serum results could be invalid.

Serum amylase level is frequently determined during an acute attack.

List on the laboratory slip the drugs the patient is receiving that increase the serum amylase level.

FACTORS AFFECTING LABORATORY RESULTS

Narcotic drugs can cause false positive levels.

IV fluids with glucose can result in false negative levels.

Contamination of the specimen with saliva can occur through coughing, sneezing, or talking when the tube is opened. This could cause false positive results.

NURSING IMPLICATIONS WITH RATIONALE

Decreased level (↓ 60 U/dl)

Know that dextrose solution in water administered intravenously can decrease the serum amylase level, causing a false negative result.

Recognize that several clinical problems can be present with decreased and increased serum amylase. Examples of these are: burns, advanced chronic pancreatitis and acute or chronic exacerbation pancreatitis, and chronic alcoholism and acute alcoholic intoxication.

Identify drugs that give false negative levels.

Determine when the patient has ingested food or sweetened fluids. Blood should not be drawn until 2 hours after eating, since sugar can decrease the serum amylase level.

Elevated level (↑ 160 U/dl)

Know the disease entities related to increased levels, especially acute pancreatitis, abdominal surgery (partial gastrectomy, biliary resection), diabetes mellitus, cancer of the pancreas, acute alcoholic intoxication, and benign prostatic hypertrophy (BPH).

Label the laboratory slip (for serum amylase) with the drugs the patient is receiving or has received in the last 24 hours. Morphine, demerol, codeine, Talwin, aspirin, and hydrodiuril can cause a false positive serum amylase level.

Check serum amylase levels for several days after abdominal surgery. Surgery of the stomach or gallbladder might cause trauma to the pancreas and cause excess amylase to be released.

Report symptoms of severe pain when pancreatitis is suspected. The physician may want to draw a serum amylase level before a narcotic is given. An elevated level may indicate an acute pancreatitis.

Explain to the patient that blood is drawn for determining whether the severe pain is due to a pancreatic problem or to another cause.

Ask the patient if he has had pancreatitis before and has taken narcotic–analgesics. A report should be given to the physician.

Report elevated serum amylase results occurring beyond 3 days. If the serum amylase levels remain elevated beyond 3 days (72 hours), pancreatic cell destruction could still be occurring.

AMYLASE (Urine)

NORMAL RANGE
Adult: 35–260 Somogyi U/hour, 6.5–48.1 U/L (SI units), 260–950 Somogyi U/24 hours.

DESCRIPTION
Amylase is an enzyme that is produced by the pancreas, salivary glands, and liver and is excreted by the kidneys. When there is an inflammation of the pancreas or salivary gland, more amylase goes into the blood and more amylase is excreted in the urine. The urine levels of amylase could remain elevated for a week, whereas the serum amylase level tends to remain elevated for a short time (peaks in 24 hours and returns to normal in 48 to 72 hours).

The urine amylase test is ordered at 1 hour, 2 hour, or 24 hour timed intervals, with the 2 hour urine specimen the most commonly ordered. The urine amylase level usually rises in 24 hours, so that several 2 hour urine specimens may be ordered. With acute pancreatitis, a value of 900 Somogyi units/hour is not unusual.

If the expected time for finding an elevated serum amylase has passed, the physician may order a 2 hour urine amylase test. A 24 hour specimen may be within normal range while a 2 hour specimen shows an increase.

One drawback of urine amylase as well as serum amylase values is their relation to renal function. A diminished renal function could lead to a decrease in urine amylase and increased serum amylase.[8,11,27,30,36]

CLINICAL PROBLEMS
Decreased level *(↓ 35 Somogyi U/hour, or ↓ 260 Somogyi U/24 hours):* diminished renal function; see Amylase—Serum.

Increased level *(↑ 260 Somogyi U/hr, or ↑ 950 Somogyi U/24 hours):* acute pancreatitis, choledocolithiasis; see Amylase—Serum.

PROCEDURE
A timed urine collection is required; thus the exact beginning and end of the urine collection should be recorded (date, hour, and minute—e.g., 2/10/83, 9:02 A.M. to 2/10/83, 11:05 A.M.). (First the patient voids and the urine is discarded.)

The urine specimen should be refigerated or kept on ice. There is a question as to whether refrigeration is needed during the urine collection time; however, it is suggested that one refrigerate. No preservative is needed. Post a sign on the patient's door, by the bed, and/or on the Kardex saying that a 2 hour or 24 hour urine specimen is being collected.

FACTORS AFFECTING LABORATORY RESULTS
Fecal material or toilet paper contamination.
Diminished urine output.
Drugs that increase or decrease amylase levels.
Prolonged urine collection time.

NURSING IMPLICATIONS WITH RATIONALE

Decreased level (↓ 35 Somogyi U/hour, or ↓ 260 Somogyi U/24 hours)
Check urinary output for 8 hours and 24 hours, BUN (blood urea nitrogen), and serum
creatinine levels. A decrease in urine output and an increase in BUN and serum
creatinine levels indicate poor kidney function. A decreased urine output could
result in a decreased urine amylase.
Explain to the patient the importance of collecting urine at a specified time. The
patient should use a urinal or bedpan and should be instructed that all urine should
be saved.
Encourage the patient to drink water during the test unless water intake is restricted
due to medical reasons. A decreased urine output could result in no 2 hour specimen
or a possible false result.

Increased level (↑ 260 Somogyi U/hour, or ↑ 950 Somogyi U/24 hours)
Explain to the patient the purpose for collecting a 2 hour or 24 hour urine specimen. A
2 hour urine specimen with an elevated amylase level could indicate pancreatitis 24
hours after an acute onset. Urine amylase levels will remain elevated longer than
serum amylase levels.
Check urinary output and give fluids if the urine output is decreased. Encouraging
fluids during the test should help in securing a urine specimen.
Check the serum amylase level(s) and compare with the urine amylase level. A low
serum amylase level and an increased urine amylase level could indicate that the
acute problem is no longer present.
Instruct the patient not to discard urine in the toilet during collection time. Inform the
family that the urine is being saved. Post notices of urine collection.
List on the laboratory slip the drugs the patient is receiving that can increase amylase
levels—e.g., narcotics.
Notify the physician when the patient is having severe abdominal pain. The physician
may want to order a 2 hour or 24 hour urine specimen the next day.
Tell the patient not to put toilet paper or feces in the urine specimen, since contamination would occur.

ANTIBIOTIC SUSCEPTIBILITY (SENSITIVITY) TEST

NORMAL RANGE
Adult: organism—sensitive, intermediate, resistant.
Child: same as adult.

DESCRIPTION
See Cultures.
It is important to identify not only the organism responsible for the infection but also
the antibiotic(s) which will inhibit the growth of the bacteria. The physician orders a

culture and sensitivity test (C and S) when a wound infection is suspected or for a possible urinary tract infection or other suspected infections. The choice of antibiotic depends on the pathogenic organism and its susceptibility to the antibiotics, as demonstrated by its inhibition zone on the agar plate.

There are two methods employed to test antibiotic susceptibility: tube dilution and disc diffusion (also called agar diffusion), with the latter being the most commonly used method. A filter paper containing small antibiotic discs is placed in a Petri dish streaked with the single type of bacteria. If bacteria surround the disc, the organism is resistant to the antibiotic. If the bacteria growth around the disc is inhibited, the organism is susceptible to the antibiotic. Recently, the term *minimal inhibitory concentration* (MIC) has been used to express (in μg/ml) the lowest concentration of the antibiotics that will prevent visible growth of a cultured microorganism.

With the tube dilution method, bacteria are cultured in several tubes having various concentrations of antibiotic. The lowest concentration of antibiotic that inhibits the growth of the organism is the choice of antibiotic concentration for the patient.[4,9,11,27,30,36]

CLINICAL PROBLEMS
Resistant: non-effective antibiotic.
Sensitive: effective antibiotic.

PROCEDURE
It takes approximately 24 hours for bacterial growth on agar and 48 hours for the completed test results.

The specimen for C and S should be taken to the laboratory within 30 minutes of collection or else refrigerated.

The specimen should be handled with care, preventing contamination and bacterial transmission (see Culture Procedure).

FACTORS AFFECTING LABORATORY RESULTS
Antibiotics and sulfonamides could cause a false negative reaction.

NURSING IMPLICATIONS WITH RATIONALE

Explain to the patient that the specimen is being collected to identify the causative organism, or give a similar response.

Collect specimen for C and S before preventive antibiotic therapy is started. Antibiotic therapy started before specimen collection could cause an inaccurate result.

Record on the laboratory slip the antibiotic(s) the patient is receiving, the dosages, and for how long the antibiotic(s) has (have) been taken.

Check lab report for C and S result. If the patient is receiving an antibiotic and the lab report shows the organism is resistant to that antibiotic, the nurse should notify the physician.

ANTINUCLEAR ANTIBODIES (ANA) (Serum)
Anti-DNA Antibody, Anti-DNP Antibody

NORMAL RANGE
Adult: negative.

DESCRIPTION

The antinuclear antibody (ANA) test was developed for assessing tissue-antigen antibodies and is frequently used for diagnosing systemic lupus erythematosus (SLE; autoimmune collagen disease), along with other clinical problems. ANAs are immunoglobulins (IgM, IgG, IgA) which react with the nuclear part of leukocytes and are tested by the immunofluorescent method. They form antibodies against DNA, RNA, and others. Two antinuclear antibodies, anti-DNA (anti-deoxyribonucleic acid) and anti-DNP (anti-D-nucleoprotein) are almost always present with SLE. Anti-DNA will fluctuate according to the disease process, with remission, and with exacerbation. It is normally present (95 percent) in lupus nephritis. Radioimmunoassay is used in detecting anti-DNA.

The total ANA is frequently positive for active SLE, but can also be positive in systemic sclerosis, scleroderma, rheumatoid arthritis, cirrhosis of the liver, leukemia, infectious mononucleosis, and ulcerative colitis.

With a negative test result, the diagnosis of SLE is inclusive, however many times the test is repeated. A titer >1:25 is considered positive for SLE. The ANA test should be compared with other tests for lupus.[8,9,11,14,27,30,31,34,36]

CLINICAL PROBLEMS

Normal: rheumatic fever, cranial arteritis.

Elevated—Positive: *(>1:10):* systemic lupus erythematosus (SLE—most frequent cause), progressive systemic sclerosis, scleroderma, leukemia, rheumatoid arthritis, cirrhosis of the liver, infectious mononucleosis, myasthenia gravis. *Drug influence:* antibiotics—penicillin, streptomycin, tetracycline. Antihypertensives: hydralazine (Apresoline), methyldopa (Aldomet); anti-TB: paraaminosalicylic acid (PAS), isoniazid (INH); diuretics—acetazolamide (Diamox), thiazides (Diuril, Hydrodiuril); oral contraceptives; procainamide (Pronestyl); trimethadione (Tridione).

PROCEDURE

Collect 2 to 5 ml of venous blood in a red-top tube.

There is no food or drink restriction.

Drugs the patient receives that can cause a false positive titer should be withheld with the physician's permission or, if given, should be listed on the laboratory slip.

FACTORS AFFECTING LABORATORY RESULTS

Certain drugs cause false positive results (see *Drug Influence* above).

The aging process can cause a slight positive ANA titer.

NURSING IMPLICATIONS WITH RATIONALE

Elevated—Positive Titer

Relate clinical problems and drugs to positive ANA results. With SLE, the ANA titer may fluctuate according to the severity of the disease. Certain drugs can increase the titer level.

Report and record on the chart the drugs the patient is taking that could influence a positive ANA test.

Explain to the patient that the test is to check on antibodies present in the blood. Further explanation may be needed.

Instruct the patient that he may eat and drink before the blood test.

Assess for signs and symptoms of lupus erythematosus—i.e., skin rash over the cheeks and nose, joint pain.

Promote rest during an acute phase.

ANTISTREPTOLYSIN O (ASO) (Serum)

NORMAL RANGE
   Adult: <160 U/dl. Todd
   Child: *Newborn:* Similar to mother's. *Infant:* <60 U/dl. *Preschool:* <150 U/dl. *School age:* < 200 U/dl.

DESCRIPTION
   The beta-hemolytic streptococcus secretes an enzyme known as streptolysin O, which is capable of lysing red blood cells. Streptolysin O acts as an antigen and stimulates the immune system to develop antistreptolysin O (ASO) antibodies. A high titer of ASO indicates that streptococci are present and may cause rheumatic fever or acute glomerulonephritis. Increased serum ASO levels can also indicate a recent strep-tococcal infection.
   The ASO antibodies appear approximately 1 to 2 weeks after the infection and their level peaks 3 to 4 weeks after onset. It may remain elevated for months. Many school-age children have a higher ASO titer level than do preschool children or adults.
   Approximately 80 percent of patients with acute rheumatic fever (ARF) have an elevated ASO titer (>250 Todd units). The ASO titer for ARF and acute glomerulone-phritis (AGN) may go as high as 500 to 5000 Todd units, depending on the disease's severity and duration. There can be positive ASO levels which are not related to ARF and AGN, frequently indicating a streptococcal infection.
   Other streptococcal antigens are: antideoxyribonuclease (ADNase—titer >10) and antistreptococcal hyaluronidase (ASH—titer >128).[8,11,20,27,31,34,36]

CLINICAL PROBLEMS
   Decreased level *(<12 U/dl):* antibiotic therapy.
   Elevated level (>160 U/dl:) acute rheumatic fever, acute glomerulonephritis, strep-tococcal upper respiratory infections, rheumatoid arthritis (mildly elevated), hyper-globulinemia with liver disease, collagen disease (mildly elevated).

PROCEDURE
   Collect 5 to 10 ml of venous blood in a red-top tube.
   There is no food or drink restriction.
   Repeated ASO testing is advisable to determine the highest level of increase (once or twice a week).

FACTORS AFFECTING LABORATORY RESULTS
   Antibiotic therapy decreases the antibody response.
   Increased level in healthy persons (carriers).

NURSING IMPLICATIONS WITH RATIONALE

Elevated level (>160 U/dl)
Check serum ASO levels when the patient is complaining of joint pain in the extremi-ties. An elevated level (>500 U/dl) could be indicative of acute rheumatic fever, and a slight elevation (>170 U/dl) could be indicative of rheumatoid arthritis.
Explain to the patient that the ASO test is a test to determine whether a streptococcal infection could be present.
Instruct the patient that food and drink are not restricted.
Check the urinary output when the serum ASO is elevated. A urinary output of less than 600 ml/24 hours may be associated with acute glomerulonephritis.

ARTERIAL BLOOD GASES (ABGs) (Arterial Blood—Overview)
Blood Gases

NORMAL RANGE

Adult: *pH:* 7.35-7.45. *PCO$_2$:* 35-45 mmHg. *PO$_2$:* 75-100 mmHg. *HCO$_3$:* 24-28 mEq/L. *BE:* +2 to -2 (±2 mEq/L).

Child: *pH:* 7.36-7.44. *PCO$_2$, PO$_2$, HCO$_3$:* similar to adult.

DESCRIPTION

See also *pH; PCO$_2$; PO$_2$; Bicarbonate, Base Excess.*

Determination of arterial blood gases (ABGs) is usually ordered to assess disturbances of acid–base balance due to a respiratory disorder, cardiac failure, drug overdose, renal failure, uncontrolled diabetes mellitus, and other metabolic disorders.

A pH under 7.35 indicates acidosis and a pH over 7.45 indicates alkalosis. To determine whether the acidosis has a respiratory cause, the PCO$_2$ should be checked. An elevated PCO$_2$ with a low pH indicates respiratory acidosis. If the PCO$_2$ is normal and the bicarbonate and base excess are decreased, metabolic acidosis is indicated. Likewise, the type of alkalosis can be determined by checking the PCO$_2$ and the HCO$_3$.[8,17,30,36]

CLINICAL PROBLEMS

See *Clinical Problems* for pH.

PROCEDURE

Notify the laboratory that blood gases are to be sent.

Collect 1 to 5 ml of arterial blood in a heparinized needle and syringe, remove the needle, make sure there is no air in the syringe, and apply an airtight cap over the tip of the syringe. Some laboratories require only 0.5 ml of blood.

Place the syringe with arterial blood in an ice bag (to minimize the metabolic activities of the sample) and deliver it immediately to the laboratory. A gas analyzer machine is used for analyzing ABGs.

Indicate on the ABGs slip whether the patient is receiving oxygen and the rate of flow.

Apply pressure to the puncture site for 2 to 5 minutes.

There is no food or drink restriction.

Be sure the blood is not collected from the same arm used for the IV infusion.

FACTORS AFFECTING LABORATORY RESULTS

Hemolysis of the blood sample. No ice around the blood sample and exposure to air.

Drugs that increase and decrease pH levels (see pH—*Clinical Problems*).

NURSING IMPLICATIONS WITH RATIONALE

Explain to the patient the purpose for the arterial blood test. Explanation could be brief, such as "to determine the acid–base status of the body fluids," or a similar response.

Explain to the patient the procedure for the ABGs test. Explanation could include the following: "Blood will be taken from an artery in the arm or groin; hand pressure will be applied to the puncture site for 2 to 5 minutes to stop bleeding."

Instruct the patient that food and drinks are not restricted.

Decreased and Elevated levels

See especially pH; also PCO$_2$, PO$_2$, HCO$_3$.

Note: Interpretation of results will be more meaningful when the pH, PCO$_2$, and HCO$_3$ are evaluated as a group. Looking at a single result may be misleading.

ASCORBIC ACID (VITAMIN C) (Plasma and Blood)

NORMAL RANGE
    Adult: 0.6–1.6 mg/dl (plasma), 34–91 μmol/L (SI units–plasma), 0.7–2.0 mg/dl (blood), 40–114 μmol (SI units-blood).
    Child: 0.6–1.6 mg/dl (plasma).

DESCRIPTION
    See Ascorbic Acid Tolerance.
    Ascorbic acid (vitamin C) is a water-soluble vitamin found in fresh fruits and vegetables. Deficiencies of vitamin C still occur, but the severe deficiency known as scurvy is rare.
    Vitamin C is important for the formation of collagen substances and certain amino acids, in wound healing, and in withstanding the stresses of injury and infection. Since vitamin C is vitally important to the body's defense mechanisms in dealing with stress due to injury and disease, the patient's ascorbic acid level should be known. This test can also be used to determine whether the ascorbic acid therapy is adequate. Excess ingestion of vitamin C is not considered toxic, as is excess ingestion of vitamins A and D, since excess vitamin C is excreted in the urine.[11,14,27,28]

CLINICAL PROBLEMS
    Decreased level *(↓ 0.6 mg/dl plasma):* scurvy, low vitamin C diet, malabsorption, pregnancy, infections, cancer, severe burns.
    Elevated level *(↑ 1.6 mg/dl plasma):* excess vitamin C ingestion. *Causes of false positive readings:* clinitest, serum creatinine, serum uric acid, serum bilirubin, serum ALT and AST, blood glucose, serum cholesterol. *Causes of false negative readings:* test for occult blood in stool, serum triglycerides.

PROCEDURE
    Collect 5 ml of venous blood in a gray-top tube.
    There is no food or drink restriction.

FACTORS AFFECTING LABORATORY RESULTS
    High doses of ascorbic acid can cause inaccurate results.

NURSING IMPLICATIONS WITH RATIONALE

Recognize the functions of ascorbic acid in maintaining the state of wellness. Ascorbic acid has been taken by persons in large doses (>1 g) to prevent colds. This has not been medically proven effective.

Answer the patient's questions concerning the importance of vitamin C. It helps with the healing process. It is not medically proven to prevent colds, but some people feel it helps.

Decreased level (↓ 0.6 mg/dl)

Relate vitamin C deficit to certain clinical problems—e.g., infections, burns. Vitamin C is lost during severe infections and burns.

Teach the patient to eat foods rich in vitamin C—i.e., oranges, grapefruits, strawberries, cantaloupe, pineapple, broccoli, cabbage, spinach, kale, turnips (all excellent to good sources). Approximately 25 percent of the population has an ascorbic acid deficit in the body.

Elevated level († 1.6 mg/dl)
Record on the patient's chart a habit of taking high doses of vitamin C continuously.
High doses of ascorbic acid can cause false positive laboratory results (see *Clinical Problems* above).

ASCORBIC ACID TOLERANCE (Blood and Urine)
Vitamin C Tolerance

NORMAL RANGE
Adult: *Blood:* >1.6 mg/dl. *Urine:* 4, 5, or 6 hour sample. Oral: 10 percent of administered amount. IV: 30–40 percent of administered amount.
Child: not usually done.

DESCRIPTION
The ascorbic acid tolerance test is useful for determining the degree of ascorbic acid deficiency. Patients having severe burns, infections, or malignancy frequently have an ascorbic acid deficiency even when they are receiving vitamin C or have a diet adequate in vitamin C. With an ascorbic acid deficit, wound healing and recovery are prolonged.
The blood and urine tests are normally done together.[11]

CLINICAL PROBLEMS
Decreased level *(<1.6 mg/dl [blood], <30 percent IV [urine]):* infections, burns, cancer.
Elevated level *(>1.6 mg/dl [blood], >40 percent IV [urine]):* excess vitamin C administration.

PROCEDURE
Foods high in ascorbic acid should be omitted for 24 hours before the test (i.e., fruits and vegetables). Water can be given.
Have the patient void and discard the urine before beginning the test.
Administer ascorbic acid, orally (11 mg/kg of body weight in a glass of water) or intravenously (10 mg/kg of body weight in saline solution).
Collect 5 ml of venous blood in a gray-top tube 4 to 6 hours after the ascorbic acid is administered.
Collect a 4, 5, or 6 hour urine specimen in a bottle containing acetic acid. The bottle should be kept on ice or refrigerated and taken to the laboratory immediately at the end of the specified time.

FACTORS AFFECTING LABORATORY RESULTS
Oral high potency vitamin supplements.
Ascorbic acid in intravenous fluids.
Inaccurate urine collection time and inaccurate labeling.

NURSING IMPLICATIONS WITH RATIONALE

Explain to the patient that the purpose of the test is to determine whether there is a vitamin C deficiency in the body.
Explain to the patient that for 24 hours he should not eat foods high in ascorbic acid—i.e., oranges or orange juice, grapefruit, strawberries, or green vegetables. Drinking water is permissible.

Have the patient void and discard the urine.

Administer ascorbic acid orally or intravenously according to body weight.

Instruct the patient that all urine should be saved for 4, 5, or 6 hours (according to the order or laboratory policy) in a bottle kept on ice or refrigerated. Following collection time, the urine specimen should be taken immediately to the laboratory.

Explain to the patient that blood will be drawn 4 to 6 hours after the ascorbic acid is administered.

Post the time for urine collection on the chart or Kardex or by the bedside. Visitors should not discard the patient's urine.

ASPARTATE AMINOTRANSFERASE (AST) (Serum)
Serum Glutamic Oxaloacetic Transaminase (SGOT)

NORMAL RANGE

Adult: 5–40 U/ml (Frankel) 4–36 IU/L, 16–60 (Karmen) U/ml U/L at 30 °C, 8–33 (SI units) at 37 °C.

Newborns: four times the normal level.

Child: similar to adults.

DESCRIPTION

AST/SGOT is an enzyme found mainly in the heart muscle and liver, with moderate amounts in skeletal muscle, the kidneys, and the pancreas. Its concentration is low in the blood except when there is cellular injury, and then large amounts are released into the circulation.

High levels of serum AST are found following an acute myocardial infarction (AMI) and liver damage. Six to ten hours after an AMI, AST leaks out of the heart muscle and reaches its peak (<200 U/L) 24 to 48 hours after the infarction. The serum AST level returns to normal 4 to 6 days later if there is no additional infarction and no liver damage. In liver disease, the serum level increases by ten times or more and remains elevated for a longer period of time.

Serum levels of AST and ALT are frequently compared, and if AST is elevated and ALT is not, then myocardial damage is suspected. Several enzymes are used (i.e., CPK, LDH, and AST) in diagnosing myocardial infarction.[8,11,14,16,27,30,31,36]

CLINICAL PROBLEMS

Decreased level *(↓ 5 Frankel units/ml):* pregnancy, diabetic ketoacidosis, beriberi. *Drug influence:* salicylates.

Elevated level *(↑ 40 Frankel units/ml):* acute myocardial infarction, hepatitis, liver necrosis, musculoskeletal diseases and trauma, intramuscular injections, acute pancreatitis, cancer of the liver, severe angina pectoris, strenuous exercise. *Drug influence:* antibiotics—ampicillin, carbenicillin, clindamycin, cloxacillin, erythromycin, gentamicin, lincomycin, nafcillin, oxacillin, polycillin, tetracycline; vitamins—folic acid, pyridoxine, vitamin A; narcotics—codeine, morphine, meperidine (Demerol); antihypertensives—methyldopa (Aldomet), guanethidine; mithramycin; digitalis preparation; cortisone; flurazepam (Dalmane); indomethacin (Indocin); isoniazid (INH); rifampin; oral contraceptives; salicylates; theophylline.

PROCEDURE

Collect 5 to 10 ml of venous blood in a red-top tube.

Draw blood before drugs are given. The enzyme will remain stable for 4 days, refrigerated.

Drugs which the patient receives that can cause false positive levels should be listed on the laboratory slip along with the dates last given.

There is no food or drink restriction.

Care should be taken to prevent hemolysis of the blood specimen.

FACTORS AFFECTING LABORATORY RESULTS

Intramuscular injections.

Hemolysis of the blood specimen.

Drugs increasing the serum AST level (see *Drug Influence* above).

Salicylates may cause false positive or negative serum levels.

NURSING IMPLICATIONS WITH RATIONALE

Elevated level (↑ 40 U/ml or ↑ 33U/L [SI units])

Relate clinical problems and drugs to elevated serum AST levels.

Hold drugs causing an elevated serum AST for 24 hours prior to the blood test, with the physician's permission. Drugs that should not be withheld should be listed on the laboratory slip and charted.

Explain to the patient the purpose of the test. Explanation could be brief—e.g., "to measure the enzyme level in the blood"—or a more detailed explanation could be given.

Do not administer intramuscular (IM) injections before the blood test. IM injections can increase the serum AST level. Few medications (e.g., Morphine) can be given intravenously without affecting the serum level.

Instruct the patient that he may eat and drink prior to the test.

Assess the patient for signs and symptoms of MI—e.g., chest and arm pain, dyspnea, or diaphoresis. Changes should be reported and charted.

B

BARBITURATE (Blood)

NORMAL RANGE
Adult: *Therapeutic:* 10–30 µg/ml (mcg/dl).
Toxic: Short-acting: 3 mg/dl (secobarbital—Seconal; pentobarbital—Nembutal).
Moderate-acting: 6 mg/dl (amobarbital—Amytal; butabarbital—Butisol). Long-acting:
9 mg/dl (phenobarbital—Luminal; mephobarbital—Mebaral).
Child: *Therapeutic:* 15–40 µg/dl (mcg/dl). *Toxic:* similar to adult.

DESCRIPTION
Barbiturate toxicity is a frequent cause of unconsciousness due to accidental or in-
tentional barbiturate overdose. Barbiturates have different effects, and those that are
short-acting tend to be more potent and toxic than the long-acting types. Phenobarbital tends to be least toxic; however, this depends on the amount taken. This long-
acting barbiturate peaks in 12 to 18 hours and its serum half-life is 5 to 6 days.
Alcohol and tranquilizers can intensify the effects of barbiturates. The three most
commonly used barbiturates are phenobarbital (used as a sedative or anticonvulsant),
secobarbital, and pentobarbital (used as a sedative for sleep). Blood barbiturate levels
should be measured on unconscious/comatose patients when the cause of unrespon-
siveness is unknown.[8,9,11,14,36]

PROCEDURE
Collect 5 to 10 ml of venous blood in a red- or green-top tube.
There is no food or drink restriction.
Urine and gastric contents may be examined for barbiturates.

FACTORS AFFECTING LABORATORY RESULTS
Alcohol and tranquilizers.
Drugs: antipyrine and theophylline (these drugs elevate the barbiturate level).

NURSING IMPLICATIONS WITH RATIONALE

Observe for signs and symptoms of barbiturate toxicity—i.e., depressed respirations,
bradycardia, and loss of consciousness.
Obtain a history from the family or a friend to determine whether the patient has been
taking a barbiturate and, if he has, which type. Report the drug history to the
physician.
Monitor the urinary output. Renal dysfunction due to renal ischemia and tubular
damage can prolong recovery. Diuretics, especially osmotic, have been used for
correcting the effects of long-lasting barbiturates.
Teach the patient not to combine alcohol with barbiturates. Alcohol intensifies the
effects of barbiturates, and respiratory distress could result.
Report to the physician if the patient is taking tranquilizers and barbiturates. The
combination of these two drugs could cause respiratory distress.
Inform the patient that it is important to keep medical appointments when taking barbiturates so that the physician can evaluate the effects of the drug and have the
blood barbiturate levels checked.

BASOPHILS (Blood)
White Blood Cell Differential Count

NORMAL RANGE
Adult: 0.4–1 percent of the total white blood cells (leukocytes): 40–100 cu mm

DESCRIPTION
Basophils are a type of polymorphonuclear granulocyte that make up the smallest proportion of white blood cells (WBC). Basophil granules contain heparin and histamine. Heparin is an anticoagulant and is liberated by the basophils. It prevents cell clumping and blood coagulation during an inflammatory process. There is an increased number of basophils during the healing process.

It is thought that basophils, like eosinophils, are under the influence of the adrenal glands. Increase in adrenocortical hormones will cause a decrease in basophils.[9,14,21,36]

CLINICAL PROBLEMS
Decreased level (↓ *0.4 percent):* stress, hyperthyroidism, hypersensitivity reaction, pregnancy. *Drug influence:* steroids: Cortisone, ACTH.
Elevated level (↑ *1 percent):* inflammatory process, polycythemia vera, leukemia, Hodgkin's disease, acquired hemolytic anemia, healing stage (infection or inflammation).

PROCEDURE
Same as for Differential White Blood Cell Count.

FACTORS AFFECTING LABORATORY RESULTS
Prolonged steriod therapy.

NURSING IMPLICATIONS WITH RATIONALE

Elevated level (↑ 1 percent)
Relate elevated basophils to clinical problems, mainly the healing process.
Explain to the patient the purpose of the blood test. Explanation may be brief, such as "to determine if there is an increase in certain types of white blood cells."
Assess the patient for signs and symptoms of healing—e.g., normal vital signs, ability to increase movement at the injured site, or decreased edema.

BENCE–JONES PROTEIN (Urine)

NORMAL RANGE
Adult: random—negative to trace.

DESCRIPTION
Bence–Jones protein is a low molecular protein which passes through the glomeruli of the kidney into the urine. It has a lower molecular weight than the smallest plasma protein. Increased amounts of Bence–Jones protein are commonly found in the urine of persons with multiple myeloma and is also associated with other bone tumors, hyperparathyroidism, amyloidosis, leukemia, and metastatic carcinoma.

There are two methods of testing for Bence–Jones proteinuria. The classic method is the heat coagulability test; the protein coagulates at temperatures between 45° and

70° and disappears at 100°C. It will reappear when the urine is cooled. The urine electrophoresis is the newer method and is considered reliable.[8,9,11,27,34]

CLINICAL PROBLEMS

Positive: multiple myeloma (70–80 percent have positives), lymphosarcoma, osteomalacia, tumor metastasis to bone, leukemia, amyloidosis, hyperparathyroidism. *Drug influence:* tetracycline (outdated).

PROCEDURE

Collect the urine sample and send it to the laboratory.

Heat method: the urine specimen is heated to between 45° and 70°C, and if coagulation occurs, it is heated to 100°C. If it disappears at the high temperature and recoagulates as it cools, then the test is positive.

Electrophoresis of urine and serum is considered accurate and is used in many institutions.

The dipstick method for albumin will not detect the Bence–Jones protein.

There is no food or drink restriction.

FACTORS AFFECTING LABORATORY RESULTS

Outdated tetracycline.

NURSING IMPLICATIONS WITH RATIONALE

Positive Test

Relate the positive result of the test with clinical problems, especially multiple myeloma.

Explain to the patient that the urine test is to determine whether there is a specific protein in the urine. A more detailed explanation may be needed.

Inform the patient that he may eat and drink water before the test.

Answer questions the patient may have regarding the urine test—for instance, concerning the methods used in the laboratory for testing the urine.

BICARBONATE (HCO₃), BASE EXCESS (BE) (Arterial Blood)

NORMAL RANGE

Adult: *Bicarbonate:* 24–28 mmol/L (SI units), 21–28 mmol/L (SI units). *Base excess:* + 2 to −2 (±2 mEq/L)

Newborn: *Base excess:* +4 to −4.

Child: *Base excess:* +2 to −2.

DESCRIPTION

Bicarbonate (HCO₃) is an alkaline substance which comprises over half of the total buffer base in the blood. The term *base excess* refers to bicarbonate and other base substances in the blood which are able to bind excess hydrogen. When there is a deficit of bicarbonate and other bases or an increase in nonvolatile acid (such as lactic acid), metabolic acidosis occurs. If a bicarbonate excess is present, then metabolic alkalosis results. The bicarbonate plays a very important role in maintaining the pH between 7.35 and 7.45.[8,17,27,31]

CLINICAL PROBLEMS

Decreased level *(↓ 24 mEq/L [bicarbonate]):* diabetic ketoacidosis, severe diarrhea, starvation/malnutrition, acute/chronic renal failure, shock, burns, acute myocardial infarction, acute alcoholic intoxication, toxic effects of carbon monoxide. *Drug in-*

fluence: acetazolamine (Diamox), ammonium chloride, paraldehyde, sodium citrate, calcium chloride.

Elevated level (↑ *28 mEq/L [bicarbonate]):* peptic ulcer, severe vomiting, gastric suction, hypokalemia (potassium deficit), fistula of stomach and duodenum. *Drug influence:* sodium bicarbonate, potassium oxalate.

PROCEDURE
Same as for Arterial Blood Gases and pH.

FACTORS AFFECTING LABORATORY RESULTS
Same as for Arterial Blood Gases and pH.

NURSING IMPLICATIONS WITH RATIONALE

Explain to the patient the purpose of the test. Explanation may be brief, such as "to determine the acid–base status of the blood."

Explain to the patient the procedure for the ABGs test. Explanation could include: "Blood will be taken from an artery in the arm or groin; hand pressure will be applied to the puncture site for 2 or more minutes to control bleeding."

Instruct the patient that there is no food or drink restriction.

Decreased level (↓ 24 mEq/L; >−2)
Relate decreased levels of HCO_3 or base excess greater than −2 to clinical problems, drugs, and metabolic acidosis. When there is tissue breakdown from shock, malnutrition, etc., acid metabolites (e.g., lactic acid) are released. Another cause of metabolic acidosis is the ketone bodies (fatty acid) from diabetic ketoacidosis.

Assess for signs and symptoms of metabolic acidosis, such as rapid, vigorous breathing (Kussmaul breathing); flushed skin; restlessness; and decreased bicarbonate and base excess levels.

Elevated level (↑ 28 mEq/L; >+2)
Relate an elevated bicarbonate level or base excess greater than +2 to clinical problems and metabolic alkalosis. With severe vomiting and gastric suction, hydrogen and chloride (hydrochloric acid) are lost, causing an alkalotic state. Drugs containing sodium bicarbonate taken in excess or over a long period of time could cause metabolic alkalosis.

Assess the patient for signs and symptoms of metabolic alkalosis, such as shallow breathing, vomiting, and elevated bicarbonate level and base excess.

Check other ABGs results. If the pH is low, the PCO_2 is high, and the HCO_3 is high, the acid–base imbalance is respiratory acidosis with metabolic compensation. The elevated HCO_3 is compensating for the acidotic state caused by respiratory acidosis.

BILIRUBIN (INDIRECT) (Serum)
Van den Bergh Test

NORMAL RANGE
Adult: 0.1–1.0 mg/dl, 1.7–17.1 μmol/L (SI units).

DESCRIPTION
See Bilirubin (Total and Direct).
Indirect-reacting or unconjugated bilirubin is protein-bound and is associated with increased destruction of red blood cells (hemolysis).

Elevated indirect bilirubin can occur in autoimmune or transfusion-induced hemolysis, in hemolytic processes due to sickle cell anemia, in pernicious anemia, and with malaria and septicemia. Internal hemorrhage into soft tissues and the body cavity can cause the bilirubin to rise in 5 to 6 hours. With certain clinical problems, CHF, and severe liver damage, both indirect and direct bilirubin levels will increase. Indirect bilirubin frequently increases because the damaged liver cells cannot conjugate normal amounts, which leads to increased unconjugated bilirubin.

Levels of indirect serum bilirubin may increase in hemolytic disease in newborns (erythroblastosis fetalis) to levels exceeding 20 mg/dl. The newborn's liver is immature and, when extremely high levels of bilirubin occur, irreversible neurologic damage, referred to as kernicterus, could result. In all probability, a transfusion exchange would be indicated.[8,11,27,31,36]

CLINICAL PROBLEMS

Decreased level (↓ *0.1 mg/dl*): *Drug influence:* see Bilirubin (Total and Direct).
Elevated level (↑ *1.0 mg/dl*): erythroblastosis fetalis, sickle cell anemia, transfusion reaction, pernicious anemia, malaria, septicemia, hemolytic anemias, congestive heart failure, decompensated cirrhosis, hepatitis. *Drug influence:* aspidium, rifampin, phenothiazines. See Bilirubin (Total and Direct).

PROCEDURE

There is no lab test for indirect bilirubin. Indirect bilirubin is calculated by subtracting the direct bilirubin from the total bilirubin:

$$\text{Total bilirubin} - \text{Direct bilirubin} = \text{Indirect bilirubin}$$

In newborn infants, only the total is determined, and this represents the indirect bilirubin only.

FACTORS AFFECTING LABORATORY RESULTS

Same as Bilirubin (Total and Direct).

NURSING IMPLICATIONS WITH RATIONALE

Elevated levels (↑ 1.0 mg/dl)
Relate elevated indirect bilirubin levels to clinical problems.
Check the patient's indirect serum bilirubin level and compare it with the direct bilirubin result. If the indirect bilirubin is elevated and the direct is not, then the cause is a hemolytic problem.
Explain to the patient that the test is to determine whether an anemic or blood problem could be present, or make a similar statement.
Instruct the patient not to eat before blood is drawn. Carrots, yams, or foods high in fat should not be eaten the night before.

BILIRUBIN (TOTAL AND DIRECT) (Serum)

NORMAL RANGE

Adult: *Total:* 0.1–1.2 mg/dl, 1.7–20.5 μmol/L (SI units). *Direct* (conjugated): 0.1–0.3 mg/dl, 1.7–5.1 μmol/L (SI units).
Newborn: *Total:* 1–12 mg/dl, 17.1–205 μmol/L (SI units).
Child: 0.2–0.8 mg/dl.

DESCRIPTION

Bilirubin is formed from the breakdown of hemoglobin by the reticuloendothelial system and is carried in the plasma to the liver, where it is conjugated (directly) to form bilirubin diglucuronide and is excreted in the bile. There are two forms of bilirubin in the body: the conjugated or direct-reacting (soluble) and the unconjugated or indirect-reacting (protein-bound). If the total bilirubin is within normal range, direct and indirect bilirubin levels do not need to be analyzed. If one value of bilirubin is reported, it represents the total bilirubin.

Direct or conjugated bilirubin is frequently the result of obstructive jaundice, either extrahepatic (from stones or tumor) or intrahepatic in origin. Conjugated bilirubin cannot escape in the bile into the intestine and thus backs up and is absorbed into the bloodstream. Damaged liver cells cause a blockage of the bile sinusoid, increasing the serum level of direct bilirubin. With hepatitis and decompensated cirrhosis, both direct and indirect bilirubin may be elevated.

Serum bilirubin (total) in newborns can be as high as 12 mg/dl. Jaundice is frequently present when serum bilirubin levels are greater than 3 mg/dl.[8,9,11,27,30,31,34,36]

CLINICAL PROBLEMS

Decreased level *(↓ 0.1 mg/dl [adult total]):* iron deficiency anemia. *Drug influence:* barbiturates, salicylates (aspirin)—large amounts), penicillin, caffeine.

Elevated level *(↑ 1.2 mg/dl [adult total]):* obstructive jaundice due to stones or neoplasms, hepatitis, cirrhosis of the liver, infectious mononucleosis, liver metastasis (cancer), Wilson's disease. *Drug influence:* antibiotics—amphotericin B, clindamycin, erythromycin, gentamicin, lincomycin, oxacillin, tetracyclines; sulfonamides; anti-TB—PAS, Isoniazid (INH); allopurinol; diuretics—acetazolamide (Diamox), ethacrynic Acid (Edecrin); mithramycin; dextran; diazepam (Valium); barbiturate; narcotics—codeine, morphine, meperidine (Demerol); flurazepam (Dalmane); indomethacin (Indocin); methotrexate; methyldopa (Aldomet); papaverine; procainamide (Pronestyl); steroids; oral contraceptives; tolbutamide (Orinase); vitamins A, C, and K.

PROCEDURE

Collect 5 to 10 ml of venous blood in a red-top tube.

Keep the patient NPO except for water.

Hold medications which would increase the serum bilirubin for 24 hours, with the physician's approval. If medications need to be given, those drugs should be listed on the laboratory slip and reported.

Prevent hemolysis of the blood specimen. The tube containing the blood should not be shaken.

Caution: Whenever blood is drawn for liver function tests, avoid self-contamination to prevent possible infection (such as hepatitis). Use isolation technique.

Protect the blood specimen from sunlight and artificial light, as light will reduce the bilirubin content. Blood should be sent to the lab immediately so that separation of serum from the cells can be performed as soon as possible to avoid hemolysis.

Infants can have the blood taken from the heel of the foot. Two blood microtubes should be filled.

FACTORS AFFECTING LABORATORY RESULTS

A high-fat dinner prior to the test may affect bilirubin levels.

Carrots and yams may increase the serum bilirubin level.

Hemolysis of the blood specimen can give inaccurate results. The tube should not be shaken.

A blood specimen exposed to sunlight and artificial light will degrade the bile pigments. Certain drugs (see *Drug Influence* above) can increase or decrease the serum bilirubin level.

NURSING IMPLICATIONS AND RATIONALE

Elevated level (↑ 1.2 mg/dl)

Check the serum bilirubin (total) and, if it is elevated, check the direct and indirect bilirubin levels.

Explain to the patient that the test is a liver function test, the purpose of which is to determine whether the liver can conjugate bilirubin and excrete it in the bile.

Instruct the patient that he should have nothing by mouth except water before the test. If his medications are withheld, an appropriate explanation should be given. The nurse should emphasize that fats, carrots, and yams should not be eaten the night before the blood test.

Record on the chart and Kardex the drugs the patient is taking which could increase the bilirubin level.

Check the sclera of the eyes and the inner aspects of the arm for jaundice.

BILIRUBIN AND BILE (Urine)

NORMAL RANGE
Adult: *Negative:* 0.02 mg/dl.

DESCRIPTION

Bilirubin is not normally present in urine; however, a very small quantity could be present without being detected by routine test methods. Bilirubin is formed from the breakdown of hemoglobin and is transported to the liver, where it is conjugated and is excreted as bile. Conjugated or direct bilirubin is water-soluble and is excreted in the urine when there is an increased serum level. Unconjugated or indirect bilirubin is fat-soluble and cannot be excreted in the urine.

Bilirubinuria (bilirubin in urine) indicates liver damage or biliary obstruction (e.g., stones), and a large amount has a characteristic dark amber color. When the amber-colored urine is shaken, it produces a yellow foam. It can frequently be tested by the floor nurse with a dipstick or tablet.[8,9,11,27,30,34,36]

CLINICAL PROBLEMS

Elevated level *(↑ 0.02 mg/dl):* obstructive biliary disease; liver disease—hepatitis, toxic agents; CHF with jaundice; cancer of the liver (secondary). *Drug influence:* phenothiazines—chlorpromazine (Thorazine), acetophenazine (Tindal); chlorprothizene (Taractan); phenazopyridine (Pyridium); chlorzoxazone (Paraflex).

PROCEDURE

Use either bili-Labstix or Ictotest reagent tablets for the bilirubinuria test. The bili-Labstix is dipped in urine and after 20 seconds is compared to a color chart on the bottle. For bili-Labstix and Ictotest tablets, follow the directions on the bottle.

Test urine bilirubin within 1 hour. Keep urine away from ultraviolet light.

There is no food or drink restriction.

FACTORS AFFECTING LABORATORY RESULTS

Certain drugs can give a false positive result (see *Drug Influence* above).

Exposure of urine to light for 1 hour will cause deterioration of bile pigments.

NURSING IMPLICATIONS WITH RATIONALE

Elevated level (↑ 0.02 mg/dl)
Check the serum bilirubin—total and direct—and report if it is elevated. Test the urine
for bilirubinuria.
Assess the color of the urine. If it is dark amber in color, shake the urine specimen and
note whether a yellow foam appears.
Notify the physician of amber urine with yellow foam.
Record the results of a bili-Labstix and the urine color on the patient's chart or Kardex.

BLEEDING TIME (Blood)

NORMAL RANGE
Adult: *Ivy method:* 1–6 minutes. *Duke method:* 1–3 minutes. SI units for the Ivy and
Duke methods are the same.

DESCRIPTION
Two methods, Ivy and Duke, are used to determine whether bleeding time is normal or
prolonged. Bleeding time is lengthened in thrombocytopenia (decreased platelet
count— <50,000) and inability of blood vessels to constrict. The test is frequently
performed when there is a history of bleeding (easy bruising), familial bleeding, or
preoperative screening. The Ivy technique, in which the forearm is used for the incision, is the most popular method. Aspirins and anti-inflammatory medications can
prolong the bleeding time.[8,9,11,27,30,31,36]

CLINICAL PROBLEMS
Decreased rate: Hodgkin's disease.
Prolonged rate *(6 minutes [Ivy]):* thrombocytopenic purpura, platelet abnormality,
vascular abnormalities, leukemia, severe liver disease, DIC disease, aplastic anemia,
factor deficiencies (V, VII, XI), Christmas disease, hemophilia. *Drug influence:* salicylates (aspirins, others), dextran, mithramycin, coumadin, streptokinase–streptodornase (fibrinolytic agent).

PROCEDURE
Ivy method: Cleanse the volar surface of the forearm (below the antecubital space)
with alcohol and allow it to dry. Inflate the blood pressure cuff to 40 mmHg and leave
it inflated during the test. Puncture the skin 2.5 mm deep on the forearm; start timing
with a stopwatch. Blot *blood drops* carefully every 30 seconds until bleeding ceases.
The time required for bleeding to stop is recorded in seconds.
Duke method: The area used is the earlobe.
There is no food or drink restriction.

FACTORS AFFECTING LABORATORY RESULTS
Method used; improper technique—the puncture wound might be deeper than
required. Blotting the incision area and not the blood drops can break off fibrin
particles, prolonging the bleeding time.
Aspirin and anticoagulants increase the bleeding time.

NURSING IMPLICATIONS WITH RATIONALE

Prolonged rate (>6 minutes)
Relate prolonged bleeding time to clinical problems and drugs. The nurse should be
familiar with the methods used to obtain the bleeding time.
Explain to the patient the purpose of the bleeding time test. If it is for preoperative
screening information, this should be explained.
Explain to the patient how the test is performed. In the Ivy method the forearm is
used, and in the Duke method the earlobe is used. The step-by-step method of the
procedure should be explained (see *Procedure* above). The nurse should check with
the laboratory for changes in procedure.
Allow time for the patient to ask questions.
Obtain a drug history of the last time (date) the patient took aspirin or anticoagulants.
Aspirin prevents platelet aggregation, and bleeding can be prolonged by taking
only one aspirin tablet (5 grains or 325 mg) 3 days prior to test. A history of taking
"cold medications" should be recorded, since many cold remedies contain
salicylates.
Note whether the patient has been consuming alcohol. Alcohol increases bleeding time,
and the bleeding may be difficult to stop.
Apply a dressing to the puncture wound site (Ivy method) to stop the bleeding.
Instruct the patient not to take aspirin and over-the-counter cold remedies for 3 days
before the test. If the patient takes aspirins or anticoagulants, the laboratory
should be notified and the drug names should be written on the laboratory slip.

BLOOD GASES

See Arterial Blood Gases, PH, PCO_2, PO_2, Bicarbonate.

BLOOD UREA NITROGEN (BUN) (Serum)

NORMAL RANGE
   Men: 10–25 mg/dl.
   Women: 8–20 mg/dl.
   Infant: 5–15 mg/dl.
   Child: 5–20 mg/dl.

DESCRIPTION
   Urea is formed in the liver as an endproduct of protein metabolism, circulates in the
   blood, and is excreted by the kidneys. An elevated BUN could be an indication of
   dehydration, prerenal failure, or renal failure. Dehydration from vomiting, diarrhea,
   and/or inadequate fluid intake can cause an increase in the BUN (up to 50 mg/dl). Once
   the patient is hydrated, the BUN should return to normal; if it does not, prerenal or
   renal failure should be suspected. Nephrons (kidney cells) tend to decrease during the
   aging process, and so older persons may have a higher BUN.
   A low BUN value usually indicates overhydration (hypervolemia). After a loss of 80
   percent of hepatic function, urea production will decrease.[8,9,11,17,30,31,36]

CLINICAL PROBLEMS
   Decreased level (↓ *8 mg/dl):* severe liver damage, low-protein diet, overhydration,
   malnutrition (negative nitrogen balance), IV fluids (glucose). *Drug Influence:*
   phenothiazines.

Increased level (↑ *25 mg/dl)*: dehydration; high protein intake; gastrointestinal bleeding; prerenal failure—low renal blood supply from CHF, diabetes mellitus, acute myocardial infarction, renal insufficiency/failure from shock, sepsis, kidney diseases (glomerular nephritis, pyelonephritis); licorice (excessive ingestion). *Drug influence:* nephrotoxic drugs; diuretics—i.e., hydrochlorothiazide (Hydrodiuril), ethacrynic acid (Edecrin), furosemide (Lasix), triamterene (Dyrenium); antibiotics—i.e., bacitracin, cephaloridine (high doses), gentamicin, kanamycin, chloramphenicol (Chloromycetin), methicillin, neomycin, vancomycin; antihypertensive agents—methyldopa (Aldomet), guanethidine (Ismelin); sulfonamides; propranolol; morphine; lithium carbonate; salicylates.

PROCEDURE

Collect 5 ml of venous blood in a gray-top tube.
It is preferable to have the patient remain NPO for 8 hours.

FACTORS AFFECTING LABORATORY RESULTS

The hydration status of the patient should be known. Overhydration can give a false low BUN level, and dehydration can give a false high BUN level.

Drugs (i.e., antibiotics, diuretics, and antihypertensive agents) raise the BUN level.

NURSING IMPLICATIONS WITH RATIONALE

Decreased level (↓ 8 mg/dl)

Relate any clinical problems associated with a decreased serum BUN level.

Assess the patient's dietary intake. A low protein intake and a high carbohydrate intake can decrease the BUN level.

Report on patients receiving continuous dextrose intravenously without protein intake.

Check the patient for signs and symptoms of overhydration—i.e., irritated cough, dyspnea, neck vein engorgement, and chest rales when the BUN is decreased. Overhydration (hypervolemia) causes hemodilution, diluting the urea in the blood.

Elevated level (↑ 25 mg/dl)

Relate clinical problems associated with an increased serum BUN level.

Report urinary output less than 25 ml (cc)/hour or 600 ml (cc)/day. Urea is excreted by the kidneys, and with a decreased urine output, urea accumulates in the blood.

Check vital signs. A fast pulse, decreased blood pressure, and increased respiration could indicate dehydration and, if severe enough, could lead to shock.

Determine the hydration status of the patient. If dehydration is present, the elevated BUN may be attributed to hemoconcentration. Hydrating with intravenous fluids should correct the problem.

Avoid overhydration with intravenous fluid. Rapid administration of IV fluids can overload the vascular system, especially in the aged, in children, and in heart patients, resulting in hypervolemia. This can lead to pulmonary edema.

Assess the patient's dietary intake. A high-protein diet will increase the serum BUN. Individuals on a high-protein diet for dieting purposes will have an elevated BUN level unless adequate fluids are taken.

Recognize drugs that increase the BUN—i.e., antibiotics, diuretics, antihypertensive agents, and others (see *Drug Influence* above).

Teach patients with a slightly elevated BUN to increase fluid intake. Care should be taken in forcing fluids in patients with heart and kidney problems.

BROMIDE (Serum)

NORMAL RANGE
   Adult: toxic levels—>100 mg/dl.
   Child: same as adult.

DESCRIPTION
   The use of bromides as a prescription drug for depression and sedation is seldom ordered; however, today many bromide-containing compounds in patent medicines are
   available to the public. Because of the cumulative effect of bromides, chronic bromide
   intoxication is becoming a common occurrence. Acute bromide intoxication is rare,
   since bromide can cause gastrointestinal irritation.
   The half-life of bromide is 12 days. Bromide is slowly excreted by the kidney, and the
   treatment for chronic bromide intoxication is to accelerate urinary excretion by
   chloride administration and mercurial diuretics.[9,11,14,36]

PROCEDURE
   Collect 5 ml of venous blood in a green-top tube.
   There is no food or drink restriction.
   A colorimetric test using gold chloride is an old, but still useful test. The gold chloride
   reacts with the bromide in the plasma/serum, forming a yellow/red/orange color,
   depending on the bromide concentration.

FACTORS AFFECTING LABORATORY RESULTS
   An extremely high bromide level will cause a decreased chloride level, since both are
   anions.

NURSING IMPLICATIONS WITH RATIONALE

Observe for signs and symptoms of chronic bromide intoxication—i.e., anorexia, fever,
   skin rash, motor incoordination, tremors, delirium, impaired intellectual function,
   constipation, and weight loss.
Obtain a history on over-the-counter drugs taken: when, for how long, and the daily
   quantity taken. If the bottle is available, the label should contain the ingredients in
   the medicine.
Teach patients to read labels on patent medicines. Explain the importance of contacting a physician before taking most patent medicines.
Check urine output. Bromides are excreted slowly by the kidneys, so "good" kidney
   function is extremely important.

C

CALCIUM (Ca) (Serum)

NORMAL RANGE
Adult: 4.5–5.5 mEq/L, 9–11 mg/dl, 2.3–2.8 mmol/L (SI units).
Newborn: 3.7–7.0 mEq/L, 7.4–14.0 mg/dl.
Infant: 5.0–6.0 mEq/L, 10–12 mg/dl.
Child: 4.5–5.8 mEq/L, 9–11.5 mg/dl.

DESCRIPTION
Calcium is found most abundantly in the bones and teeth (99 percent); this calcium is usually available for restoration of a normal serum calcium level. Approximately 50 percent of the calcium is ionized, and only ionized calcium can be utilized by the body; however, in most laboratories the total serum calcium level determination does not differentiate between ionized and nonionized calcium. There is a new technique available to measure ionized Ca. In acidosis, more calcium is ionized, regardless of the serum level, and in alkalosis, most of the calcium is protein-bound and cannot be ionized. Tetany symptoms are present when the pH is greater than 7.45 (alkalosis) and the serum calcium level is low.

Calcium has many functions besides making bone and teeth strong and durable. It strengthens capillary membranes. With a calcium deficit, there is an increased capillary permeability which causes fluid to pass through the capillary. Calcium is necessary for the transmission of nerve impulses and contraction of the myocardium and skeletal muscles. It causes blood clotting by converting prothrombin into thrombin.

The parathyroid hormone and vitamin D promote calcium absorption from the gastrointestinal mucosa, and parathyroid hormone also directs the bone to release calcium when there is a deficit. Calcitonin secreted from the thyroid gland lowers the serum calcium level (the kidneys excrete calcium) and increases the phosphorous levels.

A low serum calcium level is called hypocalcemia, and an increased level is called hypercalcemia. Calcium imbalances require immediate attention, for serum calcium deficit can cause tetany symptoms, unless acidosis is present, and serum calcium excess can cause cardiac arrhythmias.[5,7,8,11,17,24,30,33]

CLINICAL PROBLEMS
Decreased level *(<4.5 mEq/L [adult]):* diarrhea, malabsorption of calcium from the GI tract, laxative abuse, extensive infections, burns, lack of calcium and vitamin D intake, hypoparathyroidism, chronic renal failure due to phosphorous retention, alcoholism, pancreatitis. *Drug influence:* cortisone preparations; antibiotics—gentamicin, methicillin; magnesium products (antacids); laxative (excessive use); heparin; insulin; mithramycin; acetazolamide (Diamox); BSP (test).

Elevated level *(>5.5 mEq/L [adult]):* hypervitaminosis D; hyperparathyroidism; malignant neoplasm of the bone, lung, breast, bladder, or kidney; multiple myeloma; prolonged immobilization; multiple fractures; renal calculi; exercise; alcoholism (alcoholic binge); milk–alkali syndrome. *Drug influence:* alkaline antacids, estrogen preparations, calcium salts, vitamin D.

PROCEDURE
Collect 5 to 10 ml of venous blood in a red-top tube.
There is no food or drink restriction, unless SMA_{12} is ordered.

FACTORS AFFECTING LABORATORY RESULTS
   Drugs: thiazide diuretics, laxatives, antacids, and cortisone contribute to calcium
      excess and deficit.
   Diet: low in calcium or high in calcium and vitamin D.
   IV saline (NaCl) solution can promote calcium loss.

NURSING IMPLICATIONS WITH RATIONALE

Explain to the patient the purpose of the blood test—for instance, "to determine the
   calcium level in the blood." This blood test may be part of the SMA_{12}, and the
   explanation may include: "to determine values of various chemical substances in
   the blood."
Explain that food and drink may be restricted. It should be reported if the patient has
   consumed large quantities of milk products in the last several weeks or months or
   has been taking calcium tablets.

Decreased level (<4.5 mEq/L [adult])
Recognize clinical problems and drugs that can cause hypocalcemia—i.e., diarrhea,
   malabsorption syndrome, laxative abuse, extensive infections and burns, chronic
   renal failure, hypoparathyroidism, cortisone, heparin, insulin, and magnesium
   products.
Observe for signs and symptoms of hypocalcemia—i.e., tetany symptoms: muscular
   twitching and tremors, spasms of the larynx, paresthesia (tingling in and numbness
   of fingers), facial spasms, and spasmodic contractions.
Check serum calcium values and report abnormal results to the physician, especially if
   tetany symptoms are present.
Teach the patient to avoid overuse of antacids and to prevent the chronic laxative
   habit. Excessive use of certain antacids could cause alkalosis and does decrease
   calcium ionization. In addition, many antacids contain magnesium, which could
   lower the serum calcium level. Many laxatives contain phosphates (phosphorous)
   which have an opposing effect on calcium, causing calcium loss. Chronic use of laxatives will decrease calcium absorption from the gastrointestinal tract. Suggest
   fruits for improving bowel elimination.
Encourage the patient to consume foods high in calcium, in milk and milk products,
   and/or in protein. Protein is needed to enhance calcium absorption.
Teach the patient with hypocalcemia to avoid hyperventilation and crossing his legs,
   which could increase tetany symptoms.
Assess for positive Chvostek's and Trousseau's signs of hypocalcemia. To test for
   positive Chvostek's sign, tap the area in front of the ear and observe for spasms of
   the cheek and the corner of the lip. To test for positive Trousseau's sign, inflate the
   blood pressure cuff for several minutes and observe for carpal spasms.
Administor oral calcium supplements before or 1 to 1.5 hours after meals.
Observe for symptoms of hypocalcemia when the patient is receiving massive transfusions of citrated blood. Citrates prevent calcium ionization. The serum calcium level
   may not be affected.
Monitor the pulse regularly if the patient is receiving a digitalis preparation and
   calcium supplements. Calcium excess enhances the action of digitalis and can cause
   digitalis toxicity (nausea, vomiting, anorexia, bradycardia—arrhythmias).
Administer intravenous fluids with 10 percent calcium gluconate slowly. Calcium
   should be administered in 5 percent dextrose/water and not in a saline solution, for
   sodium promotes calcium loss. Calcium should not be added to solutions containing
   bicarbonate, since rapid precipitation will occur.

Monitor the ECG during hypocalcemia for prolonged ST segments and lengthened Q–T intervals.

Elevated level (>5.5 mEq/L [adult])
Recognize clinical problems and drugs related to hypercalcemia—i.e., hyperparathyroidism, tumors of the bone, prolonged immobilization, multiple fractures, hypervitaminosis D, and calcium salts.
Observe for signs and symptoms of hypercalcemia—i.e., lethargy, headaches, weakness, muscle flaccidity, heart block, anorexia, nausea, and vomiting.
Teach patients to avoid foods high in calcium, to be ambulatory when possible, and to increase oral fluid intake. Increased fluid intake dilutes calcium in the serum and urine and prevents calculi formation.
Promote active and passive exercises for bedridden patients. This will prevent calcium loss from the bone.
Identify symptoms of digitalis toxicity when the patient has an elevated serum calcium level and is receiving a digitalis preparation.
Give loop diuretics as ordered. Notify the physician if the patient is receiving a thiazide diuretic, for this will inhibit calcium excretion.
Check the urine pH. Calcium salts are more soluble in acid urine (pH < 6.0) than in alkaline. Encourage such acid-ash foods as cranberry juice, meats, fish, poultry, eggs, cheese, and cereals to keep the urine acidic.
Handle patients with long-standing hypercalcemia and bone demineralization gently to prevent pathologic fractures.
Monitor the rate of IV saline solutions. Sodium from saline solution promotes calcium excretion (sodium is reabsorbed by the kidney). Observe for symptoms of overhydration—i.e., a constant, irritated cough; dyspnea; neck and vein engorgement; and chest rales from use of saline.

CALCIUM (Urine)
Sulkowitch Test (Random Specimen); Quantitative (24 Hour Urine Collection)

NORMAL RANGE
Adult: Sulkowitch +1 to +2. *24 hour:* low-calcium diet—<150 mg/24 hours, <3.75 mmol/24 hours (SI units); average-Ca diet—100–250 mg/24 hours, 2.50–6.25 mmol/24 hours; high-Ca diet—250–300 mg/24 hours, 6.25–7.50 mmol/24 hours.
Child: same as adult.

DESCRIPTION
Urine calcium reflects the dietary intake of calcium, the serum calcium level, and the effects of disease entities (hypo- or hyperparathyroidism, multiple myeloma, bone tumors, etc.). Hypercalciuria (increased calcium levels in the urine) usually accompanies an increased serum calcium level. Calcium excretion fluctuates and is lowest in the morning and highest after meals.
The Sulkowitch test for urine calcium is a popular test, mainly because it roughly measures the amount of calcium in a random specimen of urine. Sulkowitch reagent is added in equal value to the sample of urine, and precipitation occurs if calcium is present. To rule out hypercalcemia and hypercalciuria, an early morning specimen should be tested. For determining hypocalcemia and hypocalciuria, a urine specimen should be taken after a meal.
A 24 hour urine specimen for calciuria is useful for determining parathyroid gland disorders. In hyperparathyroidism, the urinary calcium excretion is usually increased; it is decreased in hypoparathyroidism.[5,7,8,9,11,17,30,36]

CLINICAL PROBLEMS

Decreased level *(<100 mg/24 hours [average-Ca diet])*: hypoparathyroidism, vitamin D deficiency, hypothyroidism, chronic renal failure, malabsorption syndrome. *Drug influence:* thiazide diuretics, viomycin.

Elevated level *(>250 mg/24 hours [average-Ca diet])*: hyperparathyroidism; osteoporosis; hyperthyroidism; malignancies—bone, breast, bladder; multiple myeloma; leukemias; hypervitaminosis D; amyotrophic lateral sclerosis (ALS); renal calculi; acid–base imbalance. *Drug influence:* cholestyramine resin, sodium- and magnesium-containing drugs, parathyroid injection, vitamin D.

PROCEDURE

Collect the urine specimen for the Sulkowitch test at a specific time (in the morning or after a meal).

For a 24 hour urine collection, label the bottle with the exact date and the times that the urine collection started and ended. For the Sulkowitch test, place a label on the container with the time and date of the urine specimen.

Indicate on the laboratory slip whether the patient's calcium intake has been limited in the last 3 days or whether the patient has had an average or high calcium intake.

Preservatives are required by some laboratories; however, in most institutions, a preservative or refrigeration is not required.

FACTORS AFFECTING LABORATORY RESULTS

Discarded urine. All urine should be saved for the 24 hour urine collection.

Diet: high or low in calcium content.

Thiazide diuretics and drugs containing sodium and magnesium.

NURSING IMPLICATIONS WITH RATIONALE

Explain that the purpose for the urine collection (single random specimen or 24 hour collection) is to determine the amount of calcium excreted in the urine. A more detailed explanation may be needed.

Inform the patient and his family that urine is to be saved and should not be discarded. Inform the patient not to put toilet paper or feces in the urine.

Decreased level (<100 mg/24 hours [average-Ca diet])

Associate clinical problems and drugs with a decreased urine calcium level. The Sulkowitch test is a screening test for a rough measurement of urine calcium and for comparison of urine calcium to serum calcium. The 24 hour urine collection (quantitative test) is useful for identifying parathyroid disorders—hypoparathyroidism and hyperparathyroidism.

Observe for tetany symptoms if the patient's urine calcium is low. See Calcium (Serum) for tetany symptoms.

Have available a 10 percent solution of calcium gluconate for emergencies. When administered, IV calcium should be diluted in dextrose in water solution and not in saline solution.

For other nursing implications, see Calcium (Serum).

Elevated level (>250 mg/24 hours [average-Ca diet])

Associate clinical problems and drugs with an elevated urine calcium level—i.e., hyperparathyroidism, bone tumors, osteoporosis, hypervitaminosis D, renal calculi, drugs containing sodium and magnesium, and others.

Observe patients for symptoms of renal calculi, especially if there is a history of renal calculi. Strain the urine, if indicated, and report severe low-back pain.

Prevent the possibility of a pathologic fracture by moving the patient gently. The patient should be encouraged to do active exercises.

For other nursing implications, see Calcium (Serum).

CARBON DIOXIDE COMBINING POWER (Serum or Plasma)
CO_2 Combining Power

NORMAL RANGE
Adult: 22–30 mEq/L, 22–30 mmol/L (SI units).
Child: 20–28 mEq/L.

DESCRIPTION
The carbon dioxide (CO_2) combining power test is performed to determine metabolic acid–base abnormalities. This test measures the amount of carbon dioxide dissolved in the serum or plasma at a given temperature and pressure. The serum CO_2 acts as a bicarbonate (HCO_3) determinant, since CO_2 and HCO_3 interact in the blood. When serum carbon dioxide is low, bicarbonate is lost and acidosis results (metabolic acidosis). With an elevated serum CO_2 excess, bicarbonate is conserved and alkalosis results (metabolic alkalosis). This test is not as effective in determining respiratory acidosis and alkalosis as it is in determining metabolic acid–base disturbances.[8,9,11,30,31,36]

CLINICAL PROBLEMS
Decreased level *(↓ 22 mEq/L [adult]):* metabolic acidosis, diabetic ketoacidosis, starvation, severe diarrhea, dehydration, shock, acute renal failure, salicylate toxicity, exercise. *Drug influence:* diuretics—chlorothiazide (Diuril), hydrochlorothiazide (Hydrodiuril), triamterene (Dyrenium); antibiotics—methicillin, tetracycline; nitrofurantoin (Furadantin); paraldehyde.

Elevated level *(↑ 30 mEq/L [adult]):* metabolic alkalosis, severe vomiting, gastric suction, peptic ulcer, hypothyroidism, potassium deficit, emphysema (hypoventilation). *Drug influence:* barbiturates; steroids—hydrocortisone, cortisone; diuretics—mercurial agents, ethacrynic acid (Edecrin).

PROCEDURE
Collect 7 to 10 ml of venous blood in a green-top tube. If possible, a tourniquet should not be used, and if it is used, the fist should not be opened and closed, but kept closed without straining.

The blood sample was previously collected under oil, but now it is frequently collected in a tube containing heparin under a vacuum, making it anaerobic.

There is no food or drink restriction.

FACTORS AFFECTING LABORATORY RESULTS
Drugs that can increase or decrease the serum CO_2 level (see *Drug Influence* above).

NURSING IMPLICATIONS WITH RATIONALE

Explain to the patient that the test is to determine the acid–base balance in the body.
A more detailed explanation may be needed.

Instruct the patient that food and drink intake is not restricted.

Explain to the patient the method of collecting the blood sample (i.e., a tourniquet may or may not be used). Hospitals and institutions differ in method. It is preferable not to use a tourniquet, since stasis can cause diffusion of gases.

Decreased level (↓ 22 mEq/L)

Know that a decreased serum CO_2 is related to an acidotic state. Whenever there is excess acid in the body and the kidneys cannot excrete it, metabolic acidosis results. There are many causes of acidosis (see *Clinical Problems* above).

Assess for signs and symptoms of metabolic acidosis when the patient's serum CO_2 is decreased, especially when it is less than 15 mEq/L. Symptoms include deep, vigorous breathing (Kussmaul breathing) and flushed skin.

Report clinical findings of metabolic acidosis to the physician.

Elevated level (↑ 30 mEq/L)

Know that an increase serum CO_2 is related to an alkalotic state. Whenver there is an excess of bicarbonate in the body or a loss of acid, metabolic alkalosis occurs. There are many causes of alkalosis (see *Clinical Problems* above).

Assess for signs and symptoms of metabolic alkalosis when the patient has been vomiting or has had gastric suction for several days. Signs and symptoms include shallow breathing, a serum CO_2 greater than 30 mEq/L, and a base excess greater than +2.

CARBON MONOXIDE, CARBOXYHEMOGLOBIN (Blood)

NORMAL RANGE

Adult: *Nonsmoker:* 2.5 percent of hemoglobin. *Smoker:* 2–5 percent saturation of hemoglobin. *Heavy smoker:* 5–9 percent saturation of hemoglobin. *Toxic:* >25 percent saturation of hemoglobin.

Child: similar to adult nonsmoker.

DESCRIPTION

Carbon monoxide (CO) combines with hemoglobin to produce carboxyhemoglobin, which can occur 200 times more readily than the combination of oxygen with hemoglobin (oxyhemoglobin). When carbon monoxide replaces oxygen in the hemoglobin in excess 25 percent carbon monoxide toxicity occurs.

Carbon monoxide is formed from incomplete combustion of carbon-combining compounds, as in automobile exhaust, fumes from improperly functioning furnaces, and cigarette smoke. Continuous exposure to CO, increasing carboxyhemoglobin by more than 60 percent, leads to coma and death. The treatment for carbon monoxide toxicity is to administer a high concentration of oxygen.[8,9,11,30,36]

CLINICAL PROBLEMS

Elevated level *(↑ 2.5 percent):* smoking and exposure to smoking, automobile exhaust fumes, defective gas-burning appliances.

PROCEDURE

Collect 5 to 10 ml of venous blood in a lavender-top tube.

The most common method of analysis is performed with an IL CO oximeter, a direct-reading instrument.

There is no food or drink restriction.

FACTORS AFFECTING LABORATORY RESULTS

Heavy smoking.

NURSING IMPLICATIONS WITH RATIONALE

Determine from the patient's history (obtained from the patient, his family, or his friends) whether carbon monoxide inhalation could have occurred.

Assess for mild to severe carbon monoxide toxicity. Symptoms of mild CO toxicity are headache, weakness, malaise, dizziness, and dyspnea with exertion. Symptoms of moderate to severe toxicity are severe headache, bright red mucous membranes, and cherry red blood. When carboxyhemoglobin exceeds 40 percent, the blood's residue is brick red.

Identify individuals that might be a candidate for carbon monoxide poisoning. Persons complaining of continous headaches or who are living (24 hours a day) in a house with an old heating system in the winter should have a blood carbon monoxide test performed.

Explain to the patient that the blood test is to determine the carbon monoxide concentration in the blood, or give a similar response.

CARCINOEMBRYONIC ANTIGEN (CEA) (Blood)

NORMAL RANGE
Adult: <2.5 ng/ml.
Child: not normally done; assumed to be low (level) after the child is several months old.

DESCRIPTION
Carcinoembryonic antigen (CEA) has been found in the gastrointestinal epithelium of embryos and has been extracted from tumors in the adult GI tract. Originally, the CEA test was to detect colon cancer, especially adenocarcinoma. However, elevated levels have been obtained in various organ malignancies and in benign diseases when inflammation and tissue destruction are present. CEA should never be used as the sole criterion for diagnosis.

The CEA test is a nonspecific test; however, elevated levels have been found in approximately 70 percent of patients with known cancer of the large intestine and pancreas. The primary role of the CEA test is to monitor the treatment of colon and pancreatic carcinoma; it is also used for follow-up studies once cancer has been diagnosed. If the levels fall below 2.5 ng/ml following treatment, the cancer is most likely under control. A CEA test may be ordered at 30 to 90 day intervals, and if a significant CEA level reoccurs, the physician may resume chemotherapy treatments or consider another form of therapy. CEA test results over 10 ng/ml are suggestive of a tumor.[8,9,11,27,30,31]

CLINICAL PROBLEMS
Elevated level *(> 2.5 ng/ml):* cancer of the GI tract—esophagus, stomach, small and large intestine, rectum; cancer of the liver, pancreas, lung, breast, cervix, bladder, testis, kidney; leukemia; pulmonary emphysema; cirrhosis of the liver; bacterial pneumonia; chronic ischemic heart disease; acute pancreatitis; acute renal failure; peritoneal fluid; ulcerative colitis; chronic cigarette smoking; neuroblastoma; inflammatory diseases; surgical trauma.

PROCEDURE
Collect 10 to 15 ml of venous blood in a lavender-top tube. The blood should fill the tube to capacity. A radioimmunoassay (RIA) procedure is used.

Heparin should not be administered for 2 days before the test, since it interferes with the results.

There is no food or drink restriction.

FACTORS AFFECTING LABORATORY RESULTS
Heparin interferes with the result of the CEA test.
Prevent hemolysis.

NURSING IMPLICATIONS WITH RATIONALE

Elevated level (>2.5 ng/ml)
Relate clinical problems to elevated CEA levels. CEA levels over 2.5 ng/ml do not always indicate cancer, nor do levels below 2.5 ng/ml indicate an absence of cancer. The CEA test is not a screening test, but is used for management of cancer treatment.

Explain to the patient the purpose of the test. Explanation can be as brief as "It's for determining response to treatment," or a more detailed explanation may be needed.

Instruct the patient that he may eat and drink before the test.

Hold heparin injections for 2 days before the test, with the physician's permission. If heparin is given, this fact should be noted on the laboratory slip.

CAROTENE (Serum)

NORMAL RANGE
Adult: 40–200 µg/dl (mcg/dl), 0.74–3.72 µmol/L (SI units).
Child: 40–130 µg/dl.

DESCRIPTION
Carotene is a fat-soluble vitamin found in yellow and green vegetables and fruits. After absorption from the intestine, carotene is stored in the liver and can be converted to vitamin A, according to body needs. When fat absorption is decreased, the serum carotene level is decreased, which is indicative of fat malabsorption syndrome.

There are various causes of serum carotene deficit, such as poor diet, malabsorption, high fever, and pancreatic insufficiency. This test is used mostly for screening purposes. When the deficit is less than 30 µg/dl, malabsorption syndrome is suspected.[8,11,27,30]

CLINICAL PROBLEMS
Decreased level *(↓ 40 µg/dl [adult]):* malabsorption syndrome, pancreatic insufficiency, protein malnutrition, febrile illness, severe liver disease, cystic fibrosis.
Elevated level *(↑ 200 µg/dl [adult]):* hyperlipidemia, diabetes mellitus, chronic nephritis, hypothyroidism, diet high in carrots, hypervitaminosis A (slight elevation), pregnancy, hypocholesterolemia.

PROCEDURE
Collect 5 to 10 ml of venous blood in a red-top tube. Protect from light.

Foods rich in carotene—yellow and green vegetables, vegetable juice, and fruits—should be omitted for 2 to 3 days before the test (check laboratory procedure). If the physician wishes to check the serum carotene level for determining the absorption ability, a diet high in carotene will be ordered for several days. Water is permitted.

NPO, a diet low in carotene, or a diet high in carotene should be recorded on the laboratory slip.

FACTORS AFFECTING LABORATORY RESULTS
Mineral oil will interfere with carotene absorption.
Foods rich in carotene can affect the serum results.

NURSING IMPLICATIONS WITH RATIONALE

Decreased level (↓ 40 μg/dl)
Relate clinical problems to serum carotene deficit. The most frequent cause is malabsorption syndrome, often with a serum level below 30 μg/dl. There are various causes of low serum carotene (see *Clinical Problems* above), but the test is primarily for screening purposes to determine intestinal absorption disorders.
Explain to the patient that his diet will be high or low in carotene, depending on the physician's clinical assumptions and orders. Drinking water is permitted.
Explain to the patient that the test is to determine whether there is a vitamin (carotene) deficiency.
Answer the patient's questions concerning what foods to avoid or to eat before the test. Vegetables and fruits are rich in carotene.

Elevated level (↑ 200 μg/dl)
Relate clinical problems to elevated serum carotene levels. Hyperlipidemia and an excess carrot consumption are the two most frequent causes of serum carotene excess.

CATECHOLAMINES (Urine)

NORMAL RANGE
    Adult: <100 μg/24 hours (higher with activity), <0.59 μmol/24 hours (SI units), 0–14 μg/dl (random), epinephrine <10 ng/24 hours, norepinephrine <100 ng/24 hours.
    Child: level less than adult due to weight differences.

DESCRIPTION
    Catecholamines are hormones (epinephrine and norepinephrine) secreted by the adrenal medulla. Catecholamine production increases after strenuous exercise; however, urinary levels are 3 to 100 times greater than normal in cases of pheochromocytoma (tumor of the adrenal medulla). In some psychiatric patients, the urine catecholamine level increases only slightly. In children, this test may be used to diagnose malignant neuroblastoma.
    Certain drugs, coffee, and bananas cause elevated catecholamine levels.[11,27,30,34]

CLINICAL PROBLEMS
    Elevated level *(>100 μg/24 hours):* pheochromocytoma; severe stress—septicemia, shock, burn, peritonitis; malignant neuroblastoma; acute myocardial infarction (first 48 hours); chronic ischemic heart disease; cor pulmonale; carcinoid syndrome; manic depressive disorder; depressive neurosis; strenuous excercise. *Drug influence:* antibiotics—ampicillin, declomycin, erythromycin, tetracyclines; antihypertensives—methyldopa (Aldomet), hydralazine (Apresoline); vitamins—ascorbic acid (vitamin C), B complex; chlorpromazine (Thorazine); quinine or quinidine; Isuprel or epinephrine by inhalation.

PROCEDURE
Collect urine for 24 hours in a large container with a preservative (10 ml of concentrated HC1) and keep the bottle refrigerated. Some hospitals may not require a preservative.
Drugs (see *Drug influence* above), coffee, and bananas should not be taken for 3 to 7 days before the test. The number of days may vary among laboratories.
Food and drinks other than those already mentioned are not restricted.
Label the large container with the patient's name and the dates and exact times for the 24 hour urine collection—e.g., 4/10/83, 7:30 A.M. to 4/11/83, 7:30 A.M.

FACTORS AFFECTING LABORATORY RESULTS
Foods: bananas, coffee.
Certain drugs: see *Drug Influence* above.

NURSING IMPLICATIONS WITH RATIONALE

Explain to the patient that the purpose for the test is to determine the amount of a hormone (catecholamine) excreted in the urine.
Post on the patient's door and/or bed and Kardex the dates and times of urine collection.
Explain to the patient and family that all urine should be saved in the refrigerated container. Inform the patient that toilet paper and feces should not be put in the urine.
Instruct the patient not to eat bananas or drink coffee for 3 to 7 days before the test.
Withhold drugs for 3 days or more and record those drugs (see *Drug Influence* above) which the patient must take on the laboratory slip and progress sheet.

Elevated level (>100 μg/24 hours
Recognize causes of elevated urine catecholamines other than pheochromocytoma. These include severe stress, strenuous exercise, and acute anxiety and other psychiatric disorders. The highest levels occur in pheochromocytoma.
Check vital signs and report rising blood pressure readings.
Report to the physician and record on the nurse's notes or progress notes whether the patient has been involved in strenuous activity or has suffered from severe anxiety.
See VMA (Vanilmandelic Acid) results.

CEREBROSPINAL FLUID (CSF)
(Color, Pressure, Cell Count, Protein, Chloride, Glucose, Culture)
Spinal Fluid

NORMAL RANGE

	Color	Pressure (mm H_2O)	Cell Count (Leukocytes)— cu mm (mm^3)	Protein (mg/dl)	Chloride (MEq/L)	Glucose (mg/dl)
Adult	Clear, colorless	75–175	0–8	15–45	118–132	40–80
Child	Clear, colorless	50–100	0–8	14–45	120–128	35–75
Premature infant			0–20	<400		
Newborn	Clear		0–15	30–200	110–122	20–40
1–6 months				30–100		

DESCRIPTION

Cerebrospinal fluid (CSF), also known as spinal fluid, circulates in the ventricles of the brain and through the spinal cord. Of the 150 ml of CSF, approximately 100 ml are produced by the blood in the brain ventricles and reabsorbed back into circulation daily.

Spinal fluid is obtained by a lumbar puncture (spinal tap) performed in the lumbar sac at L3 to L4, or at L4 to L5. First CSF pressure is measured, then fluid is aspirated and placed in sterile test tubes. Data from the analysis of the spinal fluid is important for diagnosing spinal cord and brain diseases.

The analysis of spinal fluid usually includes color, pressure, cell count (leukocytes—WBC), protein, chloride, and glucose. In addition, the pH of the CSF is usually checked, and it is usually slightly lower—about one-tenth (0.1) of a point—than the pH of the serum. The CSF protein and glucose levels are lower than the blood levels; however, the CSF chloride level is higher than the serum chloride level. Normally, a culture is done to detect any organism present in the spinal fluid.[4,8,11,27,36]

CLINICAL PROBLEMS

CSF	Decreased Level	Elevated Level	Comments
Color		Abnormal color: (1) Pink or red—subarachnoid or cerebral hemorrhage; traumatic spinal tap (2) Xanthochromia (yellow color)—previous subarachnoid hemorrhage	Yellow color indicates old blood (4 to 5 days after a cerebral hemorrhage), mixture of bilirubin and blood, or extremely elevated protein levels; fluid discoloration normally remains for 3 weeks.
Pressure	Dehydration, hypovolemia	Intracranial pressure due to Meningitis, subarachnoid hemorrhage, brain tumor, brain abscess, encephalitis	Slight elevation can occur with holding breath or tensing of muscles.
Cell count (lymphocytes)		<500 mm³: viral infections—poliomyelitis, aseptic meningitis; syphilis of CNS; multiple sclerosis; brain tumor; abscess; subarachnoid hemorrhage (40 percent or more monocytes) >500 mm³: ↑ granulocytes, purulent infection	WBC differential count may be ordered to identify the types of leukocytes.

CLINICAL PROBLEMS

CSF	Decreased Level	Elevated Level	Comments
Protein		Meningitis: TB, purulent, aseptic Guillain–Barre syndrome Subarachnoid hemorrhage Brain Tumor Abscess Syphilis Drug influence: anesthetics, acetophenetidin, chlorpromazine (Thorazine), phenacetin, salicylates (aspirin), streptomycin, sulfonamides	Protein and cell counts usually increase together.
Chloride	Tuberculosis meningitis Bacterial meningitis		IV saline or electrolyte infusion could cause an inaccurate result. Syphilis, brain tumors and abscess, and encephalitis do not affect the CSF chloride level.
Glucose	Purulent meningitis Presence of fungi, protozoa, or pyogenic bacteria Subarachnoid hemorrhage Lymphomas Leukemia	Cerebral trauma Hypothalamic lesions Diabetes (hyperglycemia)	Brain abscess or tumor and degenerative diseases have little effect on the CSF glucose. The CSF glucose is usually two-thirds of the blood glucose. The blood glucose level is determined for comparative reasons.
Culture		Meningitis	Generally done when meningitis is suspected.

PROCEDURE
Check the hospital procedure for a lumbar puncture (spinal tap). The physician performs the procedure.

Collect a sterile lumbar puncture tray, an antiseptic solution (i.e., Betadine, or iodine), a local anesthetic (i.e., lidocaine), sterile gloves, and tape.

Place the patient in a "fetal" position, with the back bowed, the head flexed on the chest, and the knees drawn up to the abdomen.

Label the three test tubes 1, 2, and 3.

The physician checks the spinal fluid pressure, using a manometer attached to the needle. The physician collects a total of 10 to 12 ml of spinal fluid—3 ml in a no. 1 tube, 3 ml in a no. 2 tube, and 3 ml in a no. 3 tube. The first tube could be contaminated (with blood from the spinal tap) and should *not* be used for cell count, culture, or protein determination.

Label the tubes with the patient's name, date, and room number. Take the test tubes immediately to the laboratory. Do not refrigerate—especially the tube for culture.

There is no food or drink restriction.

Queckenstedt procedure: The Queckenstedt procedure is performed during a lumbar puncture when spinal block is suspected. Temporary pressure is applied to the jugular veins while the CSF pressure is monitored. Normally, the CSF pressure will rise when the jugular veins are compressed. In partial or total CSF block, the pressure fails to rise with jugular vein compression; *OR* it takes 15 to 30 seconds for CSF pressure to drop after compression is released.[8,36]

FACTORS AFFECTING LABORATORY RESULTS

Refrigeration can affect the results of the culture.

A traumatic spinal tap could cause the presence of blood in the fluid specimen, which could be mistaken for a clinical problem.

Certain drugs could cause a false increased CSF protein level (see "Drug influence" under *Clinical Problems* above)

IV fluid containing chloride could invalidate the CSF chloride level determination.

Hyperglycemia could increase the CSF glucose level.

NURSING IMPLICATIONS WITH RATIONALE

Explain to the patient the purpose of the test. Explanation may be brief, such as, "to analyze the spinal fluid content." A more detailed explanation may be needed.

Explain the procedure for the lumbar puncture to the patient by giving a step-by-step detailed explanation. Inform the patient that you or a designated person will remain with him during the procedure.

Answer the patient's questions concerning the test. Questions you cannot answer should be referred to appropriate persons.

Do not mix the numbers on the test tube specimens. The first tube may have some RBC because of the needle insertion. For culture, the second or third test tube is used. For protein and cell count, the third specimen tube is used.

Instruct the patient to relax and take deep and slow breaths with his mouth open. Hold the patient's hand to give reassurance, unless this is opposed by the patient.

Check the vital signs before the procedure and afterwards at specified times—i.e., 1/2, 1, 2, and 4 hours.

Assess for changes in the neurologic status after the procedure—i.e., ↑ temperature, ↑ BP, irritability, numbness and tingling in the lower extremities, and nonreactive eye pupils.

Instruct the patient to remain flat in bed in the prone or supine position for 4 to 8 hours following the lumbar puncture. Headaches are common due to spinal fluid leaking from the site of the lumbar puncture, which can occur if the patient is in an upright position.

Administer an analgesic as ordered to relieve a headache if it occurs.

Be supportive of the patient before, during, and after the lumber puncture.

CERULOPLASMIN (Cp) (Serum)

NORMAL RANGE
   Adult: 23–50 mg/dl, 230–500 mg/L (SI units).
   Infant: <23 mg/dl, or may be normal.
   Child: similar to adult.

DESCRIPTION
   Ceruloplasmin (Cp) is a copper-containing glycoprotein known as one to the alpha$_2$-globulins in the plasma. Ceruloplasmin is produced in the liver and binds with copper. Copper plays a crucial role in enzyme performance and uses Cp as its vehicle for transporting purposes. The principle role of ceruloplasmin is not clearly understood, except that when there is a serum deficit, there is an increased urinary excretion of copper and increased depositing of copper on the cornea, brain, liver, and kidney, causing damage and destruction of the organs. A deficit of ceruloplasmin or hypoceruloplasmin can result in Wilson's disease (hepatolenticular degeneration), commonly seen between the ages of 7 and 15 and in early middle age.
   Ceruloplasmin levels are frequently low at birth. Oral contraceptives and pregnancy can increase the serum ceruloplasmin levels.[11,14,27,34]

CLINICAL PROBLEMS
   Decreased level *(↓ 23 mg/dl [adult]):* Wilson's disease (hepatolenticular degeneration), protein malnutrition, nephrotic syndrome, newborns and early infancy.
   Elevated level *(↑ 50 mg/dl [adult]):* cirrhosis of the liver; hepatitis; pregnancy; Hodgkin's disease; cancer of the bone, stomach, lung; myocardial infarction; rheumatoid arthritis; infections and inflammatory process; exercise. *Drug influence:* oral contraceptives, estrogen drugs.

PROCEDURE
   Collect 5 ml of venous blood in a red-top tube.
   There is no food or drink restriction.
   Withhold drugs containing estrogen for 24 hours before the blood test, with the physician's permission.

FACTORS AFFECTING LABORATORY RESULTS
   Estrogen therapy and exercise could cause an elevated serum ceruloplasmin level.
   In Wilson's disease with severe liver damage, a normal serum level could result.

NURSING IMPLICATIONS WITH RATIONALE

Decreased level (↓ 23 mg/dl)
Relate hypoceruloplasmin (serum ceruloplasmin deficit) to Wilson's disease. The serum level is frequently below 15 mg/dl and is commonly seen after the age of 7.
Assess for signs and symptoms of Wilson's disease—i.e., abnormal muscular rigidity (dystonia), tremors of the fingers, dysarthria, and mental disturbances.
Explain to the patient that the test is for determining a certain protein deficiency. Further explanation may be needed.
Instruct the patient that he may eat or drink before the test.
Check the cornea of the eye for a discolored ring (Kayser–Fleisher ring) from copper deposits.

Elevated level (↑ 50 mg/dl)
Relate clinical problems of liver disorders, cancer, infections, inflammations, and drugs to hyperceruloplasmin (serum ceruloplasmin excess).

Note whether the patient has been exercising in the last 24 hours, since a slight elevation could be due to strenuous exercise.

CHLORIDE (Cl) (Serum)

NORMAL RANGE
Adult: 95–105 mEq/L, 95–105 mmol/L (SI units).
Newborn: 94–112 mEq/L.
Infant: 95–110 mEq/L.
Child: 98–105 mEq/L.

DESCRIPTION
Chloride is an anion found mostly in the extracellular fluid. Serum chloride is like an orphan to some physicians, being frequently ignored or not considered of importance. Chloride plays an important role in maintaining body water balance, osmolality of body fluids (with sodium), and acid–base balance. It combines with hydrogen ion to produce the acidity (hydrochloric acid, or HCl) in the stomach.

For maintaining acid–base balance, chloride competes with bicarbonate for sodium. When the body fluids are more acidic, the kidneys excrete chloride and sodium, and bicarbonate is reabsorbed. In addition, chloride shifts in and out of red blood cells in exchange with bicarbonate (HCO_3 shifts out of the RBC to the extracellular fluid as Cl shifts in).

Most of the chloride ingested is combined with sodium (sodium chloride—NaCl or "salt"). The daily required chloride intake is 2 g. Hypochloremia is the name for a serum chloride deficit. Hyperchloremia means serum chloride excess.[5,8,11,17,18,22,30]

CLINICAL PROBLEMS
Decreased level *(↓ 95 mEq/L [adult]):* vomiting, gastric suction; diarrhea; hypokalemia (↓ K), hyponatremia (↓ Na); low-sodium diet; continuous IV 5 percent dextrose/water; gastroenteritis, colitis; adrenal gland insufficiency (Addison's disease); diabetes acidosis; heat exhaustion; hyperaldosteronism; acute infections; burns; excessive diaphoresis (sweating/perspiration); metabolic alkalosis. *Drug influence:* diuretics—mercurials, thiazides, loop; bicarbonates.
Elevated level *(↑ 105 mEq/L [adult]):* dehydration; hypernatremia (↑ Na); hyperparathyroidism; cancer of the stomach; multiple myeloma; adrenal gland hyperactivity; head injury; eclampsia; cardiac decompensation; excessive IV saline (0.9 percent NaCl); kidney dysfunction—glomerulonephritis, acute renal failure, pyelonephritis; hyperventilation; metabolic acidosis. *Drug influence:* acetazolamide, ammonium chloride, boric acid, cortisone preparations, ion exchange resins, triamterene (prolonged use—dyrenium).

PROCEDURE
Collect 5 to 10 ml of venous blood in a red- or green-top tube.'
There is no food or drink restriction. This test may be combined with other tests (e.g., for serum electrolytes), so the patient may be required to take nothing by mouth (NPO). Check with the laboratory.

FACTORS AFFECTING LABORATORY RESULTS
Drugs: see *Drug Influence* above.

NURSING IMPLICATIONS WITH RATIONALE

Explain to the patient that the purpose of the test is to determine the chloride (electrolyte) level in the blood.

Decreased level (↓ 95 mEq/L [adult])

Relate clinical problems and drugs to hypochloremia. Severe vomiting, continuous gastric suction, and excessive diaphoresis could cause a considerable chloride loss. Other causes should be considered—diabetic acidosis (ketone bodies replacing the chloride ions), severe diarrhea, gastroenteritis, Addison's disease, burns, and potent diuretics.

Assess for signs and symptoms of hypochloremia—i.e., hyperexcitability of the nervous system and muscles, tetany (twitching), tremors, slow and shallow breathing, and decreased blood pressure due to fluid and chloride loss.

Inform the physician when the patient is receiving intravenous dextrose in water continuously. If no other solutes are given, the body fluids will be diluted and the patient will not receive the daily required chloride intake.

Teach the patient not to drink only plain water if there is a serum chloride deficit. Encourage the patient to drink fluids containing sodium and chloride—e.g., broth, tomato juice, Pepsi Cola.

Check the serum potassium and sodium levels. Chloride is frequently lost with sodium and potassium (plentiful in the GI tract). With vomiting, potassium, hydrogen, and chlorides are lost, causing hypokalemic–hypochloremic alkalosis. Both potassium and chloride must be replaced, for if potassium is given and not chloride, hypokalemic alkalosis will persist.

Instruct the patient to drink and eat foods rich in chloride—i.e., broth, seafoods, milk, meats, eggs, and table salt.

Observe for symptoms of overhydration when the patient is receiving several liters of normal saline (0.9 percent NaCl) for sodium and chloride replacement. Sodium holds water, and if there is a history of heart or kidney disorder, water accumulation could occur. Symptoms of overhydration include a constant, irritated cough; dyspnea; neck and hand vein engorgement; and chest rales.

Elevated level (↑ 105 mEq/L [adult])

Relate clinical problems and drugs to hyperchloremia. Dehydration/hypovolemia causes hemoconcentration, and this results in elevated electrolyte levels. Other common causes include head injury, hyperventilation, cancer of the stomach, eclampsia, and cardiac decompensation. See *Drug Influence* above.

Assess for signs and symptoms of hyperchloremia (similar to acidosis)—i.e., weakness, lethargy, and deep, rapid, vigorous breathing.

Instruct the patient to avoid drinking or eating salty foods. Encourage the patient not to use the salt shaker and some salt substitutes.

The patient should read labels, for some salt substitutes contain calcium chloride, calcium gluconate, and/or potassium chloride.

Notify the physician if the patient is receiving intravenous fluids containing normal saline. Check for symptoms of overhydration.

Monitor daily weights and intake and output to determine whether fluid retention is present due to sodium and chloride excess.

CHLORIDE (Sweat)
Screening (Silver Nitrate); Iontophoresis (Pilocarpine)

NORMAL RANGE
    Adult: <60 mEq/L.

Child: <50 mEq/L; marginal—50-60 mEq/L; abnormal—>60 mEq/L (possible cystic fibrosis).

DESCRIPTION

Sodium and chloride concentrations in sweat are higher in persons with cystic fibrosis, even though there usually is not an increased amount of sweat. Sweat chloride is considered more reliable than sweat sodium for diagnostic purposes. Some false negatives of sweat sodium have been reported in persons with cystic fibrosis.

There are two types of sweat chloride tests used: (1) screening tests; which use silver nitrate on agar or filter (special) paper and require contact with hand (palm or fingers), and (2) iontophoresis, in which pilocarpine is placed on the forearm to increase sweat gland secretion. A positive screening test is usually validated with iontophoresis, since the chloride level in the palm of the hand is usually higher than anywhere else. Some physicians feel that the screening should be routine in all children; however, others disagree.[11,14,20,27,34]

CLINICAL PROBLEMS

Elevated level *(>60 mEq/L):* cystic fibrosis, asthma.

PROCEDURE

Screening Test *(silver nitrate):* Wash the child's hand and dry it. For 15 minutes, keep the hand from contacting any other part of the body.

Moisten the test paper containing silver nitrate compound with distilled water (*not saline*).

Press the child's hand on the paper for 4 seconds.

A positive result occurs when the excess chloride combines with the silver nitrate to form white silver chloride on the paper.

A heavy hand imprint is left by the child with cystic fibrosis.

Iontophoresis *(pilocarpine*—usually performed by lab personnel): Electrodes are placed on the skin of the forearm to create a small electric current for transporting pilocarpine (a stimulating drug) into the skin to induce sweating.

Sweat is collected and weighed. Chloride is measured.

There is no food or drink restriction.

FACTORS AFFECTING LABORATORY RESULTS

Unwashed hands for the screening test.

Use of saline solution to moisten the test paper.

NURSING IMPLICATIONS WITH RATIONALE

Explain the procedures (screening or iontophoresis or both) to the child and family. Answer questions if possible or refer them to the physician or laboratory personnel.

Explain to the child and family that the tests are not painful.

Remain with the child during the procedure. Give comfort and reassurance as needed.

Elevated level (>60 mEq/L)

Associate an elevated sweat chloride to cystic fibrosis. With cystic fibrosis, sweat chloride levels could be two to five times greater than normal.

Obtain a familial history of cystic fibrosis, when indicated.

Determine whether the child has washed and dried his hands before the screening test is performed. Dried sweat can leave a chloride residue, thus causing a false positive result.

CHOLESTEROL (Serum)

NORMAL RANGE
Adult: 150–250 mg/dl (may increase with age), 3.90–6.50 mmol/L (SI units).
Infant: 70–175 mg/dl.
Child: 120–240 mg/dl.

DESCRIPTION
Cholesterol is a blood lipid synthesized by the liver and is found in red blood cells, cell membranes, and muscles. About 70 percent of cholesterol is esterified (combined with fatty acids), and 30 percent is in the free form. Cholesterol is used by the body (1) to form bile salts for fat digestion and (2) for the formation of hormones by the adrenal glands, ovaries, and testes. Thyroid hormones and estrogen decrease the concentration of cholesterol, and an oophorectomy increases it.

Serum cholesterol levels can be used as an indicator of liver function since it is synthesized by the liver, but serum cholesterol can also be used as an indicator of atherosclerosis and coronary artery disease. Hypercholesterolemia can cause plaque deposits in the coronary arteries, thus contributing to myocardial infarction. High serum cholesterol levels can be due to a familial (hereditary) tendency, biliary obstruction, and/or dietary intake.[8,9,11,27,30,31,34,36]

CLINICAL PROBLEMS
Decreased level *(↓ 150 mg/dl [adult]):* hyperthyroidism, Cushing's syndrome (adrenal hormone excess), starvation, malabsorption, anemias, acute infections. *Drug influence:* corticosteroids—cortisone; thyroxine; antibiotics—kanamycin, neomycin, paramomycin, tetracycline; nicotinic acid; estrogens; glucagon; heparin; salicylates (aspirin); PAS; colchicine; oral hypoglycemic agents.

Elevated level *(↑ 250 mg/dl [adult]):* acute myocardial infarction, atherosclerosis, hypothyroidism, biliary obstruction, biliary cirrhosis, cholangitis, familial hypercholesterolemia, uncontrolled diabetes mellitus, nephrotic syndrome, pancreatectomy, pregnancy (third trimester), Type II hyperlipoproteinemia, heavy stress periods, high-cholesterol diet (animal fats). *Drug influence:* aspirin; corticosteroids—cortisone; steroids—anabolic agents and androgens; oral contraceptives; epinephrine and norepinephrine; bromides; phenothiazines—chlorpromazine (Thorazine), trifluoperazine (Stelazine); vitamins A and D; sulfonamides; diphenylhydantoin (Dilantin).

PROCEDURE
Keep the patient NPO (food, fluids, and medications) for 12 hours. The patient may have water. Medications and food may be permitted prior to the test in some institutions. The nurse should check with the physician and laboratory.

Collect 5 to 10 ml of venous blood in a red-top tube.

List drugs that are not withheld on the laboratory slip.

FACTORS AFFECTING LABORATORY RESULTS
Aspirin and cortisone could cause decreased or elevated serum cholesterol levels.

A high-cholesterol diet before the test.

Severe hypoxia could increase the serum cholesterol level.

Hemolysis of the blood specimen may cause an elevation of the serum cholesterol level.

NURSING IMPLICATIONS WITH RATIONALE

Decreased level (↓ 150 mg/dl)

Relate clinical problems and drugs to hypocholesterolemia. Certain antibiotics can produce a temporary reduction of cholesterol levels.

Elevated level (↑250 mg/dl)
Relate clinical problems and drugs to hypercholesterolemia. An elevated cholesterol level can indicate liver disease as well as coronary artery disease.

Hold drugs which could increase the serum level for 12 hours before the blood is drawn, with the physician's permission.

Explain to the patient the purpose of the test. Explanation could be brief such as, "to determine the blood cholesterol level" or a more detailed explanation could be given.

Instruct the patient that he is not to eat or drink fluids except water for 12 hours before the blood is drawn. Institutions' NPO policies may differ.

Instruct the patient with hypercholesterolemia to decrease his intake of foods rich in cholesterol—i.e., bacon, eggs, butter, fatty meat, seafood, and cocoanut.

Answer questions regarding cholesterol and the blood test. The nurse may wish to explain the purposes of cholesterol in the body.

Teach the patient with severe hypercholesterolemia to keep medical appointments for follow-up care.

CHOLINESTERASE (Red Blood Cells or Plasma)
Acetylcholinesterase (True Cholinesterase of Blood Nerve Tissue—RBC); Pseudocholinesterase (Serum)

NORMAL RANGE
Adult: 0.5–1.0 units (RBC), 3–8 units/ml (plasma), 6–8 IU/L (RBC), 8–18 IU/L at 37°C (plasma).
Child: similar to adult.

DESCRIPTION
There are two different cholinesterases (CHS): *acetylcholinesterase* (true cholinesterase), found in the red blood cells (erythrocytes) and nerve tissue, and *pseudocholinesterase*, or serum cholinesterase (PCHE). Cholinesterase is an enzyme which breaks down acetylcholine at the nerve synapse and neuromuscular junction.

Decreased cholinesterase levels may indicate insecticide poisoning due to excess exposure to organic phosphate agents, liver disorders (hepatitis and cirrhosis), or an acute infection. This test is not used for assessment of liver function.[2,9,14,27,30,36]

CLINICAL PROBLEMS
Decreased level (↓ 0.5 unit): insecticide poisoning; liver disorders—hepatitis, cirrhosis, obstructive jaundice; malnutrition; acute infections; anemias; carcinomatosis.
Elevated level (↑ 1.0 unit): nephrotic syndrome.

PROCEDURE
Collect 5 to 10 ml of venous blood in a green-top tube.
There is no food or drink restriction.

FACTORS AFFECTING LABORATORY RESULTS
Nonheparinized tube for cholinesterase–red blood cell test.

NURSING IMPLICATIONS WITH RATIONALE

Decreased level (↓ 0.5 pH unit)
Explain to the patient that the purpose for the test is to determine the value of a specific enzyme in the blood.

Obtain a history of the patient's exposure to insecticides—kind, length of time, and amount. Excessive exposure to organic phosphate can cause acute or chronic toxicity, and the acetylcholinesterase level would be decreased.

Report to the physician and record on the chart if the patient has not been eating or has an acute infection.

CLOT RETRACTION (Blood)

NORMAL RANGE

Adult: 1 to 24 hours (retraction of clot).
Child: similar to adult.

DESCRIPTION

The clot retraction (shrunken clot) test is useful in determining whether bleeding disorders are due to a decreased platelet count. Other factors can also influence the test result—i.e., fibrinogen concentration, red cell mass, thrombin, and temperature. This is a simple test (the rate and degree of contraction of a blood clot are measured) in which a clot of blood in a test tube will diminish in size because of fluid (serum) separating from the red cells. Platelets are responsible for the shrinkage of the blood clot. Frequently, when there is a platelet deficit, clot retraction will be slower and the clot formation will be softer.

In 1 hour, the clot should be one-half of its original size (volume). The retraction should be near completion in 4 hours and definitely completed in 24 hours.[8,9,27,30,36]

CLINICAL PROBLEMS

Decreased clot formation: thrombocytopenia (decreased platelets); thrombasthenia (abnormal platelets); anemia—pernicious, folic acid, aplastic; Waldenstrom's macroglobulinemia.

PROCEDURE

Collect 5 ml of venous blood in a red-top tube.
There is no food or drink restriction.

FACTORS AFFECTING LABORATORY RESULTS

High hematocrit can cause poor clot retraction.
Decreased fibrinogen can cause red blood cells to spill out of the serum when retraction begins—poor cell retraction.
Anticoagulants can inhibit clot formation.

NURSING IMPLICATIONS WITH RATIONALE

Decreased or Poor Clot Formation

Explain to the patient that the purpose of the test is to determine how soon the blood will form a firm clot.

Explain that food and drinks are not restricted. This may differ in some laboratories.

Report to the physician if bleeding time is prolonged.

Note when the blood clot begins to separate from the tube wall. This usually begins to happen within 30 minutes to 1 hour. Note the length of time required for clot retraction (clot shrinking and fluid release).

Check the consistency of the clot. Soft clots and shapeless clots may be due to abnormal or decreased platelets.

Check the patient's hemoglobin, hematocrit, and platelet count. A high hematocrit due to hemoconcentration or polycythemia may cause decreased clot retraction. Clot retraction is influenced by the number of functional platelets, and not necessarily by the total count.

COAGULATION TIME (CT) (Blood)
Lee–White Clotting Time, Venous Clotting Time (VCT)

NORMAL RANGE
Adult: Three tube method: 5–15 minutes (average 8 minutes).
Child: similar to adults.

DESCRIPTION
The coagulation time (CT), or the Lee–White test (clotting time), one of the oldest tests of coagulation, determines the time it takes for venous blood to clot in a glass test tube. CT or the Lee–White test should not be used as a screening test for diagnosing bleeding conditions, since it is not sensitive enough to detect mild to moderate coagulation problems, only severe ones. In addition, it is not specific for any one of the 13 coagulation factors. With a normal CT, there could still be a clotting problem.

CT is commonly used to monitor and regulate patients receiving heparin therapy so as to keep the clotting time at approximately 20 minutes. Three glass test tubes are used and tilted at 30 second intervals to enhance clotting.[8,9,11,27,30,34,36]

CLINICAL PROBLEMS
Decreased time (↓ *5 minutes*): eclampsia. *Drug influence:* Steroids—cortisone, epinephrine (adrenalin).

Prolonged time (↑ *15 minutes*): afibrinogenemia, hyperheparinemia, severe coagulation factor deficiencies, toxic effects of venom, heat stroke. *Drug influence:* anticoagulants, heparin; antibiotics—carbenicillin, tetracycline; azathioprine (Imuran); mithramycin.

PROCEDURE
A glass syringe and glass test tubes should be used. Plastic test tubes could lengthen the clotting time by 20 to 40 minutes.

Test timing begins when blood enters the glass syringe. When using a plastic syringe, timing is started when the blood enters the glass test tube. Laboratory procedure differs from one institution to another and should be checked.

For the Lee–White test, three glass test tubes at 37 °C are used. Each tube should have 1 ml of venous blood, and the tubes should be tilted every 15 to 30 seconds to enhance clotting through the contact of the blood with the glass tube surface. When a firm clot has formed, the time should be recorded.

FACTORS AFFECTING LABORATORY RESULTS
Use of plastic test tubes.

Poor venipuncture procedure—i.e., red blood cells hemolyzed in the syringe as blood is drawn from the vein.

Improper tilting of test tubes and timing of blood samples.

Drugs causing prolonged clotting time (see *Drug Influence* above).

Due to difficulty in standardizing the technique, there are other tests of choice, such as the activated partial thromboplastin time (APTT).

NURSING IMPLICATIONS WITH RATIONALE

Decreased time (↓ 5 minutes)
Relate decreased clotting time to certain drugs—i.e., cortisone and adrenalin.

Prolonged (increased) time (↑ 15 minutes)
Relate prolonged or increased clotting time to clinical problems and drugs. Frequently, prolonged CT does not occur until there is a severe clotting problem. CT may be normal in mild hemophilia.
Explain to the patient the purpose of the CT test. The explanation will most likely be "to monitor heparin therapy and to adjust dosage as needed."
Explain to the patient the procedure for the test. Explanation could be brief, such as, "Blood will be drawn before heparin is given." A more detailed explanation might be needed.
Instruct the patient he may eat and drink before the blood is drawn.
Assess for signs and symptoms of bleeding due to a prolonged CT. Symptoms could include bleeding under the skin or from the nose, mouth, or rectum.

COLD AGGLUTININS (Serum)
Cold Hemagglutinin

NORMAL RANGE
Adult: 1:8 antibody titer, >1:16 significantly increased, >1:32 definitely positive.
Child: similar to adult.

DESCRIPTION
Cold agglutinins (CAs) are antibodies which agglutinate red blood cells at temperatures between 0° and 10°C. The walls of the red blood cell contain lipoid material which acts as the antigen or receptor for the antibody (CA). At body temperature (37°C), CAs rarely agglutinate the red blood cells, and so the blood sample is placed in a warmed (37°C) collecting tube.
Usually, persons have CA titers of 1:8. Elevated titers (> 1:32) are found frequently in patients with primary atypical pneumonia or with other clinical problems, such as influenza, pulmonary embolism, and cirrhosis. The cold agglutinins test is often done during the acute and convalescence phases of illness.[8,9,11,20,30,36]

CLINICAL PROBLEMS
Elevated level (>1:32 titer): primary atypical pneumonia, influenza, cirrhosis of the liver, lymphatic leukemia, multiple myeloma, pulmonary embolism, acquired hemolytic anemias, malaria, infectious mononucleosis, frostbite.

PROCEDURE
Collect 7 ml of venous blood in a red-top tube. The needle, syringe, and collecting tube should be warmed to 37°C before the venipuncture. The warmed syringe or tube should be put in a warm bath and taken immediately to the laboratory. The blood sample should not be refrigerated.
If it is impossible to keep the blood sample warmed to 37°C, then the laboratory will rewarm the sample for 30 minutes before the serum is separated from the cells.
There is no food or drink restriction.

FACTORS AFFECTING LABORATORY RESULTS
Antibiotic therapy may cause inaccurate results.
Elevated cold agglutinins may interfere with typing and cross-matching.
Improper blood collection procedure.

NURSING IMPLICATIONS WITH RATIONALE

Elevated level (>1:32 antibody titer)
Relate elevated cold agglutinin levels to clinical problems, particularly primary
    atypical penumonia.
Explain to the patient the purpose of the test. Explanation could be brief, such as, "to
    determine the antibody titer in the blood," or a similar response.
Explain to the patient the procedure for the blood test (see *Procedure* above).
Instruct the patient that food and drinks are not restricted.
Answer the patient's questions concerning the significance of the test. Answers might
    include: "most persons have an antibody titer level, but some have higher levels,
    such as older adults and those with viral infections; high titers may persist for
    years, and the test may be repeated at a later date."

COMPLEMENT C3 TEST (Serum)
C3 Component of the Complement System

NORMAL RANGE
    Adult: *Male:* 80–180 mg/dl. *Female:* 76–120 mg/dl. *Blacks:* 90–220 mg/dl.
    Child: Usually not performed.

DESCRIPTION
    C3 is the most abundant component of the complement system, (a group of 11
    proteins). Complements contribute about 10 percent of the total plasma proteins. The
    complement system has an important role in the immunologic system and the comple-
    ments' components are activated when IgG and IgM antibodies are combined with
    their specific antigens. With activation, the components, especially C3 and C4, func-
    tion as enzymes.
    The total complement system and C3 are decreased in lupus erythematosus,
    glomerulonephritis, and acute renal transplant rejection. Following onset of an acute
    or chronic inflammatory process or acute tissue destruction (necrosis), the total
    complement (C) may be temporarily elevated. C3 and C4 of the complement system are
    best known, and the others (C1, C2, and C5 to C9) are still under study and intense
    research.[8,9,27,30,31,36]

CLINICAL PROBLEMS
    Decreased level *(↓ 80 mg/dl [nonblack male]):* systemic lupus erythematosus (SLE);
    glomerulonephritis; acute poststreptococcal glomerulonephritis; acute renal trans-
    plant rejection; cirrhosis of the liver; multiple sclerosis (slightly lower); protein
    malnutrition; anemias—pernicious, folic acid; septicemia (gram-negative); bacterial
    endocarditis.
    Elevated level *(↑ 180 mg/dl [nonblack male]):* acute rheumatic fever; rheumatoid ar-
    thritis; early SLE; malignant neoplasms of the esophagus, stomach, colon, rectum,
    pancreas, lungs, breast, cervix, ovary, prostate, and bladder.

PROCEDURE
Collect 5 to 10 ml of venous blood in a red-top tube.
Take the blood sample to the laboratory immediately.
There is no food or drink restriction.

FACTORS AFFECTING LABORATORY RESULTS
Heat can destroy complement components.
C3 is unstable and the serum value may decrease if the sample is left standing for 1 to 2 hours at room temperature.

NURSING IMPLICATIONS WITH RATIONALE

Explain to the patient the purpose of the test. Explanation could be brief, such as, "to determine the concentration of a protein component in the blood."
Instruct the patient that food and drinks are not restricted.

Decreased level (↓ 80 mg/dl)
Relate a decreased C3 level to clinical problems, such as lupus and kidney involvement (see *Clinical Problems* above).
Check the serum C3 value with other laboratory studies that are ordered for diagnostic purposes related to a specific health problem.

Elevated level (↑ 180 mg/dl)
Relate an elevated C3 level to an acute or chronic inflammatory process and tissue necrosis. Examples are rheumatic fever, rheumatoid arthritis, and malignancies with metastasis.

COMPLEMENT C4 (Serum)
C4 Component of the Complement System

NORMAL RANGE
Adult: *Males:* 15–60 mg/dl. *Females:* 15–52 mg/dl. *Blacks:* 16–66 mg/dl.
Child: Usually not performed.

DESCRIPTION
See Complement C3.
C4 is the second most abundant component of the complement system (a group of 11 serum proteins). When C4 is activated, its serum level is extremely low. C3 and C4 are frequently compared, and if C4 is in the normal range and C3 is decreased, then the C3 is the active component. C4 is significantly decreased in lupus nephritis.
An elevated serum C4 level is indicative of an acute inflammatory process; however, a well (healthy) person may have an elevated C4 level. With cancer, the C4 level is usually increased (with links to the stage of the disease), but the serum level drops significantly in the terminal phase of the malignancy.[10,14,27,31]

CLINICAL PROBLEMS
Decreased level *(↓ 15 mg/dl [nonblack male]):* lupus nephritis, systemic lupus erythematosus (C4 decreased time is longer than C3 decreased time), acute post-streptococcal glomerulonephritis (C4 usually lower than C3), cirrhosis of the liver, bacterial endocarditis.

Elevated level (↑ 60 mg/dl [nonblack male]): rheumatoid spondylitis; juvenile rheumatoid arthritis; cancer of the esophagus, stomach, colon, rectum, pancreas, lung, breast, cervix, ovary, prostrate, and bladder.

PROCEDURE

Collect 5 to 10 ml of venous blood in a red-top tube.
Take the blood sample to the laboratory immediately.
There is no food and drink restriction.

FACTORS AFFECTING LABORATORY RESULTS

Heat will decrease complement C4.
C4 is unstable and the serum level will decrease if it remains at room temperature for more than 1 to 2 hours.

NURSING IMPLICATIONS WITH RATIONALE

Explain to the patient the purpose of the test. Explanation may be brief, such as, "to determine a protein component in the blood."
Instruct the patient that food and drinks are not restricted.

Decreased level (↓ 15 mg/dl)

Relate a decreased serum C4 level to clinical problems. With lupus nephritis and post-streptococcal glomerulonephritis, the serum C4 level is extremely low.
Compare the serum C3 and C4 results to determine which component of the complement system is involved.

Elevated level (↑ 60 mg/dl)

Relate an elevated serum C4 level to clinical problems. An increased serum level occurs with cancer; however, in the terminal stage, the serum level is frequently decreased.

COOMBS DIRECT (Blood—RBC)
Direct Antiglobulin Test

NORMAL RANGE

Adult: negative.
Child: negative.

DESCRIPTION

The direct Coombs test detects antibodies attached to red blood cells (RBC) which may cause cellular damage. This test can identify a weak antigen–antibody reaction even when there is no visible red blood cell agglutination. A positive Coombs test reveals antibodies present on RBC, but the test does not identify the antibody responsible.
This test is useful for diagnosing early erythroblastosis fetalis of newborns, auto-immune hemolytic anemia, hemolytic transfusion reaction, and some drug sensitizations—i.e., to levodopa and Aldomet.
The direct Coombs Test is also known as the direct antiglobulin test, a method of detecting in vivo sensitization of red blood cells.[8,9,11,27,30]

CLINICAL PROBLEMS

Negative: *Drug influence:* heparin.
Positive *(+1 to +4):* erythroblastosis fetalis (hemolytic disease of newborns); acquired hemolytic anemia (autoimmune); transfusion reactions (blood incompatibility); leu-

kemias—lymphocytic, myelocytic; systemic lupus erythematosus. *Drug influence:* antibiotics—cephaloridine (Loridine), cephalothin (Keflin), penicillin, streptomycin, tetracycline, aminopyrine (Pyradone); chlorpromazine (Thorazine); diphenylhydantoin (Dilantin); ethosuximide (Zarontin); hydralizine (Apresoline); isoniazid (INH); Levodopa; methyldopa (Aldomet); procainamide (Pronestyl); quinidine; rifampin (Rifadin); sulfonamides.

PROCEDURE

Collect 5 ml of venous blood in a red-top tube. Venous blood from the umbilical cord of a newborn may be used.

There is no food or drink restriction.

FACTORS AFFECTING LABORATORY RESULTS

Certain drugs may cause a positive test result (see *Drug Influence* above).

NURSING IMPLICATIONS WITH RATIONALE

Positive test ($\gamma+1$)

Explain to the patient the purpose of the test. Explanation could be brief, such as, "to determine the presence of antibodies in the blood."

Report the drugs patient is receiving which could produce a positive direct Coombs test—i.e., antibiotics, Dilantin, sulfonamides, Thorazine, Aldomet, and others (see *Drug Influence* above).

Observe for signs and symptoms of whole blood transfusion reactions—i.e., chills, fever (slight temperature elevation), and rash.

Observe the newborn for symptoms of erythroblastosis fetalis, especially if the condition is suspected. The main symptom is jaundice of the skin, nails, and sclera.

COOMBS INDIRECT (Serum)

NORMAL RANGE

Adult: negative.

Child: negative.

DESCRIPTION

The Coombs indirect test can detect free antibodies in the patient's serum and identify certain red cell antigens. This test is always done in cross-matching blood for transfusions in order to prevent transfusion reaction to incompatible blood due to minor blood type factors. As a result of previous transfusions, a recipient's blood may contain specific antibody (antibodies) that could cause a transfusion reaction.

The indirect Coombs test is also known as the indirect antiglobulin test, a method of detecting in vitro sensitization of red blood cells.[8,11,27,34]

CLINICAL PROBLEMS

Positive *(+1 to +4):* incompatible cross-matched blood, specific antibody (previous transfusion), anti-Rh antibodies (detected during pregnancy), nonspecific autoantibody (acquired hemolytic anemia). *Drug influence:* same as for the direct Coombs test (see Coombs Direct).

PROCEDURE
   Collect 5 ml of venous blood in a red-top tube. The blood bank will use the serum from
   the recipient's blood and select the compatible blood for proper transfusion.
   There is no food or drink restriction.

FACTORS AFFECTING LABORATORY RESULTS
   Drugs causing positive results—see *Clinical Problems: Drug Influence* under Coombs
   Direct.

NURSING IMPLICATIONS WITH RATIONALE

Explain to the patient the purpose of the test. Explanation could be brief, such as, "to
   determine if there are any antibodies in the blood which could cause a transfusion
   reaction."
Obtain a history of previous transfusions and report any previous transfusion reactions.
Report any drugs the patient is receiving which could cause a positive result. Record
   drug information on the patient's chart in the nurse's notes or progress notes.

COPPER (Cu) (Serum)

NORMAL RANGE
   Adult: *Male:* 70–140 μg/dl (mcg/dl), 11–22 μmol/L (SI units). *Female:* 80–155 μg/dl,
   12.6–24.3 μmol/L (SI units).
   Newborn: 20–70 μg/dl.
   Child: 30–150 μg/dl.
   Adolescent: 90–240 μg/dl.

DESCRIPTION
   Copper is required for hemoglobin synthesis. Approximately 90 percent of the copper
   is bound to α_2-globulin, referred to as ceruloplasmin, which is the means of copper
   transportation in the body. In hepatolenticular disease (Wilson's disease), the serum
   copper level is less than 20 μg/dl and the urinary copper level is greater than 100 μg/24
   hours. There is a decrease in copper metabolism with Wilson's disease, and excess
   copper is deposited in the brain (basal ganglia) and liver, causing degenerative
   changes. A low-copper diet and D-penicillamine will promote copper excretion.
   Hypercupremia (excess copper) can be observed during pregnancy, anemias, leukemia,
   collagen disease, and thyroid diseases. Serum copper and serum ceruloplasmin tests
   are frequently ordered together and compared. Both show decreased levels with
   Wilson's disease.[9,14,34]

CLINICAL PROBLEMS
   Decreased level *(70 μg/dl [male]):* hepatolenticular disease (Wilson's disease), protein
   malnutrition, chronic ischemic heart disease.
   Elevated level *(140 μg/dl [male]):* cancer of the bone, stomach, large intestine, liver,
   lung; Hodgkin's disease; leukemias; hypothyroidism; hyperthyroidism; pernicious
   anemia; iron deficiency anemia; rheumatoid arthritis; systemic lupus erythematosus;
   pregnancy; cirrhosis of the liver.

PROCEDURE

Collect 5 ml of venous blood in a red-top tube or green tube (heparinized).
There is no food or drink restriction.
Note: A test for urinary copper may be requested simultaneously with the blood test.

FACTORS AFFECTING LABORATORY RESULTS

A diet low or high in copper before the blood test.
Metallic contamination of collection tubes or equipment.

NURSING IMPLICATIONS WITH RATIONALE

Decreased level (↓ 70 μg/dl)

Relate the clinical problems of decreased levels to the patient's low serum copper level
and his complaints.
Explain to the patient that the test is to determine the amount of copper in the body.
Instruct the patient that he may eat and drink before the test.
Explain to the patient with Wilson's disease that he should avoid foods rich in copper—i.e., organ meats, shellfish, mushrooms, whole-grain cereals, bran, nuts, and
chocolate. Canned foods should be omitted. A low-copper diet and D-penicillamine
promote copper excretion.
Assess for signs and symptoms of hepatolenticular disease (Wilson's disease)—i.e.,
rigidity, dysarthria, dysphagia, incoordination, and tremors.
Check for a Kayser–Fleischer ring (dark ring) around the cornea. This is a copper de-
posit which the body has not been able to metabolize.
Compare the serum copper level with the serum ceruloplasmin level if both have been
ordered. If hepatolenticular disease is present, the serum levels will be decreased.

Elevated level (↑ 140 μg/dl)

Relate the clinical problems of elevated levels to the patient's elevated serum copper
level and his complaints. The serum copper test is not the most effective diagnostic
test for hypercupremia; there are many conditions which cause hypercupremia.
However, the test can be used with other tests for diagnostic purposes.

CORTICOTROPIN, CORTICOTROPIN-RELEASING FACTOR (CRF) (Plasma)
ADRENOCORTICOTROPIC HORMONE (ACTH)

NORMAL RANGE

Corticotropin (or ACTH) is measured by bioassay and immunoassay procedures:
ACTH—8 A.M. to 10 A.M., up to 80 pg/ml.

DESCRIPTION

Corticotropin, or ACTH, is stored and released from the anterior pituitary gland under
the influence of corticotropin-releasing factor (CRF), synthesized from the hypothalamus, and plasma cortisol. When plasma cortisol is decreased, CRF is released and
so is ACTH. Stress due to surgery, physical trauma, emotional trauma, bacterial infections also increases the ACTH level. The plasma ACTH level is highest in the morning
and lowest in the evening.
Several tests are performed to determine whether there is an increased or decreased
secretion of cortiosteroids (cortisol is the major one) from the adrenal glands. One
cause of excess secretion is a hyperactive pituitary gland, which could be due to a
pituitary tumor. Synthetic cortisol (dexamethasone or Decadron) is given to suppress

ACTH, and if an extremely high dose is needed for suppression, then there is pituitary involvement.

Another test is the ACTH stimulation test, which is a screening test to determine whether there is a corticosteroid deficit known as Addison's disease. ACTH is given and, for a normal test result, the plasma cortisol level should double in 1 hour. If the plasma cortisol level remains the same or gets lower, Addison's disease or adrenal gland insufficiency is the cause.[9,14,30,31,36]

CLINICAL PROBLEMS

Decreased level: Cancer of the adrenal gland, adrenal cortical hyperfunction (Cushing's syndrome). *Drug influence:* steroids—cortisone, prednisone, decadron.

Elevated Level: stress—trauma, physical or emotional, pyrogens; adrenal cortical hypofunction; pituitary neoplasm.

PROCEDURE

Collect two tubes of 15 ml of venous blood in a green-top tube (heparinized blood). Send immediately on ice to the laboratory. The technologist will separate the plasma and whole blood; the former will be frozen within 15 minutes. Radioimmunoassay is the method of choice.

There is no food or drink restriction.

FACTORS AFFECTING LABORATORY RESULTS

Drugs: oral contraceptives, estrogen, etc.

Physical activity prior to the blood test.

Obesity can cause an elevated serum level.

Inaccurate labelling of blood specimen—i.e., with the wrong time.

NURSING IMPLICATIONS WITH RATIONALE

Decreased level

Recognize that steroid drugs (cortisone, prednisone) decrease ACTH secretion. With a decrease in ACTH, there will be a decrease in corticosteroids.

Explain to the patient the purpose for the ACTH stimulation test. Explanation could be brief, such as, "to determine if there is a hormone deficiency" (see *Description* above).

Elevated level

Relate elevated plasma ACTH levels to clinical problems. Adrenal gland insufficiency or a pituitary tumor will increase ACTH secretion.

Explain to the patient the purpose of the ACTH suppression test. Explanation could be brief, such as, "to determine the function of the pituitary gland" (see *Description* above).

Instruct the patient to avoid physical activity and stress.

CORTISOL (Plasma)
Hydrocortisone, Compound F

NORMAL RANGE

Adult: 8 A.M.–10 A.M.: 5–23 µg/dl (mcg/dl), 138–635 nmol/L (SI units). 4 P.M.–6 P.M. (approximately one-half the levels of the peak time, 8 A.M.–10 A.M.): 3–13 µg/dl, 83–359 nmol/L (SI units).

Child: 8 A.M.–10 A.M.: 15–25 µg/dl. 4 P.M.–6 P.M.: 5–10 µg/dl.

DESCRIPTION

Cortisol is a potent glucocorticoid released from the adrenal cortex in response to ACTH stimulation. Cortisol affects carbohydrate, protein, and lipid metabolism; acts as an anti-inflammatory agent; helps with maintenance of blood pressure; inhibits insulin action; and stimulates glucogenesis in the liver.

Levels of plasma cortisol are higher in the morning and lower in the afternoon. When there is adrenal or pituitary dysfunction, the diurnal variation in cortisol function ceases (Cushing's syndrome) and there is no variation.[8,11,27,30,31]

CLINICAL PROBLEMS

Decreased level *(↓ 5 µg/dl [adult, 8 A.M.–10 A.M.]):* anterior pituitary hypofunction, adrenal cortical hypofunction (Addison's disease), respiratory distress syndrome (low birth weight newborns), hypothyroidism, exercise (slight decrease). *Drug influence:* androgens, Dilantin.

Elevated level *(↑ 23 µg/dl [adult, 8 A.M.–10 A.M.]):* cancer of the adrenal gland, benign tumor on the adrenal cortex, adrenal cortical hyperfunction (Cushing's syndrome), stress, pregnancy, obesity, acute myocardial infarction, acute alcoholic intoxication, diabetic acidosis, hyperthyroidism. *Drug influence:* oral contraceptives, estrogens, spironolactone (Aldactone), triparanol.

PROCEDURE

Collect 5 to 10 ml of venous blood in a green-top (heparinized) tube. Tube color varies among institutions.

Write the date and time the blood was drawn on the laboratory slip. If the patient has taken estrogen or oral contraceptives in the last 6 weeks, the drug(s) should be listed on the laboratory slip. It is advisable not to do the test for at least 2 months after the medication is stopped. Otherwise, the result will be invalid, and repeating the test will be costly in both time and money.

Advise the patient to rest in bed for 2 hours before the blood is drawn.

There is no food or drink restriction.

FACTORS AFFECTING LABORATORY RESULTS

Drugs causing serum cortisol levels to increase or decrease—i.e., oral contraceptives, estrogen, etc.

Physical activity prior to the blood test.

Obesity can cause an elevated serum level.

Inaccurate labelling of the blood specimen—i.e., with the wrong time.

NURSING IMPLICATIONS WITH RATIONALE

Inform the patient that he should be on bed rest for 2 hours prior to the test. Physical activity affects the cortisol level.

Obtain a history on drugs taken prior to hospital admission or the test. Oral contraceptives and estrogen taken 6 weeks or less before the test can cause false positive results.

Explain to the patient the purpose of the test. Explanation can be brief, such as, "to determine the cortisol level in the blood." A more detailed explanation may be needed.

Instruct the patient that food and drinks are not restricted.

Mark on the chart or Kardex if the patient is receiving or has received drugs that can affect the test results.

Decreased level (↓ 5 μg/dl)
Relate the decreased serum cortisol level of the patient to clinical problems.
Observe for signs and symptoms of Addison's disease (adrenal cortical insufficiency). Symptoms are anorexia, vomiting, abdominal pain, fatigue, dizziness, trembling, and diaphoresis.

Elevated level (↑ 23 μg/dl)
Relate the increased serum cortisol level of the patient to clinical problems.
Observe for signs and symptoms of Cushing's syndrome (excess adrenal cortical hormone). Symptoms are fat deposits in the face (moonface), neck, and in the back of the chest; irritability; mood swings; bleeding under the skin; muscle wasting; and weakness.

C-REACTIVE PROTEIN (CRP) (Serum)

NORMAL RANGE
Adult: not usually present; >1:2 titer, positive.
Child: not usually present.

DESCRIPTION
C-reactive protein (CRP) appears in the blood during an acute inflammatory process and tissue destruction. CRP is a nonspecific test ordered for diagnostic reasons similar to those for the erythrocyte sedimentation rate test (ESR), but CRP precedes ESR during inflammation and necrosis and returns to normal sooner. Serum CRP is also found in many of our body fluids—i.e., pleural, peritoneal, and synovial.

The test for CRP is positive in rheumatoid arthritis, acute rheumatic fever, myocardial infarction, bacterial infection, cancer metastasis,, and pregnancy (third trimester) and with oral contraceptives and intrauterine contraceptive devices. It is frequently used to monitor acute inflammatory phases of rheumatoid arthritis and rheumatic fever so that early treatment can be initiated before progressive tissue damage occurs. Serum CRP is elevated approximately 24 hours after the acute onset and disappears when the condition subsides.[8,9,11,27,30,34,36]

CLINICAL PROBLEMS
Normal level: *Drug suppression:* steroids (cortisone, prednisone), salicylates (aspirin).
Elevated level: rheumatoid arthritis, rheumatic fever, acute myocardial infarction, cancer (breast and with metastasis), Hodgkin's disease, systemic lupus erythematosus, bacterial infections, late pregnancy, intrauterine contraceptive devices. *Drug influence:* oral contraceptives.

PROCEDURE
Collect 5 ml of venous blood in a red-top tube. Avoid heat, since CRP is thermolabile. Keep the patient NPO except for water for 8 to 12 hours before the test. Laboratory policies on NPO could vary and should be checked.

FACTORS AFFECTING LABORATORY RESULTS
Pregnancy (third trimester).
Oral contraceptives and intrauterine contraceptive devices.

NURSING IMPLICATIONS WITH RATIONALE

Elevated level (>1:2 titer)

Recognize that an elevated serum CRP level is associated with an active inflammatory process and tissue destruction (necrosis). The CRP test is nonspecific; however, the CRP is elevated during acute rheumatic fever, rheumatoid arthritis, and acute myocardial infarction.

Explain to the patient that the purpose of the test is to determine whether there is an inflammation present or to monitor the effectiveness of the treatment, or give a similar response.

Instruct the patient that he should not eat or drink (except water) for 8 to 12 hours before the blood is drawn. Check the laboratory policy.

Assess for signs and symptoms of an acute inflammatory process. Symptoms may include pain and swelling in joints, heat, redness, increased body temperature.

Notify the physician of a recurrence (exacerbation) of an acute inflammation. The physician may wish to order a serum CRP test.

Check the results of the serum CRP level. If the titer is decreasing, the patient is responding to treatment and/or the acute phase is declining. CRP may be compared to ESR. The serum CRP level will elevate and return to normal faster than the ESR level.

CREATINE PHOSPHOKINASE (CPK) (Serum)
Creatine Kinase (CK)

NORMAL RANGE
  Adult: *Male:* 5–35 μg/ml (mcg/ml), 15–120 IU/L, 55–170 U/L at 37°C (SI units). *Female:* 5–25 μg/ml, 10–80 IU/L, 30–135 U/L at 37°C (SI units).
  Newborn: 10–300 IU/L at 30°C.
  Child: *Male:* 0–70 IU/L at 30°C. *Female:* 0–50 IU/L at 30°C

DESCRIPTION
  Creative phosphokinase (CPK), also known as creatine kinase (CK), is an enzyme found in high concentration in the heart and skeletal muscles and in low concentration in the brain tissue. Serum CPK/CK is frequently elevated due to skeletal muscle disease, acute myocardial infarction, cerebral vascular disease, vigorous exercise, intramuscular injections, and electrolyte imbalance–hypokalemia. CPK/CK has two types of isoenzymes: M, associated with muscle, and B, associated with the brain. Electrophoresis separates the isoenzymes into three subdivisions, MM (in skeletal muscle and some in the heart), MB (in the heart), and BB (in brain tissue). When CPK/CK is elevated, a CPK electrophoresis is done to determine which group of isoenzymes is elevated. The isoenzyme CPK-MB could indicate damage to the myocardial cells when its value is greater than 5 percent of the total CPK.

  Serum CPK/CK and CPK-MB rise within 4 to 6 hours after an acute myocardial infarction (AMI), reach a peak in 18 to 24 hours (>6 times the normal value), and then return to normal within 3 to 4 days, unless new necrosis or tissue damage occurs. If medication for AMI has to be given parenterally, (for instance, morphine), it would be better to give it IV than IM so that mild muscle injury (from IM) would not elevate the CPK level; however, injections have little or no effect on CPK-MB. Test samples to check serum levels of CPK/CK should be drawn before an IM injection, or one should wait at least 1 hour after the IM injection.[9,11,16,27,30,31,32,36]

CLINICAL PROBLEMS

Decreased level (↓ 15 IU/L [adult male]): heredity, pregnancy (second trimester).

Elevated level (↑ 120 IU/L [adult male]): total CPK/CK is elevated in all of the following clinical problems. *CPK-MM isoenzyme:* muscular dystrophy, delirium tremens, dermatomyositis, crushed injury/trauma, surgery and postoperative state, vigorous exercise, hypokalemia, hemophilia and Christmas Disease, progressive systemic sclerosis, tetanus, toxic effects of venom. *CPK-MB isoenzyme:* acute myocardial infarction, severe angina pectoris, hypokalemia (heart muscle), cardiac defibrillation (50 percent of patients), acute myocarditis, cardiac surgery. *CPK-BB isoenzyme:* cerebral thrombosis, embolism, and hemorrhage (CVA); subarachnoid hemorrhage; cancer of the brain; toxic psychoses; acute brain injury; pulmonary embolism and infarction. *Others (General—Elevated):* diabetes acidosis, hypothyroidism, heat stroke, carbon monoxide toxicity, influenza (acute), acute pancreatitis (severe). *Drug influence:* amphotericin B; IM injections—ampicillin, carbenicillin, chlorpromazine (Thorazine); clofibrate; salicylates (aspirin)—high doses.

PROCEDURE

Collect 5 ml of venous blood in a red-top tube.

Note on the laboratory slip the number of times the patient has received IM injections in the last 24 to 48 hours.

Prevent hemolysis of the blood sample.

There is no food or drink restriction.

FACTORS AFFECTING LABORATORY RESULTS

Intramuscular injections can cause an elevated serum level of total CPK/CK.

Vigorous exercise elevates the levels.

Trauma and surgical intervention elevate serum levels.

NURSING IMPLICATIONS WITH RATIONALE

Elevated level (↑ 120 IU/L)

Relate elevated serum CPK/CK and isoenzymes (CPK-MM, CPK-MB, and CPK-BB) to clinical problems. The CPK-MB is useful in making the differential diagnosis of myocardial infarction.

Explain to the patient the purpose of the test. Explanation could be brief, such as, "to determine the enzyme concentration in the blood." A detailed explanation may be needed.

Indicate whether the patient has received an intramuscular (IM) injection in the last 24 to 48 hours on the laboratory slip, chart, and Kardex.

Instruct the patient that he may eat and drink before the test.

Assess the patient's signs and symptoms of an acute myocardial infarction (AMI). Symptoms include pain; dyspnea (SOB); diaphoresis (excess perspiration); cold, clammy skin; pallor; and arrhythmia.

Check the serum CPK/CK level at intervals and notify the physician of serum level changes. The serum CPK/CK may be repeated every 6 to 8 hours during the acute phase. When the CPK/CK and CPK-MB are highly elevated, there may be extensive muscle damage to the myocardium. For AMI, also check results of the AST (SGOT) and LDH tests.

CREATININE (Serum)

NORMAL RANGE
  Adult: 0.6–1.2 mg/dl, 53–106 μmol/L (SI units).
  Infant to 6 years: 0.3–0.6 mg/dl, 27–54 μmol/L (SI units).
  Older child: 0.4–1.2 mg/dl, 36–106 μmol/L (SI units).

DESCRIPTION
  Creatinine, a by-product of muscle catabolism, is derived from the breakdown of muscle creatine phosphate. The amount of creatinine produced daily is proportional to the muscle mass; the larger the muscle mass, the higher the serum creatinine levels. Glomeruli filter creatinine from the blood, and it is not reabsorbed by the renal tubules.
  Serum creatinine is considered a more sensitive and specific indicator of renal disease than BUN. It rises later and is *not influenced by diet or fluid intake.* A slight BUN elevation could be indicative of hypovolemia (fluid volume deficit); however, a serum creatinine of 2.5 mg/dl could be indicative of renal impairment. BUN and creatinine are frequently compared. If BUN increases and serum creatinine remains normal, dehydration (hypovolemia) is present; and if both increase, then renal disorder is present.[8,11,16,27,29,34,36]

CLINICAL PROBLEMS
  Decreased level (↓ *0.6 mg/dl [adult]):* pregnancy, eclampsia.
  Elevated level (↑ *1.2 mg/dl [adult]):* acute and chronic renal failure; shock (prolonged); systemic lupus erythematosus; cancer of the intestine, bladder, testis, uterus, prostate; leukemias; Hodgkin's disease; essential hypertension; acute myocardial infarction; diabetic nephropathy; congestive heart failure (long-standing); diet rich in creatinine—i.e., beef (high), poultry and fish (minimal effect). *Drug influence:* antibiotics—amphotericin B, cephalosporin (Ancef, Keflin), gentamicin, kanamycin, methicillin; ascorbic acid; barbiturates; lithium carbonate; mithramycin; methyldopa (Aldomet); glucose; protein; ketone bodies (↑); phenolsulfenphthalein (PSP) and bromsulphalein (BSP) tests; triamterene (Dyrenium).

PROCEDURE
  Collect 5 to 10 ml of venous blood in a red-top tube.
  List any drugs the patient is taking which could elevate the serum level on the laboratory slip.
  There is no food or drink restriction.

FACTORS AFFECTING LABORATORY RESULTS
  Certain drugs (see *Drug Influence* above) may increase the serum creatinine level.
  Roast beef consumed in large quantities.

NURSING IMPLICATIONS WITH RATIONALE

Elevated level (↑ 1.2 mg/dl)
Relate the elevated creatinine levels to clinical problems. A high serum creatinine level
  indicates renal disease, since the kidneys normally excrete creatinine.
Explain to the patient that the purpose of the test is to determine how well the kidneys
  are excreting creatinine, or give a similar response.
Instruct the patient that there is no food or water restriction prior to the test.
Hold medications (see *Drug Influence* above) for 24 hours before the test, with the
  physician's permission. Certain medications (i.e., antibiotics) cannot be withheld, so
  these should be listed on the laboratory slip and noted on the patient's chart.

Check the amount of urine output in 24 hours. Less than 600 ml/24 hours can indicate renal insufficiency. Creatinine is excreted by the kidneys, and a continuous decrease in urine output could result in an increased serum creatinine level.

Compare the BUN and creatinine levels. If both are increased, the problem is most likely kidney disease.

Suggest to the patient that he should eat less beef, poultry, and fish if his serum creatinine is extremely elevated. Normally, food does not have an effect on the serum creatinine level.

CREATININE CLEARANCE (Urine)
Creatinine (Urine)

NORMAL RANGE
Adult: *Creatinine clearance:* 100–120 ml/minute (mean value). *Urine creatinine:* Male: 20–26 mg/kg/24 hour, 0.18–0.23 mmol/kg/24 hour (SI units). Female: 14–22 mg/kg/24 hour, 0.12–0.19 mmol/kg/24 hour (SI units).
Child: *Creatinine clearance:* Male: 98–150 ml/minute. Female: 95–123 ml/minute.

DESCRIPTION
Creatinine is a metabolic product of creatine phosphate in skeletal muscle, and it is excreted by the kidneys. Creatinine clearance is considered a reliable test for estimating glomerular filtration rate (GFR), since glomeruli filter creatinine without appreciable reabsorption from the renal tubules. With renal insufficiency, the GFR is decreased and the serum creatinine is increased. GFR decreases with age, and with the older adult, the creatinine clearance may be diminished to as low as 60 ml/minute.

The creatinine clearance test consists of a 12 or 24 hour urine collection and a blood sample. However, if renal failure is known, the test is unnecessary.

The formular for calculating creatinine clearance test is:

$$\text{Creatinine clearance} = \frac{\text{Urine creatinine (mg/dl)} \times \text{Urine volume (dl)}}{\text{Serum creatinine (mg/dl)}}.$$

A creatinine clearance less than 40 ml/minute is suggestive of moderate to severe renal impairment.[8,11,27,30,31,34,36]

CLINICAL PROBLEMS
Decreased level *(↓ 100 ml/minute [adult]):* mild to severe renal (kidney) impairment, hyperthyroidism, progressive muscular dystrophy, amyotrophic lateral sclerosis (ALS). *Drug influence:* Phenacetin, steroids (anabolic), thiazides.

Elevated level *(↑ 120 ml/minute &adult?):* hypothyroidism, hypertension (renovascular), exercise. *Drug influence:* ascorbic acid, steroids, levodopa, methyldopa (aldomet), PSP test.

PROCEDURE
Avoid meats, poultry, fish, tea, and coffee for 6 hours beforee the test and during test, with the physician's permission.

Blood: collect 5 to 10 ml of venous blood in a red-top tube the morning of the test.

Urine: Have the patient void and discard the urine before the test begins. Note the time. Save all urine during the specified time (12 hour or 24 hour) in a urine container without any preservative and refrigerate or keep on ice. Encourage water hourly— 100 ml/hour, if possible—during the collection period. Label the container with the exact time and date the urine collection started and ended. Another kidney function should not be scheduled prior to this test (e.g., PSP).

FACTORS AFFECTING LABORATORY RESULTS
Phenacetin decreases the creatinine clearance.
Toilet paper and feces will contaminate the urine.

NURSING IMPLICATIONS WITH RATIONALE

Decreased level (↓ 100 ml/minute)
Relate a decreased creatinine clearance to decreased renal function.
Explain to the patient the purpose of the test. Explanation can be brief, such as, "to determine kidney function." A more detailed explanation may be needed.
Explain to the patient the procedure for blood and urine collection. Blood is drawn in the morning. The patient voids and the urine is discarded. Then all urine is saved for 12 hours or 24 hours in a urine container. Toilet paper and feces should not be in the urine.
Inform the physician of medications the patient is receiving which could cause false test results.
Instruct the patient not to eat meats, poultry, fish, tea, or coffee for 6 hours before the test or during the test, according to the physician's orders.
Encourage water intake throughout the test—approximately 100 ml/hour

CROSS-MATCHING (Blood)
Blood Typing Tests, Compatibility Test for RBC, Type and Cross-match

NORMAL RANGE
Adult: compatibility—absence of agglutination (clumping) of cells.

DESCRIPTION
The four *major* blood types (A, B, AB, and O) belong to the ABO blood group system. Red blood cells (RBC) have either antigen A, B, or AB, or none, on the surface of the cells. Type A has A antigen, B has B antigen, AB has A and B antigens, and O does not contain an antigen. These antigens are capable of producing antibodies.
The reciprocal antibody is found in the plasma—e.g., group A person will have anti-B antibody, group B will have anti-A antibody, group AB will have no antiantibody, and group O will have both anti-A and anti-B antibodies. The AB blood person is the universal recipient (can accept all blood), since there are no antibodies, and the O blood person is the universal donor (can give blood to all types). However, no more than 1 unit (500 ml) of O blood should be received by an A, B, or AB blood recipient, to prevent risks of transfusion reaction. Rh typing should be done in conjunction with ABO typing.
The compatibility of donor and recipient bloods is determined by major and minor cross-matching. Cross-matching is not a simple test, but could be comprised of a battery of tests which could take 45 minutes to complete, depending on the laboratory methods and the equipment available. "Major cross-match" is when the donor's red blood cells are combined with the recipient's serum, and if agglutination (clumping) or hemolysis (rupture of red blood cells) occurs, then the donor's blood is incompatible with the patient's blood. Antibody screening is routinely done on donor's blood, which now eliminates the minor cross-match testing.[8,9,11,30,36]

PROCEDURE
   Collect 10 ml of venous blood in a red-top tube.
   There is no food or drink restriction.

FACTORS AFFECTING LABORATORY RESULTS
   None reported.
   Previous received incompatible blood can make blood cross-matching difficult.

NURSING IMPLICATIONS WITH RATIONALE

Explain to the patient that the purpose of taking the blood sample is to type and cross-match blood for transfusion purposes.

Observe the patient for signs and symptoms of fluid volume deficit (hypovolemia). Shocklike symptoms that may be present are tachycardia (pulse > 100), tachypnea (rapid breathing), pale color, clammy skin, and low blood pressure (late symptoms). It usually takes 45 minutes to type and cross-match blood, and so crystalloid solutions (saline, lactated Ringer's) might be given rapidly to replace fluid volume until a transfusion can be administered.

Obtain a history from the blood donor as to past and present diseases, drugs being taken, travel outside of the United States, and other factors, as indicated on the questionnaire.

Check the donor's vital signs and weight. In some institutions, the donor needs to weigh 110 pounds or more to give blood.

Check the date of the unit of blood. Outdated blood is 21 days old or older. Older blood should not be given to a patient having hyperkalemia.

Monitor the recipient's vital signs before and during transfusions. An increase of 1.1 °C during transfusion can be indicative of a transfusion reaction.

Start the blood transfusion at a slow rate for the first 15 minutes and observe for adverse reactions.

Flush the transfusion set with normal saline if other intravenous solutions are ordered to follow the blood.

CRYOGLOBULINS (Serum)

NORMAL RANGE
   Adult: negative.
   Child: negative.

DESCRIPTION
   Cryoglobulins are serum globulins (protein) that precipitate from the plasma at 4 °C and return to a dissolved status when warmed. They are present in IgG and IgM groups and are usually found in such pathologic conditions as leukemia, multiple myeloma, systemic lupus erythematosus (SLE), rheumatoid arthritis, and hemolytic anemia.[9,11,27,34,36]

CLINICAL PROBLEMS
   Elevated level *(> 2 percent precipitation):* collagen diseases—systemic lupus erythematosus (SLE), rheumatoid arthritis, polyarteritis nodosa; Hodgkin's disease;

lymphocytic leukemia; multiple myeloma; acquired hemolytic anemias (autoimmune); cirrhosis (biliary); Waldenstrom's macroglobulinemia.

PROCEDURE

For the qualitative test, collect 5 ml of venous blood in a red-top tube; for the quantitative test, collect 5 to 10 ml of venous blood in a red-top tube.

The blood sample should not be refrigerated before it is taken to the laboratory.

There is no food or drink restriction.

FACTORS AFFECTING LABORATORY RESULTS

None reported.

NURSING IMPLICATIONS WITH RATIONALE

Explain to the patient that the purpose of the test is to identify serum globulins that may be present in the blood.

Explain that food and drinks are not restricted.

Elevated level

Recognize clinical problems that cause the presence of cryoglobulins, such as autoimmune diseases, collagen diseases, and leukemia.

Observe for signs and symptoms of lupus erythematosus—i.e., "butterfly" rash (erythematosus rash on the cheeks and the bridge of the nose), arthritis, and urinary insufficiency.

Observe for signs and symptoms of rheumatoid arthritis—i.e., pain and stiffness in the joints (especially in the A.M.); swollen, red, tender joints; joint deformities; and inability to make a fist and flexion contractures.

Compare serum cryoglobulins with other laboratory tests.

CULTURES (Blood, Sputum, Stool, Throat, Wound, Urine)

NORMAL RANGE

Adult: negative or no pathogen.

Child: same as adult.

DESCRIPTION

Also see Antibiotic Susceptibility Test.

Cultures are taken to isolate the microorganism which is causing the clinical infection. Most culture specimens are obtained using sterile swabs with medium (solid or broth), a sterile container (cup) with a lid, and a sterile syringe with a sterile bottle of liquid medium. The culture specimen should be taken immediately to the laboratory after collection (no longer than 30 minutes), for some organisms will die if not placed in the proper medium and incubated.

Most specimens for culture are either blood, sputum, stool, throat secretions, wound exudate, or urine. It usually takes 24 to 36 hours to grow the organisms and 48 hours for the growth and culture report.[4,8,9,11,27,30]

CLINICAL PROBLEMS

Specimen	Clinical Condition or Organism
Blood	Bacteremia
	Septicemia
	Postoperative shock
	Fever of unknown origin (FUO)
Sputum	Pulmonary tuberculosis
	Bacterial pneumonia
	Chronic bronchitis
	Bronchiectasis
Stool	Salmonella species
	Shigella species
	Enteropathogenic *Escherichia coli*
	Staphylococcus species
Throat	B. hemolytic streptococcus (rheumatic fever)
	Thrush (Candida species)
	Tonsillar infection
	Staphylococcus aureus
Wound	Staphylococcus species: *Staph. aureus*
	Pseudomonas aeruginosa
	Proteus species
	Bacteroides species
	Klebsiella species
	Serratia species
Urine	*Escherichia coli (E. coli)*
	Klebsiella species
	Pseudomonas aeruginosa
	Serratia species
	Shigella species
	Yeasts: Candida species

PROCEDURE

The specimen for culture should be taken to the laboratory *immediately* after collection.

The specimen should be obtained before antibiotic therapy is started. If the patient is receiving antibiotics, the drug(s) should be listed on the laboratory slip.

Collection containers or tubes should be sterile. Aseptic technique should be used during collection. Contamination of the specimen could cause false positive results and/or transmission of the organisms.

Hand washing is essential before and after collection of the specimen.

Blood: Cleanse the patient's skin according to the institution's procedure. Usually the skin is scrubbed first with iodine (Betadine). Iodine can be irritating to the skin, so it is removed and an application of benzalkonium chloride or alcohol is applied. Cleanse the top(s) of the culture bottle(s) with iodine and leave it or them to dry. The bottle(s) should contain a culture medium. Collect 5 to 10 ml of venous blood and place in the sterile bottle. The institution may require that the needle be passed over a flame before injecting the blood into the bottle. Special vacuum tubes containing a culture medium for blood may be used instead of a culture bottle. (Check with the laboratory for the specific techniques used; there may be variations due to the new types of media available.)

Sputum: *Sterile container or cup:* Obtain sputum for culture early in the morning, before breakfast. Instruct the patient to give several deep coughs to raise sputum. Tell the patient to avoid spitting saliva secretion into the sterile container. Saliva and post-nasal drip secretions can contaminate the sputum specimen. Keep a lid on the sterile container. The container *should not* be completely filled and should be taken immediately to the laboratory. The sputum sample should not remain for hours by the patient's bedside unless one needs a 24 hour sputum specimen (in this case, an extra sterile container should be left). *Acid-fast bacilli (TB culture):* A special container may be used for collecting a sputum specimen for detecting tercule bacilli. Follow the instructions on the container. Collect 5 to 10 ml of sputum and take the sample immediately to the laboratory or refrigerate the specimen. Three sputum specimens may be requested, one each day for 3 days. Check for proper labeling.

Stool: Collect approximately 1 inch diameter feces sample. Use a sterile tongue blade and place the tool specimen in a sterile container with a lid. The suspected disease or organism should be noted on the laboratory slip. The stool specimen should not contain urine. The patient should not be given barium or mineral oil, which can inhibit bacteria growth.

Throat: Use a sterile cotton swab or a polyester-tipped swab. The sterile throat culture kit could be used. Swab the inflamed or ulcerated tonsillar and/or postpharyngeal areas of the throat. Place the applicator in a culturette tube with its culture medium. If the patient gags or coughs, stand by the side of the patient to collect the specimen. Take the throat culture specimen immediately to the laboratory. Do *not* give antibiotics before taking the culture.

Wound: Use a culture kit containing a sterile cotton swab or a polyester-tipped swab and a tube with culture medium. Swab the exudate of the wound and place the swab in the tube containing a culture medium. Wear sterile gloves when there is an excess amount of purulent drainage.

Urine: *Clean-caught (midstream) urine specimen:* Clean-caught urine collection is the most common method for collecting a urine specimen for culture. There are non-catheterization kits giving step-by-step instructions. Catheterizing for urine culture is seldom ordered. Usually the patient collects the urine specimen for culture, so a detailed explanation should be given, according to the instructions. The penis or vulva should be well cleansed. At times, two urine specimens (2 to 10 ml) are requested to verify the organism and in case of a possible contamination of the urine specimen. Collect a midstream urine specimen early in the morning or as ordered in a sterile container. The lid should fit tightly on the container and the urine specimen should be taken immediately to the bacteriology laboratory or refrigerated. Label the urine specimen with the patient's name, the date, and the exact time of collection (7/22/84 @ 8:00 A.M.). List any antibiotics or sulfonamides the patient is taking on the laboratory slip.

FACTORS AFFECTING LABORATORY RESULTS

Contamination of the specimen.

Antibiotics and sulfonamides may cause false negative results.

Urine in the stool collection.

NURSING IMPLICATIONS WITH RATIONALE

Explain to the patient that the purpose of the culture is to determine whether there is an organism (bacteria) present.

Explain the procedure for obtaining the culture specimen. Answer questions. If the patient participates in the collection of the specimen (e.g., urine), the procedure should be reviewed several times.

Hold antibiotics or sulfonamides until after the specimen has been collected. These drugs could cause false negative results. If these drugs have been given, they should be listed on the laboratory slip and recorded on the patient's chart.

Label all specimens with the patient's name, room number, and the date and time of collection.

Deliver all specimens immediately to the laboratory or refrigerate the specimen.

Handle the specimen(s) with extreme care. Aseptic technique should be used. Prevent contamination of the specimen(s) or transmission of the organism to other patients or yourself. *Be aseptic-cautious.*

Keep lids on sterile specimen containers. Sputum cups should not be uncovered by the bedside.

Suggest a culture if a pathogenic organism is suspected. Check the patient's temperature.

D

DIFFERENTIAL WHITE BLOOD CELL COUNT (Overview)
Differential Leukocyte Count

NORMAL RANGE

Polymorphonuclear granulocytes: *Adult:* (1) Neutrophils: 50–70 percent of total WBC. Segments: 50–65 percent. Bands: 0–5 percent. (2) Eosinophils: 0–3 percent. (3) Basophils: 1–3 percent. *Child* (2 weeks to 12 years): Neutrophils: 29–47 percent. Eosinophils: same as adult. Basophils: same as adult.

Mononuclear agranulocytes: *Adult:* Lymphocytes: 25–35 percent of total WBC. Monocytes: 2–6 percent. *Child* (2 weeks to 12 years): Lymphocytes: 38–63 percent. Monocytes: 4–9 percent.

DESCRIPTION

Differential white blood cell (WBC) count is part of the complete blood count (CBC). Not only is the total white blood cell (leukocyte) count needed, but the subtypes of leukocytes should be known to determine the cause of disease.

The differential WBC count is expressed as a percentage of the total number of leukocytes. Neutrophils and lymphocytes make up 80 to 90 percent of the total leukocytes.

The "relative" number of a subtype of leukocytes is expressed in terms of percentage, and the "absolute" number is expressed in cubic millimeters (cu mm, or mm^3).[8,16,21,30,31]

Polymorphonuclear leukocytes: See also Neutrophils, Eosinophil Count, and Basophils. *Neutrophils* make up the largest percentage of leukocytes. They are the first line of defense and respond to acute infections and inflammatory diseases. Immature cells (i.e., myeloblasts, metamyelocytes, and bands) increase in number during the acute phase of illness. *Eosinophils* increase in allergic and parasitic conditions. They are under the influence of adrenocortical hormones and will decrease in number during excess hormone secretion or steroid therapy. *Basophils* prevent blood clotting during inflammation and aid in the healing process. They are composed of granules which contain heparin and histamine.

Mononuclear leukocytes: See also Lymphocytes and Monocytes. *Lymphocytes* make up the second largest percentage of leukocytes. Lymphocytes increase during chronic and viral infections. They play an important part in the immune response system. They are also under the influence of adrenocortical hormones, and like eosinophils, decrease in number during excess hormone secretion or steroid therapy. Monocytes are the second line of defense and are considered stronger and live longer than neutrophils. They respond late during an acute phase of illness, but they continue to function during the chronic phase as phagocytes by ingesting dead tissue and debris.

PROCEDURE

Collect 7 ml of venous blood in a lavender-top tube.

There is no food or drink restriction.

For *Clinical Problems, Factors Affecting Laboratory Results, and Nursing Implications With Rationale,* see White Blood Cell Count, Neutrophils, Eosinophil Count, Basophils, Lymphocytes, and Monocytes.

E

EOSINOPHIL COUNT (Blood)
Type of White Blood Cell (WBC) Differential Count; the Thorn ACTH Test

NORMAL RANGE
Adult: 1–3 percent of total leukocytes (WBC), 100–300 mm^3.

DESCRIPTION
This test is part of the white cell differential count. Eosinophils are a type of polymorphonuclear granulocyte of the leukocytes (white blood cells) which increase in allergic and parasitic conditions. They occur at antigen–antibody reaction sites and are thought to detoxify harmful protein substances produced from parasites. With an increase in steroids, either produced by the adrenal glands (adrenocortical hormones) during stress or administered orally or by injection (cortisone), eosinophils decrease in number.

The Thorn test utilizes the eosinophil count to study the function of the adrenal cortex. A baseline eosinophil count is recorded and ACTH is administered. ACTH stimulates the adrenal glands to produce adrenocortical hormone, which lowers the eosinophil count. If the eosinophils are lower than the baseline count in 4 hours, then the adrenal cortex is functioning normally. If they are only slightly decreased, then Addison's disease could be the problem.[8,9,11,14,21,30,36]

CLINICAL PROBLEMS
Decreased level *(↓ 1 percent):* Stress—burns, postoperative shock; adrenal cortical hyperfunction (i.e., Cushing's syndrome); neutrophilia. *Drug influence:* ACTH; cortisone, prednisone; thyroxin.

Elevated level *(↑ 3 percent):* allergies; parasitic disease—aspergillosis, trichinosis, visceralis, hydatidosis; cancer—bone, ovary, testis, brain; hay fever; leukemia; Hodgkin's disease; phlebitis and thrombophlebitis; asthma; chronic obstructive lung disease (COLD); kidney disease—renal failure, nephrotic syndrome; gastritis.

PROCEDURE
If the eosinophil count is part of the WBC differential count, see *Procedure* under White Blood Cells and Differential White Blood Cell Count.

Individual Quantitative Eosinophil Count: Collect 7 ml of venous blood in a lavender-top tube. Record the time the blood was drawn on the laboratory slip. The normal eosinophil count is lowest in the morning and highest in the afternoon and evening.

Thorn ACTH Test: This test uses the eosinophil count to test the response to ACTH. The patient should be NPO for 12 hours before the test. Collect 7 ml of venous blood in the morning for a baseline eosinophil count. Administer 25 mg of ACTH intramuscularly. Collect a second venous blood sample 4 hours later for the eosinophil count.

FACTORS AFFECTING LABORATORY RESULTS
Steroids (various cortisone preparations), which decrease eosinophil levels.

Time of drawing the blood sample—the count is low in the morning, high in the afternoon.

NURSING IMPLICATIONS WITH RATIONALE

Explain to the patient the purpose of the test. Explanation may be brief, such as, "to determine if there is an increase or decrease in the eosinophils." A more detailed explanation may be needed.

Decreased level (↓ 1 percent)
Relate decreased eosinophils to clinical problems and drugs. Eosinophils are under the influence of the adrenal cortex. An increase in either the adrenocortical hormone or steriods (cortisone, prednisone) will decrease the eosinophils.
Explain to the patient the procedure for the Thorn ACTH test.

Elevated level (↑ 3 percent)
Relate elevated eosinophils to allergic and parasitic diseases. Recognize other clinical problems related to eosinophil elevation.
Assess the patient for signs and symptoms of allergies, such as tearing, "runny nose," rash, and more severe reactions.
Record the time the blood sample is drawn. If drawn in the afternoon or evening, the count could be slightly higher.

ERYTHROCYTE OSMOTIC FRAGILITY (Blood)
Osmotic Fragility, Erythrocyte Fragility, Red Cell Fragility

NORMAL RANGE
  Adult:

% Saline (NaCl)	% Hemolysis	
	Fresh Blood (<3 hours)	Incubated at 37°C (24 hr Blood)
0.30	97–100	85–100
0.35	90–98	75–100
0.40	50–95	65–100
0.45	5–45	55–95
0.50	0–5	40–85
0.55	0	15–65
0.60	0	0–40

Child: similar to adult.

DESCRIPTION
Water is normally exchanged between cells and extracellular fluid according to the osmolality (concentration) of fluid. Red blood cell (erythrocyte) fluid and the plasma have similar ionic concentrations, isoosmolar or isotonic. When there is an imbalance in one of the fluids, osmosis occurs. Fluid moves from the fluid with the lesser concentration to the fluid with the greater concentration. If erythrocytes are placed in a hypo-osmolar solution, fluid with less than the normal serum/plasma osmolality (<280 mOsm/L) will move into the erythrocytes, causing them to swell and eventually rupture.
The erythrocyte osmotic fragility test determines the erythrocytes' ability to resist hemolysis (red blood cell destruction) in a hypo-osmolar solution. Erythrocytes are placed in various concentrations of saline. If hemolysis occurs at a slightly hypo-

osmolar concentration of saline (0.36 to 0.73 percent solution), there is increased osmotic fragility, and if hemolysis occurs at a severely hypo-osmolar concentration of saline, there is decreased osmotic fragility. With increased fragility, the erythrocytes are usually spherical, and with decreased fragility, the erythrocytes are thin and flat.[4,8,9,11,14,30]

CLINICAL PROBLEMS

Decreased level *(<0.30 percent):*anemias—iron deficiency, folic acid deficiency, vitamin B$_6$ deficiency, sickle cell; thalassemia major and minor (Mediterranean anemia or Cooley's anemia); hemoglobin C disease;* polycythemia vera; following splenectomy; acute and subacute necrosis of the liver; obstructive jaundice.

Elevated level *(>0.46 percent):* congenital spherocytosis; transfusion; incompatibility—ABO and Rh; acquired hemolytic anemia (autoimmune); hemoglobin C disease;* chemical or drug poisonings; chronic lymphocytic leukemia; burns (thermal).

PROCEDURE

The test is usually performed on fresh blood less than 3 hours old and/or 24-hour-old blood incubated at 37°C.

Collect 7 to 10 ml of venous blood in a lavender-top tube. The tube should be filled to its capacity. A drop of blood is placed in tubes with decreasing saline concentration. Hemolysis is frequently determined by a colorimeter.

There is no food or drink restriction.

FACTORS AFFECTING LABORATORY RESULTS

Plasma pH, temperature, glucose concentration, and O$_2$ saturation of the blood affect the osmotic fragility.

Older erythrocytes have increased osmotic fragility.

A blood sample more than 3 hours old may show an increase in osmotic fragility.

NURSING IMPLICATIONS WITH RATIONALE

Explain to the patient the purpose of the test. Explanation may be brief, such as "to determine red blood cell fragility" *or* "it is a test to check the blood cells' ability to withstand a diluted solution before rupturing" *or* "this is one of the tests used to determine certain disease entities—for instance, anemias."

Explain that food, drink, and medication are not restricted.

Decreased level (<0.30 percent)

Identify clinical problems related to a decreased erythrocyte osmotic fragility. Normally, complete hemolysis occurs with 0.30 percent saline. Thin, flat cells are usually resistant to hemolysis at 0.30 percent. Examples of diseases with a decreased fragility are the anemias (except acquired hemolytic anemia), liver disease, and polycythemia vera (see *Clinical Problems* above).

Assess for signs and symptoms of anemias—e.g., fatigue, weakness, tachycardia, and dyspnea.

Elevated level (>0.46 percent)

Identify clinical problems related to an increased erythrocyte osmotic fragility—i.e., transfusion incompatibility, acquired hemolytic anemia, and chemical or drug poisoning (see *Clinical Problems* above).

Decreased or increased fragility may occur in hemoglobin C disease.

Monitor temperature when the patient receives a blood transfusion. A slightly elevated temperature is an early sign of transfusion reaction.

Observe for signs and symptoms of transfusion reactions other than changes in temperature—i.e., rash, difficulty in breathing, and an increased pulse rate.

ERTHROCYTE SEDIMENTATION RATE (ESR) (Blood)
Sedimentation (SED) Rate

NORMAL RANGE
Adult: *Under 50 years old—Westergren method:* Male: 0–15 mm/hour. Female: 0–20 mm/hour. *Over 50 years old—Westergren method:* Male: 0–20 mm/hour. Female: 0–30 mm/hour. *Cutler method:* Male: 0–8 mm/hour. Female: 0–10 mm/hour. *Wintrobe method:* Male: 0–7 mm/hour. Female: 0–15 mm/hour.
Child: *Newborn:* 0–2 mm/hour. *4–14 years old:* 3–13 mm/hour.

DESCRIPTION
The erythrocyte sedimentation rate (ESR) test (known also as the sedimentation rate or SED rate) measures the rate at which red blood cells settle in unclotted blood in millimeters per hour (mm/hour). The ESR test is nonspecific. The rate can be increased in acute inflammatory process, acute and chronic infections, tissue damage (necrosis), rheumatoid collagen diseases, malignancies, and physiologic stress situations (e.g., pregnancy). To some hematologists, the ESR test is unreliable, since it is nonspecific and is affected by physiologic factors which cause inaccurate results.

The C-reactive protein (CRP) test is considered more useful than the ESR test because CRP increases more rapidly during an acute inflammatory process and returns to normal faster than ESR. The erythrocyte sedimentation rate test is still an old stand-by used by many physicians as a rough estimate of the disease process and for following the course of illness. With an elevated ESR, other laboratory tests should be conducted to properly identify the clinical problem.[8,9,11,16,27,30,31,34,36]

CLINICAL PROBLEMS
Decreased level *(↓ 3 mm/hour):* polycythemia vera, congestive heart failure, sickle cell anemias, infectious mononucleosis, factor V deficiency, degenerative arthritis, angina pectoris. *Drug influence:* ethambutol (Myambutol); quinine; salicylates (aspirins); cortisone, prednisone.

Elevated level *(↑ 15 mm/hour [male], ↑ 20 mm/hour [female]):* rheumatoid arthritis; rheumatic fever; acute myocardial infarction; cancer of the stomach, colon, breast, liver, kidney; Hodgkin's disease; multiple myeloma; lymphosarcoma; bacterial endocarditis; gout; hepatitis; cirrhosis of the liver; acute pelvic inflammatory disease; syphilis; tuberculosis; glomerulonephritis; systemic lupus erythematosus; hemolytic disease of newborns (erythroblastosis fetalis); pregnancy (second and third trimesters). *Drug influence:* dextran, methyldopa (Aldomet), methysergide (Sansert), penicillamine (Depen), procainamide (Pronestyl), theophylline, oral contraceptives, vitamin A.

PROCEDURE
Collect 7 ml of venous blood in a lavender-top tube. Keep the specimen in a vertical position.

Take the blood specimen to the laboratory immediately. Blood should not stand, since the SED rate could increase.

If the blood specimen is refrigerated, it should be allowed to return to room temperature before it is tested.

There is no food or drink restriction.

FACTORS AFFECTING LABORATORY RESULTS

Factors increasing the SED rate—pregnancy (second and third trimesters); menstruation; drugs (see *Drug Influence* above); the presence of cholesterol, fibrinogen, and globulins.

Factors decreasing the SED rate—newborns (decreased fibrinogen level); drugs (see *Drug Influence* above); high blood sugar, serum albumin, and serum phospholipids.

NURSING IMPLICATIONS WITH RATIONALE

Decreased level (<3 mm/hour)

Relate decreased ESR levels to clinical problems and drugs (see *Drug Influence* above).

Elevated level (>15 mm/hour [male], >20 mm/hour [female])

Relate elevated ESR levels to clinical problems and drugs. The ESR test is a nonspecific test (not related to one specific clinical problem); however, it can indicate that there is an inflammatory process.

Explain to the patient the purpose of the blood test. Explanation could be brief, such as, "to determine whether an inflammation is present." A more detailed explanation may be needed.

Instruct the patient that he may eat and drink prior to the blood test.

Answer the patient's questions about the significance of an increased ESR level. An answer could be that other laboratory tests are usually performed in conjunction with the ESR test for adequate diagnosis of a clinical problem.

Notify the physician and mark the chart if the patient has been taking oral contraceptives for a long period of time. This can increase the ESR. Hold medications which can cause false positive results for 24 hours before the test. If the patient must receive the medication (as with Aldomet and Pronestyl), then notify the laboratory personnel and write on the laboratory slip the drugs taken.

Relate the *Factors Affecting Laboratory Results* to your patient.

ESTRIOL (E₃) (Urine)

NORMAL RANGE

Adult (pregnant): 30–32 weeks, 10–30 mg/24 hours; 34–36 weeks, 12–46 mg/24 hours; 38–40 weeks, 18–60 mg/24 hours.

Child: usually not performed.

DESCRIPTION

Estriol (E₃), produced largely by the placenta, with a small amount coming from the fetal adrenal glands, represents the largest portion of the total estrogen excretion. The estriol level in the urine usually increases after 2 months of pregnancy.

This test is usually done after 30 weeks of gestation in high-risk patients (hypertensives, diabetics, patients with a history of stillbirths). If the estriol level falls after the second or during third trimester of pregnancy, there may be fetal distress, and if a marked decline occurs after 35 weeks of gestation, a Cesarean section may be indicated. Two 24 hour urine collections taken 1 day apart are analyzed to make sure there is a decrease in the estriol level. A drop of 30 to 40 percent of the normal value is indicative of placenta dysfunction and/or fetal distress.[2,11,27,30,36]

CLINICAL PROBLEMS

Decreased level (*<30 to 40 percent of normal value):* fetal distress, diabetic pregnancy, pregnancy with hypertension, impending toxemia.

Elevated level *(above normal values):* urinary tract infection, glycosuria. *Drug influence:* antibiotics—ampicillin, neomycin; hydrochlorothiazide (Hydrodiuril); Mandelamine; cortisone preparation.

PROCEDURE

Collect urine for 24 hours in a large container/bottle with an added preservative (15 ml of HC1 or 1 g of boric acid).

Make sure that a preservative is in the collection container.

Label the urine bottle with the patient's name, and the date and exact times of collection—e.g., 3/2/83, 8:00 A.M.–3/3/83, 8:03 A.M.

There is no food or drink restriction.

Two 24 hour urine specimens (taken a day apart) are usually ordered, since a single determination may be subject to too much individual variation and may make interpretation difficult.

FACTORS AFFECTING LABORATORY RESULTS

Drugs (see *Drug Influence* above).

Glycosuria and urinary tract infection can cause false positive levels.

Toilet paper and feces contaminate the urine collection specimen.

NURSING IMPLICATIONS WITH RATIONALE

Explain to the patient the purpose of the test and the procedure for urine collection. A brief explanation would be, "to determine the amount of hormonal excretion in the urine." A more detailed explanation may be needed.

Post urine collection times on the patient's door and/or bed and in the Kardex.

Explain to the patient and family that all urine should be saved during the specified time.

Instruct the patient not to put toilet paper or feces in the urine.

Explain that food and drink are not restricted.

Decreased level (<30 to 40 percent of normal value)

Recognize that high-risk patients (diabetic, hypertensive, or with a history of stillbirth) may have a fall in estriol (estrogen) excretion during pregnancy. Weekly or biweekly 24 hour urine estriol levels may be ordered. These persons (at high risk) need close monitoring.

Monitoring the fetal heart rate, the patient's blood pressure, and sugar in the urine. Hypertension and diabetes could cause placental dysfunction, leading to fetal distress.

Report glycosuria and urinary tract infection during pregnancy. Both could cause a false rise in estriol excretion. Diabetic women frequently show wide swings in estriol values, which makes estriol abnormalities difficult to document until fetal distress is present.

ESTROGENS (TOTAL) (Urine—24 Hours)

NORMAL RANGE
Adult: *Female:* preovulation, 5–25 µg/24 hours; follicular phase, 24–100 µg/24 hours; luteal phase, 12–80 µg/24 hours; postmenopause, 0–10 µg/24 hours.
　　　Male: 4–25 µg/24 hours.
Child: postpuberty, same as adult.

DESCRIPTION
　　Estrogens—hormones composed of estrone, estradiol, and estriol—are produced by the ovary, by the adrenal gland, and in pregnancy by the placenta. (Also see Estriol.) This 24 hour urine test is useful for diagnosing ovarian disorders and for the analysis of tumor tissue in breast cancer. To evaluate ovarian dysfunction, the age of the patient and the phase of the menstrual cycle should be known. As indicated under *Normal Range* above, there is a biphasia pattern of estrogen excretion in a menstrual cycle.[27,30,36]

CLINICAL PROBLEMS
　　Decreased level *(<5 µg/24 hours [female]):* ovarian dysfunction, ovarian agenesis, infantilism, pregnancy (intrauterine death), menopausal and postmenopausal symptoms. *Drug influence:* phenothiazines (in some cases), tetracyclines (in some cases), vitamins.
　　Elevated level *(>100 µg/24 hours [female]):* adrenocortical tumor, adrenocortical hyperplasia, ovarian tumor, some testicular tumors, pregnancy (gradual increase from the first trimester on). *Drug influence:* phenothiazines, tetracyclines, vitamins (in some cases).

PROCEDURE
　　Collect a 24 hour urine sample in a large container (bottle) and refrigerate. The urine bottle should contain a preservative (usually boric acid).
　　Label the urine bottle with the patient's name, and the date and exact time of collection—e.g., 5/24/83, 7:02 A.M. to 5/25/83, 7:01 A.M.
　　There is no food or drink restriction.

FACTORS AFFECTING LABORATORY RESULTS
　　Certain drugs may cause a decrease or an increase in the estrogen level (see *Drug Influence* above).
　　Saving only part of the 24 hour urine sample may cause an inaccurate result.

NURSING IMPLICATIONS WITH RATIONALE

Explain to the patient the purpose of and procedure for the test.
Explain that food and drinks are not restricted.
Check to see that a preservative is in the urine container. If not, notify the laboratory.
Post the dates and times for the urine collection on the patient's door or bed and in the Kardex.
Inform the patient and family that all urine should be saved and placed in the refrigerated container. Toilet paper and feces should not be in the urine.

Decreased level (<5 µg/24 hours)
Recognize clinical problems that will cause a decreased level of estrogens in the urine (see *Clinical Problems* above).

Obtain a history of menstrual problems and the present menstrual cycle (e.g., 14 days since the last menstrual period). The phase of the menstrual cycle has an influence on the result of the test.

Teach the patient to keep accurate monthly records on the time of menstruation, how long each menstrual period lasts, and the amount of menstrual flow.

Elevated level (>100 μg/24 hours)

Recognize clinical problems related to an elevated urine estrogens level (see *Clinical Problems* above).

F

FACTOR ASSAY (Plasma—Overview)
Factors I through XIII, Coagulation Factors, Blood Clotting Factors

NORMAL RANGE
Adult and child: *Factor I* (fibrinogen): 200–400 mg/dl (minimal for clotting, 75–100 mg/dl). *Factor II* (prothrombin): minimal hemostatic level, 10–15 percent concentration. *Factor III* (thromboplastin): variety of substances. *Factor IV* (calcium): 4.5–5.5 mEq/liter, or 9–11 mg/dl. *Factor V* (proaccelerin or labile factor): minimal hemostatic level, 5–10 percent concentration. *Factor VI* not used. *Factor VII* (proconvertin or stable factor): minimal hemostatic level, 5–15 percent concentration. *Factor VIII* (antihemophilic factor [AHF], antihemophilic globulin [AHG], antihemophilic factor A [hereditary–sex–linked]): minimal hemostatic level, 30–35 percent concentration. *Factor IX* (plasma thromboplastin component [PTC], Christmas factor, antihemophilic factor B: minimal hemostatic level, 30 percent concentration. *Factor X* (Stuart factor, Prower factor): minimal hemostatic level, 7–10 percent concentration. *Factor XI* (plasma thromboplastin antecedent [PTA], antihemophilic C): minimal hemostatic level, 20–30 percent concentration. *Factor XII* (Hageman factor, glass contact factor): 0 percent concentration. *Factor XIII* (fibrinase, fibrin stabilizing factor [FSF]: minimal hemostatic level; 1 percent concentration.[4,20,21]

DESCRIPTION
Factor assays are ordered for identification of defects in the blood coagulation mechanism due to a lack of one or more plasma factors. There are 12 factors (excluding factor VI) which are important for clot formation, and these have been numbered according to the sequence of their discovery. To standardize clotting factors, the International Committee on Nomenclature of Blood Clotting Factors was established in 1954, and 12 clotting (coagulation) factors were given Roman numerals, named, and described. These factors are listed according to their Roman numeral, name, and synonyms under *Normal Range* above.

FUNCTIONS OF COAGULATION FACTORS

Factor	Name	Source, Function
I	Fibrinogen	Manufactured by the liver; essential plasma protein; split by thrombin to produce fibrin strands necessary for clot formation.
II	Prothrombin	Produced in the liver and requires vitamin K for its synthesis; prothrombin is converted to thrombin by the action of extrinsic and intrinsic thromboplastin.
III	Thromboplastin	Thromboplastic activity is found in most tissues; converts prothrombin to thrombin.
IV	Calcium	Absorbed in the GI tract from food; inorganic ion is required in all stages of coagulation—thromboplastin generation, enzymatic conversion of prothrombin to thrombin, and stabilization of the fibrin clot.

(cont.)

FUNCTIONS OF COAGULATION FACTORS (Continued)

Factor	Name	Source, Function
V	Proaccelerin (labile factor)	Formed by the liver; for acceleration of thromboplastin generation; prompt conversion of prothrombin to thrombin; deteriorates rapidly in plasma at room temperature.
VI		Not done.
VII	Proconvertin (stable factor)	Manufacturered in the liver and requires vitamin K for its synthesis; not destroyed or consumed in the clotting process; stable in heat; accelerates the conversion of prothrombin to thrombin; use of anticoagulants depresses factor VII in the plasma.
VIII	Antihemophilic factor (A)	Produced by the reticuloendothelial cells; unstable at room temperatures; required for the generation of thromboplastin; essential for the conversion of the prothrombin to thrombin; sex-linked.
IX	Plasma thromboplastin component (PTC) (Christmas factor, antihemophilic factor B)	Manufactured in the liver and requires vitamin K for its synthesis; stable in plasma and serum is not destroyed or consumed in the clotting process; essential for generating thromboplastin; sex-linked.
X	Stuart factor	Manufactured in the liver and requires vitamin K for its synthesis; stable in plasma and serum; not consumed in the clotting process; helps produce the thromboplastin-generating system.
XI	Plasma thromboplastin antecedent (PTA) (antihemophilic C)	Synthesis unknown; present in serum and plasma; consumed during the clotting process; essential for plasma thromboplastin formation.
XII	Hageman factor	Synthesis unknown; activated in contact with glass and following injury; activated factor XII stimulates factor XI to continue the clotting process; converts plasminogen to plasmin in fibrinolysis.
XIII	Fibrinase (fibrin stabilizing factor [FSF])	Synthesis unknown; enzyme (fibrinase) present in blood, tissue, and platelets and helps to stabilize fibrin strands to form a firm clot.[4,9,20,21,30]

CLINICAL PROBLEMS

A deficiency in one or more factors usually causes bleeding disorders. The associated clinical problems and the causes of these problems are outlined in the following table.

COAGULATION FACTOR DEFICIENCIES

Factor	Clinical Problems (Decreased Levels)	Rationale
I	Hypofibrinogenemia Leukemia Severe liver disease Disseminated intravascular coagulation (DIC)	Deficiency of fibrinogen and fibrinolysis
II	Hypoprothrombinemia Severe liver disease Vitamin K deficiency	Impaired liver function, vitamin K deficit

(cont.)

COAGULATION FACTOR DEFICIENCIES (Continued)

Factor	Clinical Problems (Decreased Levels)	Rationale
	Drugs: salicylates (excessive), anticoagulants, antibiotics (excessive), hepatotoxic drugs	
III	Thrombocytopenia	Low platelet count
IV	Hypocalcemia	Low calcium intake in diet
	Malabsorption syndrome	
	Malnutrition	
	Hyperphosphatemia	
	Multiple transfusions containing citrate	
V	Parahemophilia (congenital)	Congenital problem, impaired liver function
	Severe liver disease	
	Radioactive phosphorus therapy	
VII	Hepatitis	Impaired liver function, certain drugs affecting the clotting time, vitamin K deficit
	Hepatic carcinoma	
	Hemorrhagic disease of newborn	
	Vitamin K deficiency	
	Drugs: antibiotics (excessive), anticoagulants	
VIII	Hemophilia A	Congenital disorder (sex-linked) occurring mostly in males; circulating factor VIII inhibitors
	Disseminated intravascular coagulation (DIC)	
	Multiple myeloma	
	Lupus erythematosus	
IX	Hemophilia B (Christmas disease)	Congenital disorder (sex-linked) occurring mostly in males; circulating factor IX inhibitors
X	Severe liver disease	Impaired liver function; vitamin K deficit
	Hemorrhagic disease of newborns	
	Vitamin K deficiency	
	Drugs: anticoagulants	
XI	Hemophilia C	Congenital deficiency in both males and females; circulating factor XI inhibitors
	Congenital heart disease	
	Intestinal malabsorption of vitamin K	
	Liver disease	
	Drugs: anticoagulants	
XII	Liver disease	
XIII	Agammaglobulinemia	Circulating factor XIII inhibitors; mild bleeding tendency.[4,9,20,21]
	Myeloma	
	Lead poisoning	
	Poor wound healing	

PROCEDURE

Collect 10 ml of venous blood in a blue-top tube (the tube tops used may differ among laboratories). The tube(s) should be filled to capacity.

Mix the blood with an anticoagulant solution thoroughly and avoid air bubbles.

The tubes should be delivered to the laboratory immediately.

There are no food or drink restrictions.

FACTORS AFFECTING LABORATORY RESULTS

Clotted blood.

The factor assay results (factors I, V, and VIII) could be affected if the blood samples do not receive immediate attention in the laboratory.

NURSING IMPLICATIONS WITH RATIONALE

Explain to the patient the purpose of the test. Explanation could be brief, such as, "to determine if there is a clotting factor deficiency." A more detailed explanation may be needed.

Inform the patient that food and drink are not restricted.

Observe for signs of bleeding—i.e., purpura, petechiae, or frank, continuous bleeding. Report your observations and record them on the patient's chart.

Observe the venipuncture site for seeping of blood. Apply pressure to the site.

Obtain a familial history of bleeding disorders and a history of the patient's bleeding tendency.

FBS (FASTING BLOOD SUGAR)

See Glucose—Fasting Blood Sugar.

FEBRILE AGGLUTININS (Serum)

NORMAL RANGE
Adult: (febrile group—titers): *Brucella:* <1:20, <1:20–1:80 (individuals working with animals). *Tularemia:* <1:40. *Widal (Salmonella):* <1:40 (nonvaccinated). *Weil–Felix (Proteus):* <1:40.
Child: same as adult.

DESCRIPTION
Febrile agglutination tests (febrile group) identify infectious diseases causing fever of unknown origin (FUO). Isolating the invading organism (pathogen) is not always possible, especially if the patient has been on antimicrobial therapy, so indirect methods are used to detect antibacterial antibodies in the serum. Detection of these antibodies is determined by the titer of the serum in highest dilution which will cause agglutination (clumping) in the presence of a specific antigen. The test should be done during the acute phase of the disease (maybe several times) and then done about 2 weeks later. A single agglutination titer is of minimal value. These tests can be used to confirm pathogens already isolated or to identify the pathogen present late in the disease (after several weeks).

Diseases commonly associated with febrile agglutination tests are brucellosis (undulant fever), salmonellosis, typhoid fever, paratyphoid fever, tularemia, and certain rickettsial infections (typhus fever).[4,20,27,30]

CLINICAL PROBLEM

Test	Pathogen(s)	Elevated levels
Brucella	*Brucella abortus* (cattle) *B. suis* (hogs) *B. melitensis* (goats)	Brucellosis—titer >1:160
Pasteurella (tularemia)	*Pasteurella tularensis*	Tularemia (rabbit fever)—titer >1:80

Test	Pathogen(s)	Elevated levels
Widal	Salmonella O (somatic)	Salmonellosis
	Salmonella H (flagellar)	Typhoid fever
	O and H portions of the organism act as antigens to stimulate antibody production.	Paratyphoid fever: Titer: O antigen—>1:80 suspicious, >1:160 definite; H antigen—>1:40 suspicious, >1:80 definite
	Salmonella Vi (capular)	Nonvaccinated or vaccinated over 1 year before
Weil–Felix	Proteus X	Rickettsial diseases
	Proteus OX19	Epidemic typhus
		Tick-borne typhus (Rocky Mountain spotted fever)
	Proteus OX2	Boutonneuse tick fever
		Queensland tick fever
		Siberian tick fever
	Proteus OXK	Scrub typhus: titer—>1:80 significant, >1:160 definite.

PROCEDURE

Collect 5 ml of venous blood in a red-top tube. Prevent hemolysis of the blood sample. Draw blood before starting antimicrobial therapy, if possible. If the patient is receiving drugs for an elevated temperature, write the names of the drugs on the laboratory slip.

There is no food or drug restriction.

The blood sample should be refrigerated if it is not tested immediately or frozen if it is to be kept 24 hours or longer.

FACTORS AFFECTING LABORATORY RESULTS

Vaccination could increase the titer level.

Antimicrobial therapy could decrease the titer level.

Leukemia, advanced carcinomia, some congenital deficiencies, and general debilitation could cause false negative results.

NURSING IMPLICATIONS WITH RATIONALE

Explain to the patient and family the purpose of the test. Explanation might include saying that the test is to identify the organism which is causing the fever.

Avoid shaking the blood sample to prevent hemolysis.

Obtain a history of the patient's occupation, geographic location prior to the fever, and recent vaccinations. Exposure to animals and ticks could be suggestive of the causative organism.

Record on the laboratory slip and in the patient's chart whether the patient has been vaccinated against the pathogen within the last year. Vaccinations can increase the antibody titer.

Monitor the temperature every 4 hours, when elevated.

Remind the physician of the need to repeat the tests when the fever persists and/or when the titer levels are suspicious. The physician may order the tests without being reminded. Titer levels could rise four-fold in 1 to 2 weeks.

Check to determine whether the blood sample has been taken before you give antibiotics or other drug agents to combat fever and the suspected organism. Antibiotic therapy could depress the titer level.

FIBRIN DEGRADATION PRODUCTS (FDP) (Serum)
Fibrin or Fibrinogen Split Products (FSP)

NORMAL RANGE
   Adult: 2–10 µg/ml.
   Child: not usually done.

DESCRIPTION
   The fibrin degradation products (FDP) test is usually done in an emergency when the
   patient is hemorrhaging as the result of severe injury, trauma, and/or shock. Thrombin, which initially accelerates coagulation, promotes the conversion of plasminogen
   into plasmin, which in turn breaks fibrinogen and fibrin into FDP. The fibrin
   degradation (split) products act as anticoagulants, causing continuous bleeding from
   many sites. A clinical condition resulting from this fibrinolytic (clot-dissolving) activity is disseminated intravascular coagulation (DIC).[9,26,30,36]

CLINICAL PROBLEMS
   Decreased level *(↓ 2 µg/ml):* Cerebral thrombosis.
   Elevated level *(↑ 10 µg/ml):* disseminated intravascular coagulation (DIC) caused by
   severe injury, trauma, or shock; septicemia; acute myocardial infarction (AMI);
   pulmonary embolism; acute necrosis of the liver; chronic active hepatitis; acute renal
   failure; shock.

PROCEDURE
   Collect 10 ml of venous blood in a red-top tube. Handle the blood specimen carefully to
   prevent hemolysis.
   There is no food or drink restriction.

FACTORS AFFECTING LABORATORY RESULTS
   Hemolysis of the blood sample.

NURSING IMPLICATIONS WITH RATIONALE

Elevated level (↑ 10 µg/ml)
Explain to the patient and/or family that the purpose of the test is to determine the
   cause of bleeding. A more detailed explanation may be needed.
Monitor vital signs and report shock-like symptoms—i.e., tachycardia, hypotension,
   pallor, and cold, clammy skin.
Observe and report bleeding sites—the chest, the nasogastric tube, incisional or in-
   jured areas, and others.
Report progessive discoloration of the skin.
Monitor infusion rates of intravenous fluids—crystalloids, colloids, and blood.
Check urine output hourly. Report decreased urine output (<25 ml/hour) and blood-
   colored urine.
Provide comfort and support to the patient and family.

FOLIC ACID (FOLATE) (Serum)

NORMAL RANGE
   Adult: 5–20 ng/ml (bioassay), >2.5 ng/ml (RIA; serum), >140 ng/ml (RBC).
   Child: Same as adult.

DESCRIPTION

Folic acid, one of the B vitamins, is needed for normal red and white blood cell function (necessary for normal hematopoiesis) and is required for DNA production. Folic acid is present in a variety of foods; milk, eggs, leafy vegetables, beans, liver, fruits (oranges, bananas), and whole wheat bread. Dietary deficiency is the most common cause of a serum folic acid deficit, especially in children, older adults, and persons with chronic alcoholism. With a decreased folic acid intake, it takes approximately 3 to 4 weeks for folic acid deficiency to develop and 18 to 24 weeks before folic acid anemia will occur.

Usually, the serum folic acid or folate test is performed to detect folic acid anemia. With this type of anemia, the red blood cells are abnormally large, causing a megaloblastic anemia. Other causes of serum folic acid deficit are pregnancy (due to dietary deficiency and because the fetal requirement for folic acid is so great), small intestine malabsorption syndrome, and drugs.

Note: There are many types of biologically active "folic acids." "Folate" is a collective term and thus more appropriate.[8,11,18,27,30]

CLINICAL PROBLEMS

Decreased level *(<2.5 ng/ml):* folic acid anemia (megaloblastic anemia); vitamin B_6 deficiency anemia; malnutrition; malabsorption syndrome (small intestine); pregnancy; malignancies; liver diseases; celiac sprue disease; *Drug influence:* anticonvulsants—Dilantin, Mysoline; antineoplastic agents—methotrexate (folic acid antagonists), aminopterin; antimalaria agents; oral contraceptives.

Elevated level *(>20 ng/ml):* pernicious anemia.

PROCEDURE

Collect 7 to 10 ml of venous blood in a red-top tube and send it to the lab immediately. The lab will mix 1 ml of serum with 20 ng of ascorbic acid to stabilize the folate.

Prevent hemolysis of the blood sample.

If an RBC folate determination is requested, collect 7 ml of venous blood in a lavender-top tube. Send this to the lab immediately. Ascorbic acid will be added in the lab.

There is no food or drink restriction except that the patient must have no alcoholic beverages prior to the test.

FACTORS AFFECTING LABORATORY RESULTS

Drugs (see *Clinical Problems* above).

Alcohol—persons who consume large quantities of alcohol usually have poor nutritional intake (folic acid deficiency).

NURSING IMPLICATIONS WITH RATIONALE

Recognize clinical problems and drugs related to a serum folic acid deficit—i.e., malnutrition, malabsorption syndrome, pregnancy, and others.

Explain to the patient that the purpose for the test is to determine the cause of his or her clinical symptoms *or* to check the folic acid level.

Obtain a dietary history. Collaborate with the dietitian on formulating a diet high in folic acid and have the dietitian plan the diet with the patient.

Encourage the patient to eat foods rich in folic acid—i.e., liver, lean meats, milk, eggs, leafy vegetables, bananas, oranges, beans, and whole wheat bread.

Observe for signs and symptoms of folic acid deficiency—i.e., fatigue, pallor, nausea, anorexia, dyspnea, palpitations, and tachycardia.

FOLLICLE-STIMULATING HORMONE (FSH) (Urine)

NORMAL RANGE
  Adult: *Urine:* 6–50 mouse uterine units (MUU)/24 hours; postmenopausal, >50 MUU/24 hours. *Serum:* 4–30 mIU/ml (female), 4–25 mIU/ml (male).
  Child (prepubertal): *Urine:* <10 MUU/24 hours.

DESCRIPTION
  Follicle-stimulating hormone (FSH) is a gonadatropic hormone produced and controlled by the pituitary gland. FSH stimulates the growth and maturation of the ovarian follicle (which produces estrogen) in females and promotes spermatogenesis in males.
  When there is decreased gonadal function, the FSH production is increased. Ovarian neoplasms (tumors) secrete excess estrogen, which inhibits the production of FSH.[8,9,30,31,36]

CLINICAL PROBLEMS
  Decreased level *(↓ 6 MUU/24 hours [urine]):* Benign and malignant neoplasms of the ovaries; neoplasm of the adrenal gland, testes, ovary; anorexia nervosa.
  Increased level *(↑ 50 MUU/24 hours [urine])* Gonadal failure (menopause), hypopituitary function, FSH-producing pituitary tumor, Klinefelter's syndrome.

PROCEDURE
  Collect a 24 hour urine sample in a large container with the preservative boric acid.
  Some laboratories do not require a preservative if the urine container is refrigerated.
  The pH of the 24 hour urine sample should be between 5 and 6.5. To maintain an acid urine, glacial acetic acid or boric acid may be added. Check first with your laboratory.
  There is no food and drink restriction.

FACTORS AFFECTING LABORATORY RESULTS
  Alkaline urine can give an inaccurate test result.

NURSING IMPLICATIONS WITH RATIONALE

Explain to the patient the purpose of the test. Explanation could be brief, such as, "to measure the amount of a particular hormone in the urine." A more detailed explanation may be needed.

Label the container/bottle with the patient's name and the dates and exact times of the urine collection—e.g., 5/4/83, 8 A.M. to 5/5/83, 8:01 A.M.

Post a notice on the patient's door or bed and in the Kardex concerning the 24 hour urine collection.

Instruct the patient and family not to throw any urine away. Explain that all urine should be poured in the bottle with the preservative or in the bottle in the refrigerator.

Instruct the patient not to put toilet paper or feces in the urine.

Associate decreased or increased urine FSH with clinical problems. The excess production of estrogen with most ovarian tumors will decrease the production of FSH. After menopause, more FSH will be secreted to stimulate estrogen production.

FTA-ABS (FLUORESCENT TREPONEMAL ANTIBODY ABSORPTION) (Serum)

NORMAL RANGE
  Adult: nonreactive (negative).
  Child: nonreactive (negative).

DESCRIPTION
  The FTA-ABS test is the treponemal antibody test, which uses the treponemal organism to produce and detect these antibodies. This test is most sensitive, specific, and reliable for diagnosing all stages of syphilis. It is more sensitive than the VDRL test. The FTA-ABS test is useful for confirming or ruling out suspected false positive serology tests for syphilis. The limitations of this test are that the stage and activity of the disease cannot be identified, the effectiveness of the therapy cannot be measured, and the test for syphilis remains positive even after treatment for a very long time or could remain positive forever.
  TPI (*Treponema pallidum* immobilization) was the original treponemal antibody test; it is not commonly used except for checking spinal fluid for syphilis. It is considered a difficult test to perform.[4,8,11,30]

CLINICAL PROBLEMS
  Reactive: *Positive:* syphilis. *False positives (rare):* lupus erythematosus.

PROCEDURE
  This test is more complex than the other serology tests for syphilis and is not performed in all laboratories. The sample is usually sent to a special laboratory.
  Collect 5 ml of venous blood in a red-top tube.
  There is no food or drink restriction.

FACTORS AFFECTING LABORATORY RESULTS
  Medical treatment does not eliminate the treponemal antibodies. The test results may remain positive after treatment. Test results cannot be used to monitor the patient.

NURSING IMPLICATIONS WITH RATIONALE

Explain to patient that the test is to check for syphilis, or give a similar response.
Be supportive of the patient and family. Keep conversation and information confidential except for what is required by law.
Encourage the patient to have his or her sexual friend or spouse seek medical care if the test is positive.
Check the results of other serology tests for syphilis. A positive VDRL could be false positive due to acute or chronic illness. The FTA-ABS test is reliable for syphilis, giving accurate results; however, many laboratories have to send the blood sample out for testing. Ask the patient if he or she has received treatment for syphilis. Positive FTA-ABS results can occur after treatment (penicillin, erythromycin) for months or several years or for the rest of the patient's life.
Assess for signs and symptoms of syphilis. The primary stage begins with a small papule filled with liquid which ruptures, enlarges, and becomes a chancre. With secondary syphilis, a generalized rash (macular and papular) develops and is found mainly on the arms, palms, soles of the feet, and face.

FUNGAL ORGANISMS: FUNGAL DISEASE, MYCOTIC INFECTIONS
(Smear, Serum, Culture—Sputum, Bronchial, Lesion)
Actinomyces, Histoplasma, Blastomyces, Coccidioides, Cryptococcus, Candida, Aspergillus

NORMAL RANGE
Adult: under 8.
Child: same as adult.

DESCRIPTION
There are more than 45,000 species of fungi, but only 0.01 percent, or 45, are considered pathogenic to man. Fungal infections are more common today and can be classified as (1) superficial and cutaneous mycoses (dermatophytoses), (2) subcutaneous mycoses, and (3) systemic mycoses. Examples of superficial and cutaneous mycoses are tinea pedis (athlete's foot), tinea capitis (ringworm of the scalp), tinea barbae (ringworm of the beard), and tinea crusis (jock itch). Systemic mycoses (e.g., histoplasmosis, actinomycosis, and blastomycosis) are the most serious of the fungal infections.

Most fungus organisms live in the soil and can be transmitted to man and animals by way of the lungs or a break in the skin. The persons most susceptible to fungal infections are those with debilitating or chronic diseases (e.g., diabetes) or who are receiving certain kinds of drug therapy (i.e., steroids, prolonged antibiotics, antineoplastic agents, and oral contraceptives).[2,8,11,23,27]

CLINICAL PROBLEMS

Organism	Disease Entity	Comments
Actinomyces israelii	Actinomycosis	A gram-positive nonacid-fast anaerobic organism that can produce an abscess.
Histoplasma capsulatum	Histoplasmosis	The most common systemic fungal infection. It is commonly found in the eastern part of the United States and in the Mississippi and Ohio valleys. Usually the organism is carried by birds—e.g., starlings and chickens. In most patients, histoplasmosis is a localized pulmonary disease and resembles pulmonary tuberculosis.
Blastomyces dermatitidis	Blastomycosis	It causes granulomatous lesions which involve the skin or visceral organs. Histologically, it is similar to tuberculosis.
Coccidioides immitis	Coccidioidomycosis	It is commonly found in the Southwest and in the San Joaquin Valley of California. Usually the patient has respiratory symptoms and fever of unknown origin (FUO). If the infection is overwhelming, it resembles miliary tuberculosis.
Cryptococcus neoformans	Cryptococcosis Meningitis	Fungal disease usually begins as a pulmonary infection but disseminates to the CNS (brain). The organism is usually carried by pigeons. Patients with decreased immunologic resistance (such as those with acute

Organism	Disease Entity	Comments
		leukemia or Hodgkin's disease or who are receiving steroids or immunosuppressive agents) are susceptible to the disease.
Candida albicans, fungemia	Candidiosis Monilia Thrush	Patients with debilitating diseases or who are taking steroids, antineoplastic agents, or oral contraceptives are susceptible to this fungus.
Aspergillus fumigatus	Aspergillosis	Aspergillus organisms can cause severe respiratory infection. Fungus balls (aspergilloma) develop in the lung tissue. The sputum is golden brown and contains Aspergillus hyphae.[8,27]

PROCEDURE

Samples taken to test for fungi are usually not cultured by local hospitals or local private laboratories because of cost and infrequent demand. These specimens are usually sent to either the state health laboratory, large private laboratories, or the United States Public Health Service, National Communicable Disease Center, Atlanta, Georgia, 30333.

Read the directions from the special laboratory on collection of the specimen.

Organism	Tests
Actinomyces israelii	Smear and culture of material from the lesion Biopsy
Histoplasma capsulatum	Sputum culture Histoplasmin skin test Serum test: complement-fixation or latex agglutination
Blastomyces dermatitidis	Culture Smear, wet-mount examination of the material from the lesion Biopsy—histologic examination Skin test Serum test: complement-fixation (not too sensitive)
Coccidioides immitis	Culture Sputum smears Skin test Serum test: complement-fixation (sensitive), latex agglutination (very sensitive)
Cryptococcus neoformans	Culture of cerebrospinal fluid (CSF) Serum test: latex agglutination (sensitive)
Candida albicans	Smear and culture of the skin, mucous membrane, and vagina (with potassium hydroxide [KOH] solution)
Aspergillus fumigatus	Sputum culture Skin test Serum IgE level

There is no food or drink restriction.

FACTORS AFFECTING LABORATORY RESULTS

Contamination of the specimen.

NURSING IMPLICATIONS WITH RATIONALE

Associate mycotic infections with high-risk patients—i.e., those patients having chronic illnesses (such as diabetes mellitus) or debilitating diseases (such as cancer) or who are receiving prolonged antibiotics, antineoplastic agents (anticancer chemotherapy), steroids, or oral contraceptives.

Explain to the patient that the purpose of the specimen collection is to identify the organism which is causing the clinical symptoms.

Use aseptic technique when collecting a specimen for culture. Preventing the transmission of the organism is most important. Contamination of the specimen can give inaccurate results.

Obtain a history from the patient—where he lives and his occupation. Fungus organisms, (e.g., Histoplasma, Coccidioides) are more prevalent in selected parts of the country. Report if the patient works with chickens or pigeons.

Teach the patient to wear masks when exposed to chicken feces. Explain that the *H. capsulatum* spores are in the feces and can be inhaled.

Monitor the patient's temperature. With many of the fungal diseases, the temperature is elevated.

Report clinical signs and symptoms of respiratory problems—i.e., coughing up sputum, dyspnea, and chest pain.

Check the color of the sputum. Certain fungi can be identified by the color of their secretions. Golden brown sputum is characteristic of the Aspergillus organism.

Assess the neurologic status when cryptococcosis is suspected. Report headaches and changes in sensorium, pupil size and reaction, and motor function.

G

GAMMA-GLUTAMYL TRANSFERASE (Serum)

Gamma-Glutamyl Transpeptidase (GGTP, or GTP; γ-Glutamyl Transpeptidase, γGT)

NORMAL RANGE

Adult: *Men:* (10–38 IU/L. *Women:* 5–25 IU/L, 5–40 U/L at 37°C (SI units).

DESCRIPTION

The enzyme gamma-glutamyl transpeptidase transferase (GGTP or GTP) is found primarily in the liver and kidney, with smaller amounts in the spleen, prostate gland, and heart muscle. GGTP is sensitive for detecting a wide variety of hepatic (liver) parenchymal diseases. The serum level will rise early and will remain elevated as long as cellular damage persists.

The GGTP test is becoming popular for assessing alcoholism (excessive and prolonged alcohol intake) and liver damage associated with alcohol. High levels of GGTP occur after 12 to 24 hours of heavy alcoholic drinking and may remain increased for 2 to 3 weeks after alcohol intake stops. Some alcoholic rehabilitation programs are using the GGTP level as a guide to planning care as they work with the alcoholic individuals.

A serum gamma-glutamyl transpepidase determination is frequently ordered with a test for serum alkaline phosphatase (ALP). The GGTP test is considered more sensitive for liver dysfunction than the ALP test.[8,27,30,34,36]

CLINICAL PROBLEMS

Elevated level *(↑ 38 IU/L):* cirrhosis of the liver; acute and subacute necrosis of the liver; alcoholism; viral hepatitus; chronic active hepatitis; cancer—liver, pancreas, prostate, breast, kidney, lung, brain; infectious mononucleosis; hemochromatosis (iron deposits in the liver); diabetes mellitus; hyperlipoproteinemia (type IV); acute myocardial infarction (fourth day); congestive heart failure; acute pancreatitis; acute cholecystitis; epilepsy; nephrotic syndrome. *Drug influence:* diphenylhydantoin (Dilantin), phenobarbital.

PROCEDURE

Collect 10 ml of venous blood in a red-top tube.
There is no food or drink restriction.

FACTORS AFFECTING LABORATORY RESULTS

Dilantin and barbiturates can cause a false positive GGTP test.
Excessive and prolonged alcoholic intake will elevate the GGTP level.

NURSING IMPLICATIONS WITH RATIONALE

Elevated level (↑ 38 IU/L)
Explain to the patient the purpose of the test. Explanation may be brief, such as, "It is one of the tests used to determine liver function."
Compare GGTP with alkaline phosphatase (ALP), leucine aminopeptidase (LAP) and alanine aminotransferase (SGPT or ALT). The GGTP test tends to be more sensitive for detecting liver dysfunction than the others.

Report to the physician if the patient is receiving Dilantin or phenobarbital when the test is ordered. Usually these medications cannot be withheld. Note on the laboratory slip the names of the drugs (affecting GGTP levels) and the dosages the patient is receiving.

Encourage patients with an alcoholic problem to participate in Alcoholics Anonymous or a rehabilitation program.

Assess the patient's diet. Teach patients to maintain a well-balanced diet (adequate protein and carbohydrate).

Observe for signs and symptoms of liver damage—i.e., restlessness, jaundice, twitching, flapping tremors, spider angiomas, bleeding tendencies (nose and rectal bleeding) purpura, ascites, and others.

GASTRIN (Serum or Plasma)

NORMAL RANGE
   Adult: 40–200 pg/ml.
   Child: not usually done.

DESCRIPTION
   Gastrin is a hormone secreted from the pyloric mucosa which stimulates the secretion of gastric juices—mainly hydrochloric acid (HC1). Normally increased gastrin will cause hypersecretion of HC1, which in turn inhibits gastrin secretion.
   This test is usually ordered to aid in the diagnosis of pernicious anemia, Zollinger–Ellison syndrome (a condition caused by a noninsulin-producing tumor of the pancreas which secretes excess amounts of gastrin), and stomach cancer.[5,8,27,30,31,34,36]

CLINICAL PROBLEMS
   Elevated level *(↑ 200 pg/ml):* pernicious anemia, Zollinger–Ellison syndrome, malignant neoplasm of the stomach, peptic ulcer, chronic atrophic gastritis, cirrhosis of the liver, acute and chronic renal failure. *Drug influence:* calcium gluconate IV.

PROCEDURE
   Collect 10 ml of venous blood in a red-top tube.
   Food and drinks (except water) are restricted for 12 hours before the test.

FACTORS AFFECTING LABORATORY RESULTS
   IV infusion of calcium elevates the serum gastrin level.

NURSING IMPLICATIONS WITH RATIONALE

Explain to the patient that the purpose of the test is to determine the blood level of the hormone gastrin. A more detailed explanation may be needed.

Inform the patient that food and beverages are restricted, with the exception of water, for 12 hours before the test. A fasting blood sample is required, but the length of the NPO time may differ among laboratories.

Elevated levels (↑ 200 pg/ml)
Recognize clinical conditions and drugs which can elevate the serum gastrin level (see *Clinical Problems* above).

Check the patient's serum gastrin value, for in Zollinger–Ellison Syndrome, the serum level can reach 2800 to 300,000 pg/ml. High levels are present in pernicious anemia and gastritis. With fasting, gastrin secretion will be slightly elevated.

Observe for signs and symptoms of pernicious anemia—i.e., weakness, sore tongue, pallor of the gums and lips, anorexia, loss of weight, and numbness and tingling in the extremities.

GLUCOSE—FASTING BLOOD SUGAR (FBS) (Blood)

NORMAL RANGE
  Adult: *Serum and plasma:* 70–110 mg/dl. *Whole blood:* 60–100 mg/dl.
  Newborn: 30–80 mg/dl.
  Child: 60–100 mg/dl.
  Different laboratories use different methods of analysis.

DESCRIPTION
  Glucose is formed from dietary carbohydrates (CHO), and is stored as glycogen in the liver and skeletal muscles. Insulin and glucagon, two hormones from the pancreas, affect the blood glucose level. Insulin is needed for cellular membrane permeability to glucose and for transportation of glucose into the cells. Without insulin, glucose cannot enter the cells. Glucagon stimulates glycogenolysis (conversion of stored glycogen to glucose) in the liver.

  A decreased blood sugar (hypoglycemia) results from inadequate food intake or too much insulin. When elevated blood sugar (hyperglycemia) occurs, there is not enough insulin; this condition is known as diabetes mellitus. A fasting blood sugar greater than 120 mg/dl usually indicates diabetes, and to confirm the diagnosis when the blood sugar is borderline or slightly elevated, a feasting (postprandial) blood sugar and/or a glucose tolerance test may be ordered.

  Dextrostix test is a rapid, simple, semiquantitative test for distinguishing hypoglycemia from hyperglycemia. The test takes only 1 minute, requiring a drop of blood from the finger placed onto a Dextrostix. The results are compared to a color chart with values between 40 and 130 mg/dl. This is a useful test in emergency situations.[8,9,11,17,20,21,27,30,31,34,36]

CLINICAL PROBLEMS
  Decreased level *(<70 mg/dl [adult serum or plasma]):* hypoglycemic reaction (insulin excess); cancer—stomach, liver, lung; adrenal gland hypofunction; malnutrition; alcoholism; cirrhosis of the liver; strenuous exercise; erythroblastosis fetalis, (hemolytic disease); hyperinsulinism. *Drug influence:* insulin excess.

  Elevated level *(>110 mg/dl [adult serum or plasma]):* diabetes mellitus, diabetes acidosis, adrenal gland hyperfunction (Cushing syndrome), acute myocardial infarction, stress, crushed injury, burns, infections, renal failure, hypothermia, exercise, acute pancreatitis, cancer of the pancreas, congestive heart failure, acromegaly, postgastrectomy (dumping) syndrome, extensive surgery. *Drug influence:* ACTH; cortisone preparations; diuretics—thiazides (Hydrodiuril, Diuril), "Loop" (Lasix, Edecrin); anesthesia drugs; levodopa.

PROCEDURE
  Collect 5 to 10 ml of venous blood in a gray-top tube which contains sodium fluoride to diminish glycolysis. The patient should have nothing by mouth (NPO) except water for 12 hours before the test.

The most frequently used method of analysis involves enzymatic reactions—i.e., glucose oxidase and hexokinase.

Give insulin as ordered after the blood sample is taken.

FACTORS AFFECTING LABORATORY RESULTS
Drugs—cortisone, thiazide, and "loop" diuretics can cause an increase in blood sugar.

Trauma—stress can cause an increase in blood sugar.

The Clinitest for determining urine glucose (glycosuria) may be falsely positive if the patient is taking excessive amounts of aspirin, vitamin C, and certain antibiotics (Keflin), since the test is not specific for glucose but for all reducing substances.

High doses of vitamin C could cause false negative results when using Tes-tape.

NURSING IMPLICATIONS WITH RATIONALE

Explain to the patient that the purpose for the test is to determine the fasting blood sugar value. A more detailed explanation may be needed. Explain to the patient the procedure for the test. Blood is drawn between 7 and 9 A.M. The patient should have nothing by mouth after dinner the night before the test except for water, or as indicated. If the test is ordered to monitor a diagnosed diabetic, then explain that insulin is held until after the blood is drawn. After the test, the patient will receive his insulin and then his breakfast. Record on the laboratory slip and chart, the drugs the patient is receiving daily (i.e., cortisone preparation, thiazide, or "loop" diuretics) which can increase the blood sugar. Report drug information to the physician, especially if the blood sugar test level is slightly elevated.

Decreased level (<70 mg/dl [adult serum or plasma])
Recognize clinical problems associated with low blood sugar level. Excessive doses of insulin, skipped meals, and inadequate food intake are the common causes of hypoglycemia. (See *Clinical Problems* above for other causes.)

Observe for signs and symptoms of hypoglycemia—i.e., nervousness, weakness, confusion, cold and clammy skin, diaphoresis, and increased pulse rate. Observe the patient at night for insulin reaction (diaphoresis) while the patient is sleeping.

Instruct the patient to carry lumps of sugar or candy with him at all times. Most diabetic persons have warnings when hypoglycemia occurs.

Teach the patient to adhere to the American Dietetic Association (ADA) diet, as prescribed. Explain the Exchange Lists for meal planning.

Encourage the patient to contact the American Diabetic Association for literature and information concerning their meeting dates.

Explain to the patient that strenuous exercise can lower the blood sugar (BS). Carbohydrate or protein intake should be increased before exercise or immediately after exercise; the physician should be contacted for food instruction.

Encourage the patient to take insulin one-half to one hour before breakfast and to eat meals on time.

Teach patients who are not diabetic but have a hypoglycemic problem (BS <50 mg/dl) to eat food high in protein and fat and low in CHO. Too much sugar stimulates insulin secretion. Have the patient check first with the physician.

Elevated level (>110 mg/dl [adult serum or plasma])
Recognize clinical problems associated with high blood sugar levels. Diabetes mellitus, Cushing's syndrome, and stressful situations (trauma, burns, extensive surgery) are the common causes of hyperglycemia. (See *Clinical Problems* above for other causes.)

Consider drugs (such as cortisone, thiazides, and loop diuretics) as the cause of a slightly elevated blood sugar level. If blood sugar becomes too high, notify the physician—drug dosages may need to be decreased or insulin may need to be ordered or increased.

Observe for signs and symptoms of hyperglycemia—i.e., excessive thirst (polydipsia), excessive urination (polyuria), excessive hunger (polyphagia), and weight loss. If the blood sugar is greater than 500 mg/dl, Kussmaul breathing due to acidosis may be observed (rapid, deep, vigorous breathing).

Instruct the patient to test his urine before meals. A second voiding 30 minutes after the first voiding is preferred. The patient should use Tes-tape if he is taking aspirin, vitamin C, or antibiotics (such as Keflin), for these drugs can cause false positive readings with Clinitest. High doses of vitamin C may cause false negative readings with Tes-tape.

Explain to the patient that infections can increase the blood sugar level. He should seek medical advice.

GLUCOSE—POSTPRANDIAL (FEASTING BLOOD SUGAR) (Blood)
Two Hour Postprandial Blood Sugar (PPBS)

NORMAL RANGE
Adult: *Serum or plasma:* <140 mg/dl/2 hours. *Blood:* <120 mg/dl/2 hours.
Older Adult: *Serum:* <160 mg/dl/2 hours. *Blood:* <140 mg/dl/2 hours.
Child: same as adult (laboratory PPBS will differ from <120 mg/dl to <150 mg/dl).

DESCRIPTION
A 2 hour postprandial blood sugar (PPBS) or feasting sugar test is usually done to determine the patient's response to a high carbohydrate intake 2 hours after a meal (breakfast or lunch). This test is a screening test for diabetes, normally ordered if the fasting blood sugar was high normal or slightly elevated. Physicians order a single blood test taken 2 hours after a calculated carbohydrate diet is taken. A serum glucose greater than 140 mg/dl or a blood glucose greater than 120 mg/dl is abnormal, and further tests may be needed.[8,9,27,30]

CLINICAL PROBLEMS
Decreased level *(<70mg/dl:* see Glucose—Fasting.
Elevated level *(>140 mg/dl):* see Glucose—Fasting.

PROCEDURE
A high-carbohydrate meal should be taken at breakfast or lunch. Some laboratories or physicians may request that a high-carbohydrate diet be taken 2 to 3 days before the test.

Collect 10 ml of venous blood 2 hours after the patient finishes eating breakfast or lunch. If the nurse does not draw the blood, then the laboratory needs to be told when the patient finished breakfast or lunch.

Food is restricted for 8 hours before the test, but water is not.

FACTORS AFFECTING LABORATORY RESULTS
Smoking may increase the serum glucose level.
Same as for Glucose—Fasting.

NURSING IMPLICATIONS WITH RATIONALE

Explain the purpose of the test. Explanation can be brief, such as, "It is a screening test for diabetes."

Explain the procedure to the patient. Inform the patient that food will be restricted the night before the test. In the morning, the entire breakfast should be eaten, and blood should be drawn 2 hours after finishing the breakfast.

Determine the breakfast foods that the patient likes and dislikes and notify the dietary department. If the person is not hospitalized, a prepared breakfast menu with a calculated number of carbohydrates should be given.

Elevated level (>120 mg/dl [blood], >140 mg/dl [serum])
See Glucose—fasting.

GLUCOSE TOLERANCE TEST—ORAL (GTT) (Serum)

NORMAL RANGE
Adult:

Time	Serum (mg/dl)	(Blood (mg/dl)
Fasting	70–110	60–100
0.5 Hour	<160	<150
1 Hour	<170	<160
2 Hours	<125	<115
3 Hours	Fasting level	Fasting level

Child: Depends on the child's age. Infants normally have lower blood sugar levels (see Glucose—Fasting). A child age 6 or older has glucose tolerance test results similar to those of the adult.

DESCRIPTION

A glucose tolerance test is done to diagnose diabetes mellitus in persons having high-normal or slightly elevated blood sugar values. The test may be indicated when there is a familial history of diabetes, in women having babies weighing 10 pounds or more, in persons having extensive surgery or injury, and in persons with obesity problems. The test should *not* be performed if the fasting blood sugar (FBS) is over 200 mg/dl. After the age of 60, the blood glucose level is usually 10 to 30 mg/dl higher than the "normal range."

The peak glucose level for the oral GTT is one-half to one hour after the ingestion of 100 g of glucose, and the blood sugar should return to normal range in 3 hours. Blood and urine samples will be collected at specified times.

The intravenous glucose tolerance test (IV-GTT) is considered by many to be more sensitive than the oral GTT, since absorption through the GI tract is not involved. The IV-GTT is usually done if the person cannot eat or tolerate the oral glucose. The blood glucose returns to the normal range in 2 hours. However, the values for oral GTT and IV-GTT slightly differ since IV-glucose is absorbed faster.

Hyperinsulinism can be detected with the oral GTT. After an hour, the blood glucose level is usually lower than in the fasting blood sugar test. The person might develop severe hypoglycemic reactions—there is more insulin being secreted in response to the blood glucose.[8,9,11,27,30,34]

CLINICAL PROBLEMS

Decreased level *(<70 mg/dl/3 hours):* hyperinsulinism, adrenal gland insufficiency, malabsorption, protein malnutrition.

Elevated level *(>110 mg/dl/3 hours):* diabetes mellitus; latent diabetes; adrenal gland hyperfunction (Cushing's syndrome); hyperlipoproteinemia; stress; infections; extensive surgery or injury; alcoholism; acute myocardial infarction; cancer of the pancreas; insulin resistance conditions—eclampsia, cancer metastases, acidotic conditions; duodenal ulcers. *Drug influence:* steroids—corticosteroids (Cortisone, etc.); oral contraceptives; estrogens; diuretics: (Thiazide); salicylates.

PROCEDURE

Three days before the test, the person should consume 200 to 300 g of carbohydrate (CHO) daily. Persons normally eat 100 to 150 g of CHO daily.

The patient remains NPO for 12 hours before test, except for water (no food and no medications.)

Collect 5 ml of venous blood in a gray-top tube for the fasting blood sugar. Collect a fasting urine specimen. The GTT is usually *not* performed if the FBS is over 200 mg/dl.

Give 100 g of glucose, either lemon-flavored solution or glucola. Some physicians will give glucose according to body weight (1.75 g/kg), as in pediatrics.

Obtain blood and urine specimens 0.5, 1, 2, and 3 hours after glucose intake.

No coffee, tea, or smoking are allowed during the test. No food should be eaten.

Drugs which affect test results should not be taken for 3 days prior to the GTT, if possible. Some of the drugs are cortisone, oral contraceptives, salicylates, thiazide diuretics, and oral hypoglycemia agents.

FACTORS AFFECTING LABORATORY RESULTS

Drugs (see *Drug Influence* above).

Age—older adults have higher blood sugars. Insulin secretion is decreased due to the aging process.

Emotional stress, fever, infections, trauma, being bedridden, and obesity can increase the blood sugar level.

Strenuous exercise and vomiting might decrease the blood sugar. Hypoglycemic agents will decrease the blood sugar.

NURSING IMPLICATIONS WITH RATIONALE

Explain to the patient the purpose of the test. Explanation could include that the GTT determines blood sugar levels at specified times.

Explain to the patient the procedure for the test. Explain that food, alcohol, and medications are restricted for 12 hours prior to the test. Water is permitted.

Label each specimen with the date and time obtained. The actual voiding time should be recorded on the slip.

Explain to the patient that coffee, tea, and smoking are restricted during the test. Water is allowed and encouraged; however, in some institutions, only 240 ml is permitted.

Explain to the patient that he may feel weak and giddy and perspire during the 2 to 3 hours of the test. This is frequently transitory; however, the nurse should be notified and these symptoms should be recorded. They could be signs of hyperinsulinism.

Notify the laboratory of when (the exact time) the patient drank the glucose solution. Laboratory personnel will collect the blood samples at specified times.

Have the patient minimize his activities during the test. Increased activities could affect the glucose results.

Decreased level (<70 mg/dl)

Observe for signs and symptoms of hypoglycemia, especially when hyperinsulinism is suspected. Symptoms include nervousness; irritability; confusion; weakness; pale, cold, clammy skin; diaphoresis (excessive perspiration); and tachycardia.

Obtain a history from the patient as to when hypoglycemic symptoms occur (e.g., before meals). There may be periods of nervousness, "shakiness," and weakness.

Explain that eating candy to correct nervousness and weakness should be avoided since it will temporarily correct the problem (the need for glucose) but will stimulate insulin secretion.

Elevated level (>110 mg/dl)

Recognize clinical problems and drugs which can cause a positive GTT result (see *Clinical Problems* above).

Identify factors affecting glucose results—i.e., emotional stress, infection, vomiting, fever, exercise, inactivity, age, drugs, and body weight. Most of these should be reported to the physician.

Check previous fasting blood sugar results before the test. A known diabetic normally does not, and in some cases should not, have this test performed since diabetic coma may ensue.

GLUCOSE-6-PHOSPHATE DEHYDROGENASE (G6PD or G-6-PD) (Blood)

NORMAL RANGE

Adult: varies with methods used—4.3–11.8 IU/g Hb, 125–281 U/dl packed red blood cells (RBC), 251–511 U/10^6 cells, 1211–2111 mIU/ml packed RBC.
Child: similar to adult.

DESCRIPTION

Glucose-6-phosphate dehydrogenase (G6PD) is an enzyme in the red blood cells (RBC or erythrocytes). It normally assists in glucose utilization in the RBC, utilizes oxidative substances, and protects the integrity of the erythrocytes from injury.

A G6PD deficit is a sex-linked genetic defect carried by the female (X) chromosome which will, in conjunction with infection, disease, and drugs, make a person susceptible to developing hemolytic anemia. With a moderate deficiency of G6PD enzyme, there is no apparent detectable RBC abnormality except for a decrease in the life span of the RBC. Metabolites from certain drugs possessing an oxidizing action in the red blood cells will cause an increased need for G6PD for glucose metabolism. A lack of this enzyme results in hemolysis (destruction of the red blood cells) and hemolytic anemia when augmented by an oxidative drug.[4,8,9,11,27,31]

CLINICAL PROBLEMS

Decreased level (↓ value): hemolytic anemia, diabetes acidosis, infections (bacterial and viral), septicemia. *Drug influence:* acetanilid (acetylaniline), aspirin, nitrofurantoin (Furadantin), phenacetin, primaquine, thiazide diuretics, probenecid (Benemid), quinidine, quinine, chloramphenicol (Chloromycetin), sulfonamides, vitamin K, tolbutamide (Orinase). *Food:* fava beans.

PROCEDURE

The laboratory methods used will vary. Screening tests for G6PD deficiency are methemoglobin reduction (Brewer's test), glutathione stability, dye reduction, and ascorbate and fluorescent spot tests. Check with the laboratory on whether capillary or venous blood is needed.

Collect a small amount of capillary blood in a heparinized microhematocrit tube *or* collect 5 ml of venous blood in a lavender- or green-top tube. Check with the laboratory.

There is no food or drink restriction.

FACTORS AFFECTING LABORATORY RESULTS

Drugs (see *Drug Influence*).

NURSING IMPLICATIONS WITH RATIONALE

Decreased level

Explain to the patient the purpose of the test. Explanation could be brief, such as, "to determine if there is a certain enzyme deficiency in the red blood cells."

List the drugs (see *Drug Influence* above) that the patient is taking on the lab slip.

Obtain a familial history of red blood cell enzyme deficiency. Blacks are more prone to G6PD deficiency than whites; however, the degree of anemia is not as severe in blacks as it is in whites.

Observe for symptoms of hemolysis, such as jaundice of the eyes and skin.

Check for decreased urinary output. Urine should be voided at a rate of at least 25 ml/hour or 600 ml/day. Prolonged hemolysis (destruction of red blood cells) can be toxic to the kidney cells, causing kidney impairment.

Check the hemology results.

Determine how long the patient has been taking oxidative drugs (see *Drug Influence* above). Report your findings to the physician and record them on the patient's chart. Hemolysis usually occurs 3 days after the susceptible person has taken an oxidative drug. Hemolytic symptoms will disappear 2 to 3 days after the drug has been stopped.

Teach the susceptible person to read labels on patent medicines and not to take drugs which contain phenacetin and aspirin. Most of these drugs, if taken continuously, can cause hemolytic anemia.

H

HAPTOGLOBIN (Serum)

NORMAL RANGE
Adult: Varies widely—30–160 mg/dl; also 60–270 mg/dl; 0.6–2.7 g/L—(SI units).
Newborn: 0–10 mg/dl (absent in 90 percent).
Infant (1–6 months): 0–30 mg/dl, then gradual increase.

DESCRIPTION
Haptoglobins are alpha$_2$-globulins normally in the plasma. These globulin molecules combine with free (released) hemoglobin during red blood cell destruction (hemolysis). A decreased level of serum haptoglobin indicates hemolysis. Haptoglobins are decreased in severe liver disease, hemolytic anemia, and infectious mononucleosis and are elevated in inflammatory diseases, steroid therapy, acute infections, and malignancies. A hemolytic process may be masked in persons taking steroids.[11,14,27,31,34,36]

CLINICAL PROBLEMS
Decreased level *(<30 mg/dl):* hemolysis; anemias—pernicious, vitamin B$_6$ deficiency, hemolytic, sickle cell; severe liver disease—hepatic failure; chronic hepatitis; thrombotic thrombocytopenic purpura; disseminated intravascular coagulopathy; malaria.
Elevated level *(>160 mg/dl):* inflammation; acute infections; cancer—lung, large intestine, stomach, breast, liver; Hodgkin's disease; ulcerative colitus; chronic pyelonephritis (active stage); rheumatic fever; acute myocardial infarction. *Drug influence:* steroids (cortisone).

PROCEDURE
Collect 5 to 10 ml of venous blood in a red-top tube.
There are no food or drink restrictions.
Haptoglobin levels can be measured by electrophoresis, radioimmunodiffusion, or spectrophotometry.

FACTORS AFFECTING LABORATORY RESULTS
Steroids and inflammation may cause false results. Hemolysis could occur, but the serum haptoglobin level may not indicate this.

NURSING IMPLICATIONS WITH RATIONALE

Explain to the patient that the purpose of the test is to determine whether there is a clinical problem related to red blood cell destruction, or give a similar response. The test may be requested in a patient with a suspected transfusion reaction.
Explain that there is no food or drink restriction.

Decreased level (<30 mg/dl)
Associate a decreased serum haptoglobin level with conditions causing hemolysis—i.e., hemolytic anemias, severe liver disease, and others (see *Clinical Problems* above).
Assess the patient's vital signs. Report abnormal vital signs, especially if the patient is having breathing problems. The oxygen capacity of hemoglobin may be reduced, causing a change in breathing pattern.
Assess the patient's urinary output. Excessive amounts of free hemoglobin may cause renal damage.

Elevated level (<160 mg/dl)

Associate an elevated serum haptoglobin level with clinical problems—i.e., infections, inflammation, cancer, steroid therapy, and others (see *Clinical Problems* above).

Check the serum haptoglobin level. The haptoglobin level may be masked by steroid therapy and inflammation. If hemolysis is suspected, the serum level may be normal instead of low due to steroids or inflammation. Notify the physician of the findings.

HEMATOCRIT (HCT) (Blood)

NORMAL RANGE

Adult: *Male:* 40–54 percent, 0.40–0.54 (SI units). *Female:* 36–46 percent, 0.36–0.46 (SI units).

Child: *Newborn:* 42–54 percent. *1 to 3 Years Old:* 29–40 percent. *4 to 10 Years Old:* 36–38 percent.

DESCRIPTION

The hematocrit (Hct) is the volume (in ml) of packed red blood cells found in 100 ml (1 dl) of blood, expressed as a percentage. For example, a 36 percent hematocrit would indicate that 36 ml of red blood cells were found in 100 ml of blood, or 36 vol/dl. The purpose of the test is to measure the concentration of red blood cells (erythrocytes) in the blood.

Low hematocrit levels are found most frequently in anemias and leukemias, and elevated levels are found in dehydration (a relative increase) and polycythemia vera. The hematocrit can be an indicator of the hydration status of the patient. As with hemoglobin, an elevated hematocrit level could indicated hemoconcentration due to a decrease in fluid volume and an increase in red blood cells.[8,9,11,27,30,31,36]

CLINICAL PROBLEMS

Decreased level *(↓ 40 percent [male], ↓ 36 percent [female]):* acute blood loss; anemias— aplastic, hemolytic, folic acid deficiency, pernicious, sideroblastic, sickel cell; leukemias—lymphocytic, myelocytic, monocytic; Hodgkin's disease; lymphosarcoma; malignancy of organs; multiple myeloma; cirrhosis of the liver; protein malnutrition; vitamin deficiencies—thiamine, vitamin C; fistula of the stomach or duodenum; peptic ulcer; chronic renal failure; pregnancy; systemic lupus erythematosus; rheumatoid arthritis (especially juvenile). *Drug influence:* antineoplastic agents; antibiotics— chloramphenicol, penicillin; radioactive agents.

Elevated level *(↑ 54 percent [male], ↑ 46 percent [female]):* dehydration/hypovolemia, severe diarrhea, polycythemia vera, erythrocytosis, diabetic acidosis, pulmonary emphysema (later stage), transient cerebral ischemia (TIA), eclampsia.

PROCEDURE

Obtain venous or capillary blood by one of the following methods.

1. Collect 7 ml of venous blood in a lavender-top tube. Mix well. An anticoagulant is used in the tube, and the tube should be filled to the top.
2. Collect capillary blood using the microhematocrit method. Blood is obtained from a finger prick, using a capillary tube approximately 7 cm long and 1 mm in diameter with a small suction rubber ball at the end of the tube. The capillary is centrifuged for 4 to 5 minutes, and the hematocrit percentage is read by means of a calibrated reading device.

There is no food or drink restriction.

FACTORS AFFECTING LABORATORY RESULTS

If blood is collected from an extremity which has an intravenous line, the hematocrit will most likely be low. Avoid using such an extremity.

If blood is taken to check hematocrit levels immediately after moderate to severe blood loss and transfusions, the hematocrit could be normal.

Age of the patient—newborns normally have higher Hct levels due to hemoconcentration.

NURSING IMPLICATIONS WITH RATIONALE

Explain to the patient the purpose of the test, such as, "to determine the percentage of red blood cells in the blood." A more detailed explanation may be needed.

Explain the procedure of the test to the patient. If the microhematocrit method is used, explain that the finger will be cleansed with an alcohol sponge and pricked with a lancet or needle to obtain capillary blood.

Instruct the patient that food and drinks are not restricted.

Decreased level (↓ 40 percent [male], ↓ 36 percent [female])

Relate a decreased hematocrit level to clinical problems and drugs. Blood loss and anemias are the most common causes of a low hematocrit. A hematocrit of 30 percent or less with no known bleeding frequently indicates a moderate to severe anemic condition.

Assess for signs and symptoms of anemia—i.e., fatigue, paleness, and tachycardia.

Assess changes in vital signs to determine whether shock is present due to blood loss. Symtoms could include rapid pulse, rapid respirations, and normal or decreased blood pressure.

Suggest to the physician a possible need to reorder the hematocrit test after several days of moderate to severe bleeding or transfusions. A hematocrit taken immediately after blood loss and after transfusions may appear normal.

Elevated level (↑ 54 percent [male], ↑ 46 percent [female])

Relate an elevated hematocrit level to clinical problems. Dehydration and hypovolemia are common problems with hematocrit elevation due to hemoconcentration.

Assess for signs and symptoms of dehydration/hypovolemia. A history of vomiting, diarrhea, marked thirst, lack of skin turgor, and shock-like symptoms (rapid pulse and respiration rates) could be indicative of a body fluid deficit.

Administer intravenous or oral fluids according to the physician's order to reestablish body fluid volume.

Avoid rapid administration of intravenous fluids to the older adult, child, or debilitated person so as to prevent overhydration and pulmonary edema. Signs and symptoms of overhydration are constant, irritated cough; dyspnea; hand and/or neck vein engorgement; and chest rales.

Check the hematocrit daily, if ordered, when reestablishing body fluid volume. When an elevated hematocrit returns to normal, the elevation was due to hemoconcentration.

Assess changes in urinary output. A urine output of less than 25 ml/hour or 600 ml daily could be due to dehydration/hypovolemia. Once body fluids are restored, urine output should be normal.

HEMOGLOBIN (Hb or Hgb) (Blood)
Hb A$_1$, A$_2$, F (fetal hemoglobin)

NORMAL RANGE
   Adult: *Women:* 12–16 g/dl. *Men:* 13.5–18 g/dl.
   Newborn: 14–24 g/dl.
   Infant: 10–15 g/dl.
   Child: 11–16 g/dl.

DESCRIPTION
   Hemoglobin, a protein substance found in red blood cells, gives blood its red color. Hemoglobin is composed of iron, which is an oxygen carrier. Abnormally high hemoglobin levels may be due to hemoconcentration resulting from dehydration (fluid loss). Low hemoglobin values are related to various clinical problems.
   The red blood cell (RBC) count and hemoglobin (Hb or Hgb) do not always increase or decrease in value equally. For instance, a decreased RBC count and a normal or slightly decreased Hb occur in pernicious anemia, and a normal or slightly decreased RBC and a decreased Hb occur in iron deficiency (microcytic) anemia.[4,8,11,27,30,36]

CLINICAL PROBLEMS
   Decreased level (↓ *12 g/dl):* anemias—iron deficiency, aplastic, hemocytic; severe hemorrhage; cirrhosis of the liver; leukemias; Hodgkin's disease; sarcoidosis; excess intravenous fluids; cancer—large and small intestine, rectum, liver, bone; thalassemia major; pregnancy; kidney diseases. *Drug influence:* antibiotics—chloramphenicol (Chloromycetin), penicillin, tetracycline; aspirin; antineoplastic drugs; doxampram (Dopram); hydantoin derivatives; hydralazine (Apresoline); indomethacin (Indocin); MAO inhibitors; primaquine; rifampin; sulfonamides; trimethadione (Tridione); vitamin A (large doses).
   Elevated level (↑ *18 g/dl):* dehydration/hemocentration, polycythemia, high altitudes, chronic obstructive lung disease (COLD), congestive heart failure, severe burns. *Drug influence:* gentamicin, methyldopa (Aldomet).

PROCEDURE
   Venous blood: Collect 7 ml of venous blood in a lavender-top tube. The tube should be filled to its capacity.
   Capillary blood: Puncture the cleansed earlobe, finger, or heel with a sterile lancet. Do not squeeze the puncture site tightly, for serous fluid and blood would thus be obtained. Wipe away the first drop of blood. Collect drops of blood quickly in micropipettes with small rubber tops or microhematocrit tubes. Expel blood into the tubes with diluents.
   There is no food or drink restriction.
   Do not take the blood sample from a hand or arm receiving intravenous fluid. The tourniquet should be on less than a minute.

FACTORS AFFECTING LABORATORY RESULTS
   Drugs (see *Drug Influence* above).
   Taking blood from an arm or hand receiving IV fluids.
   Leaving the tourniquet on for more than a minute. Hemoglobin results could be falsely elevated due to hemostasis.
   Living in high altitudes will increase Hb levels.
   Decreased fluid intake or fluid loss will increase Hb levels due to hemoconcentration, and excessive fluid intake will decrease Hb levels due to hemodilution.

NURSING IMPLICATIONS WITH RATIONALE

Explain to the patient the purpose of the test. Explanation could be brief, such as, "to determine the amount of hemoglobin in the blood."

Explain to the patient the procedure of the test.

Inform the patient that food and drink are not restricted.

Decreased level (↓ 12 g/dl)

Recognize clinical problems and drugs that could cause a decreased hemoglobin level (see *Clinical Problems* above). Anemia is a common cause, but usually the patient is not considered anemic until his hemoglobin is below 10.5 g/dl. Hemorrhage could cause a low hemoglobin level if the blood is not replaced; however, the hemoglobin level does not decrease immediately. It may remain normal for hours or even several days.

Observe the patient for signs and symptoms of anemia—i.e., dizziness, tachycardia, weakness, dyspnea at rest. Symptoms depend on how low the hemoglobin level is (severe anemia).

Check the hematocrit level if the hemoglobin level is low.

Elevated level (↑ 18 g/dl)

Recognize clinical problems and drugs that can cause an increased hemoglobin level (see *Clinical Problems* above). Dehydration is a major transient cause of an elevated level. Once the patient is hydrated, the hemoglobin should return to the normal range.

Observe for signs and symptoms of dehydration—i.e., marked thirst, poor skin turgor, dry mucous membranes, and shock-like symptoms (tachycardia, tachypnea, and, later, decreased blood pressure).

Teach the patient to maintain an adequate fluid intake. Frequently, older adults tend to drink less fluid.

HEMOGLOBIN ELECTROPHORESIS (Blood)

Hemoglobins A_1, A_2, F, C, S

NORMAL RANGE

Adult: *Hemoglobin (Hb or Hgb) electrophoresis:* A_1, 95–98 percent total Hb; A_2, 1.5–3.5 percent; F, <2 percent; C, 0 percent; D, 0 percent; S, 0 percent.

Newborn: *Hemoglobin:* F, 40–70 percent total Hb.

Infant: *Hemoglobin:* F, 2–10 percent total Hb.

Child: *Hemoglobin:* F, 1–2 percent total Hb after 6 months.

DESCRIPTION

The normal types of hemoglobin are Hb A_1, comprising 95 to 98 percent of the total hemoglobin; Hb A_2; and Hb F (fetal). If Hb F comprises 5 percent or more of the total hemoglobin after the age of 6 months, thalassemia (Mediterranean anemia) could be a factor. There are three clinical types of thalassemia: thalassemia major (Hb F is over 50 percent), thalassemia minor (increased Hb A_2 value), and thalassemia gene (combination of abnormal hemoglobins).

To identify normal hemoglobin types (A_1, A_2, and F) and abnormal hemoglobin types (Hb C, Hb M, Hb S, and others), a hemoglobin electrophoresis is usually ordered. It is not a routine test, but it is useful for identifying 150 or more types of hemoglobin. Many abnormal hemoglobin types do not produce harmful diseases, and so usually the types causing common hemoglobinopathies are identified through electrophoresis.

Hemogloblin S: Hb S is the most common hemoglobin variant. If both genes have Hb S, sickle cell anemia will occur, but if only one gene has Hb S, then the person simply carries the sickle trait. Approximately 1 percent of the black population in the United States has sickle cell anemia, and 8 to 10 percent carry the sickle cell trait.

Sickle cell anemia symptoms are usually not present until after the age of 6 months. In some cases, Hb S is combined with another abnormal hemoglobin type, Hb C or Hb D. Hb S/C or Hb S/D produces red blood cells (erythrocytes) that sickle as with Hb S/S. Those with sickle cell anemia have low oxygen tension (also see Sickle Cell Test).

Hemoglobin C: Hb C in the homozygous state (C/C) usually produces mild hemolytic anemia; in the heterozygous state (A/C), it produces the Hb C trait. This occurs more frequently in blacks.[4,8,9,11,27,30,36]

CLINICAL PROBLEMS

Hemoglobin Type	Elevated Level
Hemoglobin F	Thalassemia (after 6 months)
Hemoglobin C	Hemolytic anemia
Hemoglobin S	Sickle cell anemia

PROCEDURE

Collect 7 to 10 ml of venous blood in a lavender-top tube. Fill the tube to its capacity. There is no food or drink restriction.

FACTORS AFFECTING LABORATORY RESULTS

Blood transfusions given 4 months before hemoglobin electrophoresis may cause inaccurate results.

Collection of the blood sample in the wrong color-top tube.

NURSING IMPLICATIONS WITH RATIONALE

Explain to the patient that the purpose of the test is to identify any abnormal hemoglobin types.

Explain to the patient that food and drink are not restricted.

Observe for signs and symptoms of sickle cell anemia. Early symptoms are fatigue and weakness. Chronic symptoms are fatigue, dyspnea on exertion, swollen joints, bones that ache, and chest pains. Afflicted persons are susceptible to infection. Sickle cell crisis is usually due to small infarcts to various organs. The crisis usually lasts 5 to 7 days and immediate care is needed for the symptoms. Normally, the hemoglobin level does not change.

Encourage the patient to seek genetic counseling if he or she has sickle cell anemia or is a carrier of the sickle cell trait.

Instruct the patient with sickle cell anemia to minimize strenuous activity and to avoid high altitudes and extreme cold. Encourage the patient to take rest periods.

Encourage the patient to stay away from persons with infections.

Suggest that the patient carry a medical alert bracelet and/or card.

HEPATITIS B SURFACE ANTIGEN (HBsAg) (Serum)
Hepatitis-associated Antigen (HAA)

NORMAL RANGE
   Adult: negative.
   Child: negative.

DESCRIPTION
   The hepatitis B surface antigen (HBsAg) test was originally called the Australia antigen test and later the hepatitis-associated antigen (HAA) test. This test is done to determine the presence of hepatitis B virus in the blood in either an active or a carrier state (as in a hepatitis B carrier). Approximately 5 percent of persons with diseases other than hepatitis B (serum hepatitis) will have a positive HBsAg test.
   The HBsAg test is routinely performed on the donor's blood to identify the hepatitis B antigen. Transmission of hepatitis B in blood transfusions has greatly diminished through HBsAg screening of the donor's blood and excluding donors with a history of hepatitis. Though transfusion-related hepatitis B has decreased, the occurrence of hepatitis B is still on the increase.
   In hepatitis B, the HBsAg in the serum can be detected 2 to 24 weeks (average, 4 to 8 weeks) after exposure to the virus. The positive HBsAg may be present 2 to 6 weeks after onset of the clinical disease. Approximately 10 percent of the patients with positive HBsAg are carriers and their tests may remain positive for years.

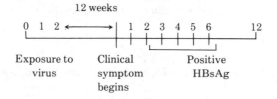

   In 75 to 90 percent of the patients, antibody to hepatitis B surface antigen (called anti-HBsAg or HBsAb) is found 2 to 12 weeks after HBsAg occurs. Anti-HBsAg can be detected for years after the acute viral infection, but it does not guarantee immunity against future hepatitis infection.[8,9,27,30,36]

CLINICAL PROBLEMS
   Elevated level *(positive):* hepatitis B, chronic hepatitis B, hemophilia, Down's syndrome, Hodgkin's disease, leukemia. *Drug influence:* drug addicts.

PROCEDURE
   The most common method for testing HBsAg is by radioimmunoassay (RIA). It is more than 75 percent sensitive in identifying the surface antigen. Immunodiffusion is 30 percent sensitive, and complement-fixation is 50 to 60 percent sensitive.
   Collect 5 ml of venous blood in a red-top tube. Careful handling of the blood sample and washing the hands are most important to keep from contacting the viral hepatitis B. There is no food or drink restriction.

FACTORS AFFECTING LABORATORY RESULTS
   None known.

NURSING IMPLICATIONS WITH RATIONALE

Explain to the patient the purpose of the test. Explanation could be brief, such as, "to determine if you have hepatitis or if you are a carrier of the hepatitis." If the person is a blood donor, the test is automatically done after the unit of blood is taken. Most of these persons do not know that the HBsAg test and other blood tests are done on donor's blood.

Obtain a history of any previous hepatitis infection and report it to the physician.

Elevated level (Positive Test)

Handle blood obtained from the patient with care, avoiding blood contact with your skin (especially if skin and nail cuts are present). This practice is necessary even though the diagnosis of hepatitis has not been confirmed. If you accidentally stick yourself with the used needle, you should, in most cases, receive gamma globulin as a preventive measure to avoid the disease.

Discard all needles and syringes used on patients having hepatitis B. Follow the hospital's isolation procedure. Again, if you accidentally stick yourself with the used needle, report immediately to the physician and nursing management.

Observe for signs and symptoms of hepatitis—i.e., lethargy, anorexia, nausea and vomiting, fever, dark-colored urine, and jaundice.

Instruct the patient to get plenty of rest; a nutritional diet, if tolerated; hard candy, if helpful; and fluids (juice and carbonated drinks).

HETEROPHILE ANTIBODY (Serum, Mono-Spot)

NORMAL RANGE
Adult: normal, <1:28 titer; abnormal, >1:56 titer.
Child: same as adult.

DESCRIPTION
Man develops antibodies called heterophiles that react with the erythrocytes (red blood cells) of animals. The concentration of the antibodies is expressed in terms of serum dilution or titer. Normally, heterophile antibodies are present in the serum at low titer (<1:28) and are known as Forssman antibodies.

A high heterophile antibody titer (>1:56) is indicative of infectious mononucleosis or serum sickness. Infectious mononucleosis is thought to be caused by the Epstein–Barre virus (EBV). To test for infectious mononucleosis, the heterophile antibodies from the patient's serum agglutinate (clump) with sheep's red blood cells. A serum dilution of 1:225 or greater is considered positive for infectious mononucleosis. With a serum dilution of 1:56 to 1:224, it is essential to ascertain if such a moderate titer is actually due to infectious mononucleosis or is due to other antibodies.

For differential diagnosis, the patient's serum antibody is tested for absorption with guinea pig kidney tissue or beef red blood cell antigens; this is followed by an agglutination test with sheep red blood cells. If the antibodies are totally absorbed by guinea pig tissue, the elevated titer is due to Forssman antibody or serum sickness and not to infectious mononucleosis. However, if the antibodies are only partially or are not absorbed by the guinea pig kidney and the remaining serum antibodies still agglutinate sheep's red blood cells, then the test is positive for infectious mononucleosis.

Forssman antibodies occur in the normal serum and are not absorbed by beef red blood cells. If the serum antibodies are completely absorbed by beef red blood cells and the treated serum will not agglutinate sheep's red blood cells, the results are positive for infectious mononucleosis or serum sickness.

Persons with infectious mononucleosis begin developing elevated heterophile antibody titers during the first 2 weeks of illness, but the highest titers are not reached until the third week. Sixty to eighty percent of persons with infectious mononucleosis have a positive heterophile antibody test.

Mono-Spot: Mono-Spot is a commercially available test for infectious mononucleosis, manufactured by Ortho Diagnostics, Raritan, N.Y. These kits are frequently used in the physician's office. Horse's red blood cells are used instead of sheep's red blood cells. When the heterophile is equal to or greater than 1:28, the Mono-Spot will be positive.[8,9,11,20,27,30,31,34]

CLINICAL PROBLEMS

Elevated level *(>1:56 titer):* infectious mononucleosis, serum sickness, viral infections.

PROCEDURE

Heterophile antibody: Collect 5 to 10 ml of venous blood in a red-top tube. There is no food or drink restriction.

Mono-Spot screening test: Collect 2 ml of venous blood in a red-top tube. Use a mono-kit and follow directions. The patient's serum is mixed with the guinea pig tissue on one spot of a glass slide, and at another spot on the slide, it is mixed with beef red cell stromata. Unwashed horse red cells are added to both spots. Observe for 1 minute for agglutination. Results of the Mono-Spot test are as follows.

1. If agglutination is stronger at the guinea pig kidney tissue spot, the test is positive for infectious mononucleosis.
2. If agglutination is stronger at the beef red cells, the test is negative for infectious mononucleosis.
3. If agglutination is present at both spots, the test is negative for infectious mononucleosis.
4. If no agglutination is present at either spot, the test is negative.

There is no food or drink restriction. Usually, in infectious mono, the white blood cell differential may have 10 to 25 percent atypical lymphocytes.

FACTORS AFFECTING LABORATORY RESULTS

Serum sickness and Forssman antibodies can cause positive titers.

NURSING IMPLICATIONS WITH RATIONALE

Explain to the patient that the purpose for the test is to determine whether infectious mononucleosis is present.

Explain to the patient the procedure for the heterophile antibody test and the Mono-Spot test.

Instruct the patient that there is no food or drink restriction.

Obtain a history of the patient's contact with any person or persons recently diagnosed as having infectious mononucleosis.

Observe for signs and symptoms of infectious mononucleosis—i.e., fever, sore throat, fatigue, swollen glands.

Determine when the symptoms (fever, fatigue, sore throat) first occurred. A repeat heterophile antibody or Mono-Spot test may be needed if the first was done too early. Elevated titers take 4 to 8 weeks to return to normal.

Encourage the patient to rest, drink fluids, and follow the physician's orders.

HUMAN CHORIONIC GONADOTROPIN (HCG) (Urine and Serum—Pregnancy Test)

NORMAL RANGE

Adult: *Urine:* single specimen (anti-HCG reagent kit). Negative: no HCG; no neutralization of antiserum; agglutination present. Positive: HCG; neutralization of antiserum; no agglutination. *Serum:* RIA test.
Child: not usually done.

DESCRIPTION

Human chorionic gonadotropin (HCG) is a hormone produced by the placenta. In pregnancy, HCG appears in the blood and urine 14 to 26 days after conception, and the HCG concentration peaks in approximately 8 weeks. After the first trimester of pregnancy, HCG production declines. HCG is not found in nonpregnant women, in death of the fetus, or after 3 to 4 days postpartum.

The immunologic test for pregnancy using anti-HCG serum is more sensitive, more accurate, less costly, and easier to perform than the older pregnancy test which used live animals. The Aschheim–Zondek test and the Friedman test are no longer used.

Certain tumors (such as the hydatidiform mole, chorionepithelioma of the uterus, and choriocarcinoma of the testicle) can cause a positive HCG test. HCG may be requested on males for the determination of testicular tumor.[8,9,11,20,30,36]

CLINICAL PROBLEMS

Decreased level *(negative):* nonpregnant, dead fetus, postpartum (3 to 4 days), incomplete abortion, threatened abortion (decreased IV serum value).
Elevated level *(positive):* pregnancy, hydatidiform mole, chorionepithelioma, choriocarcinoma. *Drug influence:* anticonvulsants, hypnotics, tranquilizers (phenothiazines), antiparkinsonism drugs.

PROCEDURE

Perform the pregnancy test 2 weeks (no earlier than 10 days) after the first missed menstrual period. There are several commercially prepared kits for the immunologic pregnancy test.

For the serum test, collect 5 ml of venous blood. Prevent hemolysis of the blood sample.

For the urine test, have the patient avoid fluid intake the evening before. Collect at least 60 ml of urine in the early A.M. and take the urine specimen immediately to the laboratory. The specific gravity (SG) of the urine should be greater than 1.014. A 24 hour urine collection may be requested—a preservative should be added to the bottle.

Slide agglutination and test tube agglutination tests are the methods most frequently used. The slide test has two stages. Stage I: mix a drop of urine and a drop of anti-HCG serum (reagent) on a slide. Wait 30 seconds. Stage II: add two drops of the prepared latex particles coated with HCG and mix. Wait 2 minutes. No agglutination within 2 minutes is a positive result, and agglutination within 2 minutes is a negative result. Follow the directions on the kit for the test tube agglutination test.

Note: there are at least three commercial kits, each of which may require some modification of procedure.

There is no food restriction.

FACTORS AFFECTING LABORATORY RESULTS

Diluted urine (specific gravity <1.010) could cause a false negative test result.
Certain drug groups can cause false positive test results (see *Drug Influence* above).
Protein and blood in the urine could cause false positive test results.
During menopause, there may be an excess secretion of pituitary gonadotropin hormone, which could cause a false positive result.

NURSING IMPLICATIONS WITH RATIONALE

Explain to the patient that the purpose of the test is to determine whether she is pregnant.

Inform the patient that she will receive the results of the test in 2 to 3 minutes or in 2 hours. (The frog, rabbit, and mice tests are usually not done, since the results are more costly and not as accurate as the new tests.)

Instruct the patient not to drink any fluids after the evening meal. Some laboratories state that fluid should not be taken after midnight. Normally, urine is concentrated in the morning; however, the specific gravity of urine should be greater than 1.014 for the test to be accurate.

Report to the physician and record on the laboratory slip any drugs the patient is taking that could cause a false positive result (see *Drug Influence* above).

Ask the patient when she had her last period. The test should be done 10 days or more after the missed period. A false negative result may occur if the test is done too early.

Collect the urine specimen (no less than 2 ounces) in the morning and take it immediately to the laboratory. If the test is performed in the physician's office, the nurse should test the urine immediately.

17-HYDROXYCORTICOSTEROIDS (17-OHCS) (Urine)
Corticoids 17-OH, Porter–Silber Chromogens

NORMAL RANGE
Adult: *Women:* 3–13 mg/24 hours. *Men:* 5–15 mg/24 hours.
Child: Lower than adult ranges. Differs with age.

DESCRIPTION
17-Hydroxycorticosteroids (17-OHCS) are groups of compounds from adrenocortical steroid hormones, cortisone, and hydrocortisone, which are excreted in the urine. The 17-OHCS test is the test most commonly used, besides the plasma cortisol test, for assessing adrenal cortical (cortex) function.

An increased urinary concentration of 17-OHCS beyond the normal range may indicate hyperadrenalism, and a decreased urinary concentration may indicate hypoadrenalism. Excretion levels vary among children, men, and women in relation to muscle mass and body weight.[4,8,11,27,30]

CLINICAL PROBLEMS
Decreased level *(↓ 5 mg/24 hours [men]):* Addison's disease, androgenital syndrome, hypopituitarism, myxedema (hypothyroidism). *Drug influence:* calcium gluconate, dexamethasone (Decadron), diphenylhydantoin (Dilantin), promethazine (Phenergan), reserpine (Serpasil).

Elevated level *(↑ 15 mg/24 hours [men]):* Cushing's syndrome, extreme stress, adrenal cancer, eclampsia, hyperpituitarism, hyperthyroidism. *Drug influence:* antibiotics— cloxacillin, erythromycin; acetazolamide (Diamox); ascorbic acid; chloral hydrate; chlordiazepoxide (Librium); chlorothiazide (Diuril); chlorpromazine (Thorazine); colchicine; cortisone; digoxin; digitoxin; estrogen; hydroxyzine (Atarax); iodides; oleandomycin (Matromycin); oral contraceptives; meprobamate (Equanil or Miltown); methenamine (Uritone); paraldehyde; quinine; quinidine; spironolactone (Aldactone).

PROCEDURE

Collect urine in a large container/bottle for 24 hours.

Keep the urine container/bottle refrigerated during the 24 hours. If the urine cannot be refrigerated, a preservative (boric acid 1 g or 10 ml of HC1) should be added to the bottle before urine collection is started. The preservative will prevent bacterial degradation of the steroids.

Withhold drugs for 3 days before the test to prevent a false positive or negative result. if this is not possible, any drugs given (see *Drug Influence* above) should be written on the lab slip and recorded in the patient's chart.

There is no food or drink restriction, except for coffee. Fluid intake should be encouraged.

FACTORS AFFECTING LABORATORY RESULTS

Drugs (see *Drug Influence* above). Cortisone can elevate the urinary levels of 17-OHCS, and dexamethasone (Decadron), a potent cortisone derivative, can decrease the 17-OHCS level. The potent cortisone drug inhibits ACTH production, which causes a decrease in adrenocortical hormone secretion.

If the 24 hour urine sample is not refrigerated or does not contain a preservative, the results of the test could be inaccurate.

NURSING IMPLICATIONS WITH RATIONALE

Explain to the patient that the purpose of the test is to determine whether there is any problem with the functioning of the adrenal gland.

Encourage the patient to drink 6 to 8 glasses of water or other fluid (except coffee) during the 24 hour test.

Explain to the patient that food is not restricted before or during the test.

Check the drugs the patient is receiving and withhold drugs (with the physician's permission) that may interfere with test results. Many times, medication cannot be withheld; in such cases, the drugs given should be listed on the lab slip and reported.

Explain to the patient and family that all urine should be saved during a 24 hour period.

Label the urine bottle with the patient's name and the date and exact time for the urine collection—e.g., 11/3, 1983, 7:20 A.M. to 11/4, 1983, 7:22 A.M.

Instruct the patient not to put toilet paper or feces in the urine.

Post a notice of urine collection on the patient's door or bed and in the Kardex.

Check the results of the plasma cortisol and 17-KS tests.

Decreased level (↓ 5 mg/24 hours [men])

Recognize clinical problems related to a decrease in 17-OHCS.

Observe for signs and symptoms of hypoadrenalism (Addison's disease). These symptoms include fatigue, weakness, weight loss, bronze coloration of the skin, postural hypotension, arrhythmia, craving of salty food, and fasting hypoglycemia. Report your findings to the physician.

Elevated level (↑ 15 mg/24 hours [men])

Recognize clinical problems related to an elevated 17-OHCS test result.

Observe for signs and symptoms of hyperadrenalism (Cushing's syndrome). These symptoms include fluid retention, "moon face," hirsutism, "buffalo hump," hypertension, hyperglycemia, petechiae, and ecchymosis. Report your findings to the physician.

5-HYDROXYINDOLACETIC ACID (5-HIAA) (Urine)
5-OH-Indoleacetic Acid, Serotonin Metabolite

NORMAL RANGE
Adult: *Qualitative random samples:* negative. *Quantitative 24 hours:* 2–10 mg/24 hours.
Child: not usually done—results would be similar to adult results.

DESCRIPTION
5-Hydroxyindolacetic acid (5-HIAA), a byproduct of serotonin, is excreted in the urine as the result of carcinoid tumors found in the appendix or in the intestinal wall. Serotonin is a vasoconstricting hormone secreted by the argentaffin cells of the gastrointestinal tract and is responsible for peristalsis. Carcinoid tumor cells, which secrete excess serotonin, are of low grade malignancy. Early removal of this type of tumor ensures an 80 to 90 percent chance of cure. There have been reports of some non-carcinoid tumors producing high levels of 5-HIAA.

Certain foods may elevate the 5-HIAA urinary levels, and certain drugs may elevate or decrease the 5-HIAA urinary levels. More than one random sample of urine for the 5-HIAA test may be needed if the patient has eaten certain foods or taken drugs which could cause false positive or false negative results. The 24 hour urine test usually follows the random urine screening test.[2,8,11,27,30,34]

CLINICAL PROBLEMS
Decreased level *(↓ 2 mg/24 hours): Drug influence (depresses 5-HIAA):* ACTH; heparin; imipramine (Tofranil); isoniazid (INH); MAO inhibitors; methyldopa (Aldomet); phenothiazines—chlorpromazine (Thorazine) and others; promethazine (Phenergan).
Elevated level *(↑ 10 mg/24 hours):* carcinoid tumors of the appendix and intestine, carcinoid tumor with metastasis (>100 mg/24 hours), sciatica pain (severe), skeletal and smooth muscle spasm. *Drug influence:* acetylaniline (Acetanilid), acetophenetidin (Phenacetin), glyceryl guaiacolate, mephenesin (Tolserol), methamphetamine (Methedrine), reserpine (Serpasil). *Foods:* banana, pineapple, avocados, plums, eggplant, walnuts.

PROCEDURE
Eliminate the foods and drugs listed above for 3 days before the test, if possible.
Qualitative random urine sample (for screening purposes): Collect a random urine sample and take it to the laboratory. If the urine sample is not tested immediately, it should be refrigerated. Collection of a random urine sample may need to be repeated to verify the results. The random urine screening test is usually done first, and if the test is positive, a 24 hour urine test for 5-HIAA is ordered.
Quantitative 24 hour urine collection: Collect urine for 24 hours in a large bottle with a preservative (12 g boric acid or 25 ml 6N HC1). Some laboratories require no preserva-preservative, but the urine should be refrigerated during the 24 hour collection time. Label the bottle and laboratory slip with the patient's name and the date and exact times of the urine collection (e.g., 6/24/84, 7:00 A.M. to 6/25/84, 7:00 A.M.).
Foods (except for those listed) and drinks are not restricted.

FACTORS AFFECTING LABORATORY RESULTS
Foods (see *Foods* above).
Drugs (see *Drug Influence* above).
A 24 hour urine sample which does not have a preservative and/or has not been refrigerated (check with the laboratory about the urine preservative and refrigeration).

NURSING IMPLICATIONS WITH RATIONALE

Explain to the patient the purpose of the test. Explanation may be brief, such as, "to determine if there is a substance (a hormone product) excreted in the urine." A more detailed explanation may be needed.

Instruct the patient not to eat bananas, pineapple, avocados, plums, eggplant, or walnuts for 3 days before the test. Foods and drinks other than those mentioned are permitted before and during the test.

Instruct the patient and family not to throw away any urine during the 24 hour collection time.

Inform the patient not to discard toilet paper or feces in the urine. The patient should urinate before having a bowel movement.

Inform the physician of any drugs the patient is taking which could cause a false positive or false negative result. These drugs should not be taken for 3 days before the test, if possible, and if they are, the names of the drugs should be listed on the laboratory slip and recorded in the patient's chart.

Check the 5-HIAA result of the random sample urine test and inform the physician if the result is unknown to him. A repeated test may be needed if the patient has taken drugs which can depress the 5-HIAA of if the test is negative. If the urine test is positive, the physician may order the 5-HIAA 24 hour urine test.

I

IMMUNOGLOBULINS (Ig) (Serum)
IgG, IgA, IgM, IgD, IgE

NORMAL RANGE

	Total Ig (99%; mg/dl)	IgG (80%; mg/dl)	IgA (15%; mg/dl)	IgM (4%; mg/dl)	IgD (0.002%; mg/dl)
Adult	900–2200	800–1800	100–400	55–150	0.5–3
12–16 yr	800–1300	700–1050	70–225	35–75	
7–11 yr	700–1700	600–1450	50–200	30–120	
4–6 yr	700–1700	550–1500	50–175	22–100	
1–3 yr	400–1500	300–1400	20–150	20–100	
6 months	225–1200	200–1100	10–90	10–80	
3 months	325–750	275–750	5–55	15–70	
Newborn	650–1450	640–1250	0–12	5–30	

DESCRIPTION

Immunoglobulins (Ig) are classes (groups) of proteins referred to as antibodies; they can be divided into five groups found in gamma globulin. Ig is produced by the action of B lymphocytes and plasma cells and, as is characteristic of all antibody actions, Ig responds to invading foreign antigens. As individuals are exposed to antigens, antibody (Ig) production occurs, and with further exposure to the same antigen, immunity results.

The five classes of immunoglobulins—IgG, IgA, IgM, IgD, and IgE—are separated by the process of immunoelectrophoresis. Of these five classes, IgG, IgA, and IgM are the important ones, since they make up most of the total gamma globulin. IgD and IgE are found only in small amounts in gamma globulin.

The immunologic functions of the immunoglobulins as follows.

IgG: IgG is the major immunoglobulin. IgG results from secondary exposure to the foreign antigen and is responsible for antiviral and antibacterial activity. This antibody passes through the placental barrier and provides early immunity for the newborn. The IgG response is longer and stronger than that of the other immunoglobulins.

IgA: This immunoglobulin is found mainly in the secretions of the respiratory, gastrointestinal, and genitourinary tracts, as well as in tears and saliva. Its purpose is to protect mucous membranes from invading organisms (viruses, certain bacteria—*E. coli* and *Clostridium tetani*). It does not pass the placental barrier and so the infant's serum value is very low.

IgM: IgM antibodies are produced 48 to 72 hours after an antigen enters the body and are responsible for primary immunity. This immunoglobulin produces antibody activity against rheumatoid factors, gram-negative organisms, and the ABO blood group. IgM activates the complement system by destroying antigenic substances. Since it does not pass the placental barrier, the serum value is low in newborns; however, it is produced early in life and the level increases after 9 months of age.

IgD: Unknown.

IgE: This immunoglobulin is present in serum and interstitial fluid and is increased during allergic reactions and anaphylaxis.[4,8,9,11,15,20,21]

CLINICAL PROBLEMS

Ig	Decreased level	Elevated level
IgG	Lymphocytic leukemia	Infections—all types
	Agammaglobulinemia	Severe malnutrition
	Pre-eclampsia	Chronic granulomatous infection
	Amyloidosis	Hyperimmunization
		Liver disease
		Rheumatic fever
		Sarcoidosis
IgA	Lymphocytic leukemia	Antoimmune disorders
	Agammaglobulinemia	Rheumatic fever
	Malignancies	Chronic infections
		Liver disease
IgM	Lymphocytic leukemia	Lymphosarcoma
	Agammaglobulinemia	Brucellosis
	Amyloidosis	Trypanosomiasis
		Relapsing fever
		Infectious mononucleosis
		Malaria
		Rubella virus in newborns
IgE		Allergic reactions (asthma)
		Skin sensitivity
		Drug influence
		Tetanus toxoid
		Tetanus antitoxin
		Gamma globulin

PROCEDURE

Collect 5 to 10 ml of venous blood in a red-top tube.

Record on the lab slip whether the patient has received any vaccination or immunization including toxoid within the last 6 months.

Record on the lab slip whether the patient has received blood transfusion, gamma globulin, or tetanus antitoxin injections in the last 6 weeks.

There is no food and drug restriction.

FACTORS AFFECTING LABORATORY RESULTS

Immunization and toxoids received in the foregoing 6 months can affect Ig results.

Blood transfusions, tetanus antitoxin, and gamma globulin received in the foregoing 6 weeks can affect Ig results.

NURSING IMPLICATIONS WITH RATIONALE

Explain to the patient the purpose of the test. Explanation could be brief, such as, "to determine the antibody (immunoglobulin) values."

Inform the patient that food and drink are not restricted.

Obtain a history from the patient concerning previous vaccination or immunization, including toxoids (tetanus) received in the last 6 months and blood transfusions or injections of gamma globulin or tetanus antitoxin received in the last 6 weeks.

Report to the physician and mark in the patient's chart and the lab slip if the patient has received recent blood transfusions, immunization, or injections of toxoids, tetanus antitoxin, and gamma globulins.

Decreased level (IgG, IgA, IgM)
Associate clinical problems with decreased immunoglobulin levels.
> Instruct the patient to avoid infections by using preventive measures—i.e., to avoid being around persons with colds, to get adequate rest, to eat "balanced" meals, and to maintain an adequate fluid intake.

Check the patient's body temperature periodically.

Elevated level (IgG, IgA, IgM, IgE)
Associate clinical problems and injections of toxoids, antitoxins, or gamma globulin to elevated immunoglobulin levesls (see *Clinical Problems* above).

IRON (Serum)

NORMAL RANGE
> **Adult:** 50–150 μg(mcg)/dl, 10–27 μmol/L (SI units).
> **Newborn:** 100–200 μg/dl.
> **6 Months–2 Years:** 40–100 μg/dl.

DESCRIPTION
See Iron-binding Capacity.
> Iron is absorbed directly from the small intestine into the blood and is coupled with plasma protein transferrin. Transferrin (beta$_1$-globulin) is responsible for iron transportation to the bone marrow for the purpose of hemoglobin synthesis. The storage compound for iron is ferritin. Iron that is not absorbed is excreted in the stools.
> Serum iron levels are elevated when there is excessive hemolysis (red blood cell destruction). A serum iron deficit may be caused by a chronic iron deficiency due to diet or due to excessive blood loss from GI or vaginal bleeding. Usually, serum iron and total iron-binding capacity are determined together.[8,9,11,27,30,31,36]

CLINICAL PROBLEMS
> **Decreased level** *(↓ 50 μg/dl):* iron deficiency anemia (microcytic anemia); chronic diseases—malignancies of the stomach, small and large intestines, rectum, and breast, and rheumatoid arthritis; protein malnutrition; malabsorption; peptic ulcer (chronic bleeding); chronic renal failure; pregnancy (midterm onward); premature (low birth weight) infants; dumping (GI) syndrome; infants on prolonged milk diet.
> **Elevated level** *(↑ 150 μg/dl):* hemochromatosis (excessive iron deposits); anemias—hemolytic, pernicious, untreated macrocytic, folic acid deficiency; hepatic necrosis (liver damage); toxic effects of lead; thalassemia. *Drug influence:* excessive iron supplements, oral contraceptives.

PROCEDURE
> Collect 5 to 10 ml of venous blood in a red-top tube. Many laboratories require 10 ml.
> Prevent hemolysis of the blood sample. Handle the blood sample with care. If hemolysis is suspected due to traumatic puncture, this should be noted on the specimen or another blood specimen should be drawn. Hemolysis will cause a false elevated reading.
> There is usually a food and drink restriction for 8 hours before the test. Check with your laboratory.

FACTORS AFFECTING LABORATORY RESULTS
> Hemolysis of the blood sample.
> Oral contraceptives may cause false elevation of the serum iron level.

NURSING IMPLICATIONS WITH RATIONALE

Explain the purpose of the serum iron test to the patient. Explanation could be brief, such as, "to determine if there is a deficit or excess of iron in the body."
Explain any food restriction.

Decreased level (↓ 50 µg/dl)
Recognize clinical problems related to a serum iron deficit. Some of the major causes are iron deficiency anemia due to diet, cancer or the gastrointestinal tract, malabsorption, excessive vaginal bleeding, chronic blood loss, and some chronic illnesses.
Encourage the patient to eat foods rich in iron—i.e., liver, shellfish, kidney, lean meat, egg yolk, dried fruits, whole grain, wines, and cereals. Milk has little or no iron. Nutritional instruction is important for preschool and adolescent children and pregnant women.
Observe for signs and symptoms of iron deficiency anemia. These include pallor, fatigue, headache, tachycardia, dyspnea on exertion.
Instruct the patient on how to take iron supplements (ferrous sulfate). Iron should be given following meals or snacks, since it irritates the gastric mucosa. Suggest orange juice, since the ascorbic acid promotes iron absorption. Iron supplements can cause constipation, and some iron preparations are available in combination with stool softeners.
Explain to the patient who is taking iron supplements that his stools will have a tarry appearance. Excessive nonabsorbed iron is excreted in the stools.
Use the Z-tract method to administer iron intramuscularly. See a pharmacology text on how to perform the Z-tract method.

Elevated level (↑ 150 µg/dl)
Recognize clinical problems and drugs related to serum iron excess. Some of the major problems are hemochromatosis, hemolytic anemia, and hepatic necrosis.
Observe for signs and symptoms of hemochromatosis—i.e., bronze pigmentation of the skin, diabetes due to iron deposits in the pancreas, arrhythmias, and heart failure. This disease is rare.
Instruct the patient not to take an excess amount of iron supplements. The patient should contact his physician to determine the proper iron dosage.

IRON-BINDING CAPACITY (IBC) (Serum)
Total Iron-Binding Capacity (TIBC)

NORMAL RANGE
  Adult: 250–450 µg(mcg)/dl.
  Newborn: 60–175 µg/dl.
  Infant (6 months–2 years): 100–350 µg/dl.
  Child: same as adult; 20–50 percent saturation.

DESCRIPTION
See Iron (Serum).
  The iron-binding capacity (IBC) is normally 2 to 3 times greater than the serum iron level. The IBC measures the amount of additional iron with which transferrin can bind. When the serum iron is decreased, the IBC is increased, and when the serum iron is increased, the IBC is decreased.

To determine the percentage saturation (of transferrin with iron), divide the serum iron by the total iron-binding capacity (TIBC).[8,11,14,27,30,31,36]

CLINICAL PROBLEMS

Decreased level *(↓ 250 µg/dl):* hemochromatosis (excess iron deposits in organs and tissues); anemias—hemolytic, pernicious, sickle cell; cirrhosis of the liver; renal failure (uremia); cancer of the GI tract; rheumatoid arthritis; infections. *Drug influence:* ACTH, steroids.

Elevated level *(↑ 450 µg/dl):* iron deficiency anemia, acute chronic blood loss, polycythemia, pregnancy. *Drug influence:* oral contraceptives, iron preparations, chloramphenicol (Chloromycetin).

PROCEDURE

Collect 5 to 10 ml of venous blood in a red-top tube. Many laboratories require 10 ml.

There usually are food and drink restriction for 8 hours before the test. Check with your laboratory.

Prevent hemolysis of the blood sample. If hemolysis is suspected from traumatic puncture, either draw a new blood sample or make a note on the laboratory slip. Hemolysis can cause an inaccurate reading.

FACTORS AFFECTING LABORATORY RESULTS

Hemolysis of the blood sample.

Drugs (especially ACTH and steroids) can decrease the TIBC, and oral contraceptives can increase the TIBC.

NURSING IMPLICATIONS WITH RATIONALE

Explain to the patient that the purpose of the test is to determine the iron-binding capacity of transferrin.

Explain to the patient that he will be NPO (must have nothing by mouth) for 8 hours before the test.

Decreased level (↓ 250 µg/dl)

Recognize clinical problems and drugs that cause a decrease in iron-binding capacity. Excess iron is bound to transferrin, which reduces the TIBC (there is less capacity to bind extra iron).

Nursing implications are similar to those for a decreased level of serum iron.

Elevated level (↑ 450 µg/dl)

Recognize clinical problems that cause an elevated iron-binding capacity. In iron deficiency, less iron is bound to transferrin, increasing the capacity to bind more iron when it becomes available.

Nursing implications are similar to those for an elevated level of serum iron.

K

KETONE BODIES, ACETONE (Urine)

NORMAL RANGE
Adult: negative test.
Child: negative test.

DESCRIPTION
See Acetone, Ketone Bodies (Serum).
Ketone bodies are produced to provide energy when carbohydrates cannot be utilized, as in diabetic acidosis and starvation/malnutrition. When these excess ketones are produced, ketosis (in the blood) results, thus exhausting the alkaline reserve (e.g., bicarbonates) of the body, causing an acidotic state. Ketonuria (ketone bodies in the urine) occurs as a result of ketosis.
In testing for ketonuria, acetest tablets are used to detect the two principle ketones (acetone and acetoacetic acid) in the urine. Ketostix can also be used, but this test method is more specific for acetoacetic acid.[8,9,11,14,27,30]

CLINICAL PROBLEMS
Positive result: diabetic acidosis (ketoacidosis), starvation/malnutrition, reducing diet (↓ CHO), fasting, severe vomiting, heat stroke, fetal death. *Drug influence:* ascorbic acid, levodopa compounds, insulin, isopropyl alcohol, paraldehyde, pyridium, dyes used for the tests—Bromsulphalein (BSP) and Phenolsulfonphthalein (PSP).

PROCEDURE
Collect a random urine specimen. Two tests are usually performed, as follows.
Acetest: Place an acetest tablet on a clean surface (preferably a white paper towel) and put a drop of fresh urine on the tablet. Wait 30 seconds, and if the tablet changes color (lavender, medium purple, or dark purple), the result is positive for ketones—mainly acetone (20 to 25 mg/dl in the urine) and acetoacetic acid (5 to 10 mg/dl in the urine). The test is usually done on the same urine used for testing for glycosuria. The clinitest is used for determining glycosuria and the acetest for ketonuria.
Ketostix: Dip a reagent stick in fresh urine. Wait 15 seconds and compare it to the color chart. This test is more sensitive to acetoacetic acid than it is to acetone.
The urine should be fresh or refrigerated in a closed container. Waiting may cause false negative results due to the instability of acetone.
There is not food or drink restriction.

FACTORS AFFECTING LABORATORY RESULTS
A low-carbohydrate diet or a high-fat diet.
Drugs causing false positive results (see *Drug Influence* above).
Urine kept at room temperature for 1 hour or more before testing.
Urinary tract infection—bacteria in the urine will cause a loss of acetoacetic acid.
Juvenile diabetics are more prone to ketonuria (ketosis) than adults.

NURSING IMPLICATIONS WITH RATIONALE

Positive Result
Relate ketonuria to diabetic acidosis (ketoacidosis), starvation, fasting, or a low-car-bohydrate diet. In severe diabetic acidosis, both ketonuria and glycosuria may be

present. This would not be true in severe vomiting, starvation, reducing diets and heat stroke for in such cases only ketonuria would be present.

Explain to the patient that the test is to determine whether an acid–base imbalance is present (such as acidosis due to a specified clinical problem), or give a similar response.

Explain to the patient that the urine should be freshly voided. Only 1 ml is needed. Acetone is lost in the urine if it stands at room temperature, since it is volatile.

Instruct the patient that food and drinks are not restricted.

Test for glycosuria as well as ketonuria, especially in diabetics.

Record the results of the acetest and clinitest on the patient's chart. If the results are abnormal, notify the physician.

Teach patient how to use the acetest and clinitest.

Answer the patient's questions concerning urine testing and diabetes mellitus.

Assess for signs and symptoms of diabetic acidosis, such as rapid, vigorous breathing; restlessness; confusion; sweet-smelling breath; and a positive clinitest and acetest.

17-KETOSTEROIDS (17-KS) (Urine)

NORMAL RANGE
   Adult: *Male:* 8–25 mg/24 hours. *Female:* 5–15 mg/24 hours. *Over 65 years old:* 4–8 mg/24 hours.
   Child: *Infant:* <1 mg/24 hours. *1–3 years old:* <2 mg/24 hours. *3–6 years old:* <3 mg/24 hours. *7–10 years old:* <4 mg/24 hours. *10–12 years old:* Male: <6 mg/24 hours. Female: <5 mg/24 hours.
   Adolescent: *Male:* 3–15 mg/24 hours. *Female:* 3–12 mg/24 hours.

DESCRIPTION
   17-Ketosteroids (17-KS) are metabolites of male hormones which are secreted from the testes and adrenal cortex. 17-KS are excreted in the urine. Men have a higher level of 17-KS than women, and children before puberty have a very low level. In men, approximately one-third of the hormone metabolites come from the testes and two-thirds come from the adrenal cortex. In women, nearly all of the excreted hormones (androgens) is derived from the adrenal cortex.
   Since most of the 17-KS is derived from the adrenal cortex and not from the testes, the 17-KS level is more useful for diagnosing adrenal cortex dysfunction. This test is also useful for determining pituitary and gonadal hormone function. Usually, plasma cortisol and 17-OHCS determinations are requested at the same time to further confirm adrenal dysfunctions.[4,8,11,14,27,30,36]

CLINICAL PROBLEMS
   Decreased level *(↓ 5 mg/24 hours [female], ↓ 8 mg/24 hours [male]):* adrenal cortical hypofunction (Addison's disease), hypogonadism, hypopituitarism, nephrosis, myxedema, severe debilitating diseases. *Drug influence:* diuretics—thiazides (Hydrodiuril and Diuril); chlordiazepoxide (Libritabs); estrogen; oral contraceptives; paraldehyde; reserpine; probenecid (Benemid); promazine; Meprobamate (Aldomet);* quinidine; quinine.
   Elevated level *(↑ 15 mg/24 hours [female], ↑ 25 mg/24 hours [male]):* ACTH therapy; adrenal cortical hyperfunction—adrenocortical hyperplasia, Cushing's syndrome, adrenocortical carcinoma; testicular neoplasm; ovarian neoplasm; hyperpituitarism;

---

* *Meprobamate may increase or decrease the 17-KS value.*

hirsutism; severe stress—burns, surgery, infectious diseases. *Drug influence:* acetazolamide (Diamox); antibiotics—chloramphenicol (Chloromycetin), cloxacillin, erythromycin; chlorpromazine (Thorazine); hydralazine; meprobamate (Aldomet),* phenothiazines; spironolactone (Aldactone); phenazopyridine; dexamethasone (Decadron).

PROCEDURE

Collect a 24 hour urine specimen in a large container and keep the urine container on
ice or refrigerated. Some laboratories require a preservative in the urine container—
i.e., 3 ml of acetic acid or 10 ml of hydrochloric acid—to prevent bacterial growth which
will cause steroid decomposition.

There is no food or drink restriction.

If possible, drugs that interfere with test results should not be given for 48 hours
before the test.

FACTORS AFFECTING LABORATORY RESULTS

Drugs (see *Drug Influence* above).

NURSING IMPLICATIONS WITH RATIONALE

Explain to the patient that the purpose of the test is to determine adrenal gland
 function *or* to determine the amount of a specific hormone being excreted.

Explain to the patient and family that all urine will be collected for 24 hours in the
 large urine container/bottle which is on ice or refrigerated. Inform the patient that
 he should not put toilet paper or feces in the urine.

Label the urine container with the patient's name and the date and exact times of urine
 collection—e.g., 3/20/83, 7:30 A.M. to 3/21/83, 7:30 A.M.

List on the laboratory slip the patient's sex and age. If the patient is a male, the
 laboratory results should be slightly higher than if the patient is a female. In addition, if the patient is over 65 years old, the test results should be low or low normal.

Post the times for urine collection on the patient's door or bed and in the Kardex.

Encourage the patient to increase fluid intake.

Decreased level (↓ 5mg/24 hours [female], ↓ 8 mg/24 hours [male])

Recognize clinical problems and drugs related to a decreased 17-KS level.

Observe for the signs and symptoms of adrenal gland insufficiency (Addison's
 disease), such as weakness, weight loss, polyuria, hopotension, increased pulse rate,
 and shock (if severe).

Record fluid intake and output. Report if the patient's urine output is greater than
 normal (>2000 ml/24 hours).

Monitor weight loss. In Addison's disease, sodium is not retained; therefore, both
 sodium and water are lost. Weight loss and dehydration usually occur.

Encourage the patient to wear an identification bracelet containing emergency information.

Elevated level (↑ 15 mg/24 hours [female], ↑ 25 mg/24 hours [male])

Recognize clinical problems and drugs related to an increased 17-KS level.

Observe for signs and symptoms of adrenal gland hyperfunction (Cushing's syndrome), such as moon faces, hirsutism, weight gain, a cervical–dorsal fat pad (buffalo hump), a bleeding tendency, hyperglycemia, and edema in the extremities.

Check serum potassium and blood glucose levels. Hypokalemia and hyperglycemia
 frequently occur; potassium supplements and insulin or a low-CHO diet may be
 indicated.

L

LACTIC (LACTATE) DEHYDROGENASE (LD OR LDH), LDH ISOENZYMES (Serum)

NORMAL RANGE

Adult: *Total LDH:* 150–450 U/ml (Wroblewski-LaDue method), 60–120 U/ml (Wacker method), 70–200 IU/L (differs among institutions). *Isoenzymes:* LDH_1, 17–27 percent; LDH_2, 27–37 percent; LDH_3, 18–25 percent; LDH_4, 3–8 percent; LDH_5, 0–5 percent. **Newborn:** 300–1500 IU/L.
Child: 50–150 IU/L.

DESCRIPTION

Lactic dehydrogenase (LDH) is an intracellular enzyme present in nearly all metabolizing cells, with the highest concentrations in the heart, skeletal muscle, liver, kidney, brain, and erythrocytes, but with different tissues having different isoenzymes. Lactic dehydrogenase has two distinct subunits—M (muscle) and H (heart)—and these subunits are combined in different formations to make five isoenzymes—LDH_1 (H, H, H, H), LDH_2 (H, H, H, M), LDH_3 (H, H, M, M), LDH_4 (H, M, M, M), and LDH_5 (M, M, M, M). Electrophoresis separates and measures the five components of serum LDH.

Serum LDH and LDH_1 (heat-stable lactic dehydrogenase) are used for diagnosing acute myocardial infarction along with other enzymatic tests, such as the creative phosphokinase (CPK) and aspartate amino transferase (AST) tests. Six hours after a myocardial infarction, LDH_1 increases, causing a reversal of the LDH_1/LDH_2 ratio. A high serum LDH (total) level occurs 6 to 12 hours after the infarction, reaches its peak in 24 to 48 hours, and remains elevated for 6 to 10 days, making it a useful test for delayed diagnosis of myocardial infarction, since a patient may not seek medical care for "indigestion" for several days.

LDH_3 is linked to pulmonary diseases, and LDH_5 is linked to liver and skeletal muscle diseases. In acute hepatitis, total LDH rises and the LDH_5 usually rises before jaundice develops and falls before the bilirubin level does.[8,9,11,14,16,30,31,32]

CLINICAL PROBLEMS

Elevated level *(↑ 450 U/ml [adults]—Wroblewski–LaDue):* acute myocardial infarction; congestive heart failure; cancer—lung, bone, intestines, liver, breast, cervix, testis, kidney, stomach, melanoma of the skin; acute leukemia; acute pulmonary infarction; infectious mononucleosis; anemias—pernicious; folic acid deficiency, sickle cell, acquired hemolytic; cerebral hemorrhage; acute hepatitis; shock; skeletal muscular diseases; heat stroke. *Drug influence:* narcotics—codeine, morphine, meperidine (Demerol).

PROCEDURE

Collect 5 ml of venous blood in a red-top tube.

Prevent hemolysis of the blood sample. Shaking the tube and extreme heat or cold can cause hemolysis.

List on the laboratory slip any narcotics or IM injections the patient received within 8 hours before the test.

There is no food or drink restriction.

FACTORS AFFECTING LABORATORY RESULTS
Narcotic drugs and intramuscular injections can elevate serum LDH levels.
Hemolysis of the blood sample can cause an elevated serum LDH level; the enzyme is
plentiful in the red blood cells (erthrocytes.)

NURSING IMPLICATIONS WITH RATIONALE

Elevated level (↑ 450 U/ml [adult]—Wroblewski–LaDue)
Explain to the patient that the purpose of the test is to detect the amount of a specific
enzyme in the blood. A more detailed explanation may be needed.
Explain that food and drinks are not restricted.
Record on the chart and lap slip any narcotics or IM injections that patient received
prior to the test. If the results are slightly elevated, the physician should be notified
of any narcotics or injections the patient received.
Obtain a history of the patient's discomfort. A complaint of severe indigestion several
days before could be indicative of a myocardial infarction. All information should be
recorded and reported.
Assess for signs and symptoms of an acute myocardial infarction (AMI)—i.e., pale or
gray color, sharp stabbing pain or heavy pressure pain, shortness of breath,
diaphoresis, nausea and vomiting, and indigestion.
Instruct the patient to notify the nurse of any recurrence of chest discomfort.

LDH ISOENZYMES

See Lactic Dehydrogenase.

LEAD (Blood)

NORMAL RANGE
Adult: *Normal:* 10–20 μg(mcg)/dl. *Acceptable:* 20–40 μg/dl. *Excessive:* 40–80 μg/dl.
Toxic: > 80 μg/dl.
Child: *Normal:* 10–20 μ/dl. *Acceptable:* 20–30 μg/dl. *Excessive:* 30–50 μg/dl. *Toxic:* > 50
μg/dl.

DESCRIPTION
Excessive lead exposure due to occupational contact is a hazard to adults, and lead
toxicity can occur in children from eating chipped lead-based paint found in old houses.
Sources of lead include lead gasoline (fumes), lead-based paint, unglazed pottery, and
"moonshine" whiskey prepared in lead containers. Most industry will accept a 40 μg/dl
blood lead level as a normal value.
Lead is usually excreted rapidly in the urine, but if excessive lead exposure persists,
the lead will accumulate in the bone and soft tissues. Chronic lead poisoning is more
common than acute poisoning. Lead colic (crampy abdominal pain) occurs in both
acute and chronic lead poisoning.[9,11,27,34,35]

CLINICAL PROBLEMS
Elevated level *(> 40 μg/dl [adult, excessive]):* lead gasoline, including fumes; lead-based
paint; unglazed pottery; batteries; lead containers used for storage; heat stroke
(mobilizes lead stored in the body).

PROCEDURE
Collect 7 to 10 ml of venous blood in a lavender- or green-top tube.
There is no food or drink restriction.
Urine may be requested for a 24 hour quantitative test; a lead-free container must be used.

FACTORS AFFECTING LABORATORY RESULTS
None reported.

NURSING IMPLICATIONS WITH RATIONALE

Elevated level (>40 μg/dl [adult, excessive])
Explain to the patient (or the parent of a child) that the test is to determine whether there is an accumulation of lead in the blood.
Explain to the patient that food and drinks are not restricted.
Obtain a history from the patient and/or parent concerning lead exposure. Record this history on the chart and report the information to the physician.
Observe for signs and symptoms of lead poisoning—i.e., lead colic (crampy abdominal pain), constipation, occasional bloody diarrhea, behavioral changes (from lethargy to hyperactivity, aggression, impulseness), tremors, and confusion.
Monitor the urinary output, for lead toxicity can decrease kidney function. A urine output of less than 25 ml/hour should be reported.
Monitor the medical treatment for removing body lead. Chelation therapy (whereby metal combines with another substance) is used, and the principal chelating agent is calcium disodium edetate (EDTA).
Provide adequate fluid intake. Adequate hydration prevents hemoconcentration.
Teach patients/clients who are exposed to lead (in their occupations) that blood levels should be monitored. These persons should definitely keep medical appointments.
Suggest to parents ways of satisfying children's hunger through the attention method or providing psychologic satisfaction that will replace that gained by eating lead chips.

LEUCINE AMINOPEPTIDASE (LAP) Serum)

NORMAL RANGE
Adult: *Male:* 80–200 U/ml, 19.2–28 U/L (SI units). *Female:* 75–185 U/ml, 18–44.4 U/L (SI units).

DESCRIPTION
The leucine aminopeptidase (LAP) enzyme is produced by the liver and tends to parallel serum alkaline phosphatase (ALP), except that the LAP level is normal in bone disease or malabsorption syndrome. LAP is not an indicator of pancreatic carcinoma, as was once thought, but is an indicator for biliary obstruction due to liver metastases and choledocholithiasis, just as alkaline phosphatase and transaminase are.
This enzyme test is not frequently ordered, but is useful as a supplement test in evaluating hepatobiliary tract disease.[14,27,34,36]

CLINICAL PROBLEMS
Elevated level *(↑ 200 U/ml):* cancer of the liver, extrahepatic biliary obstruction (stones), acute necrosis of the liver, viral hepatitis.

PROCEDURE
Collect 5 to 10 ml of venous blood in a red-top tube.
There is no food or drink restriction.

FACTORS AFFECTING LABORATORY RESULTS
None reported.

NURSING IMPLICATIONS WITH RATIONALE

Elevated level (↑ 200 U/ml)
Explain that the purpose of the test is to measure the amount of a specific enzyme
produced by the liver.
Explain to the patient that food, drinks, and medications are not restricted.
Compare LAP with other tests for liver dysfunction—i.e., the alkaline phosphatase
(ALP), alanine aminotransferase (ALT or SGPT), and gamma glutamyl transpeptidase (GGTP) tests. The leucine aminopeptidase test is frequently used to
verify the results of other laboratory tests. It is not considered as sensitive as the
other tests, and therefore it is not as commonly used.

LIPASE (Serum)

NORMAL RANGE
Adult: 0–1.5 U/ml (Cherry–Crandall method); 14–280 mIU/ml, 14–280 U/L (SI units).
Child: *Infant:* 9–105 IU/L at 37 °C. Child: 20–136 IU/L at 37 °C.

DESCRIPTION
Lipase is an enzyme secreted by the pancreas which moves to the duodenum, where it
aids in digesting fats. Lipase, like amylase, appears in the blood stream following
damage to the pancreas. Acute pancreatitis is the most common cause for an elevated
serum lipase. Lipase and amylase levels increase early in the disease, but serum lipase
can be elevated for up to 14 days following an acute episode, whereas the serum
amylase returns to normal after approximately 3 days. Serum lipase is useful for a late
diagnosis of acute pancreatitis. This enzyme is less useful for diagnosing chronic pancreatitis and carcinoma of the pancreas.[9,11,30,34,36]

CLINICAL PROBLEMS
Decreased level *(↓ 14 mIU/ml, ↓ 14 U/L [SI units, adult]):* late cancer of the pancreas,
hepatitis.
Elevated level *(↑ 280 mIU/ml, ↑ 280 U/L [SI units, adult]):* acute pancreatitis, cancer of
the pancreas (early stage), perforated ulcer, obstruction of the pancreatic duct, acute
cholecystitis (some cases), acute renal failure (early stage). *Drug influence:* codeine,
morphine; meperidine (Demerol); methylcholine; urecholine; steroids; guanethidine.

PROCEDURE
Collect 10 ml of venous blood in a red-top tube.
Food and liquids except water should be withheld for 8 to 12 hours.
Narcotics should be withheld for 24 hours prior to the test. If narcotics are ad-
ministered within the 24 hours, the drug and the time given should be written on the
laboratory slip.

FACTORS AFFECTING LABORATORY RESULTS
Most narcotic drugs elevate the serum lipase level.
Food eaten within 8 hours prior to the test—it has not been definitely proven that food interferes with serum lipase levels.
The presence of hemoglobin and calcium ions may cause a decreased serum lipase level.

NURSING IMPLICATIONS WITH RATIONALE

Elevated level (↑ 280 mIU/ml or 280 U/L)
Relate elevated serum lipase and amylase levels to acute pancreatitis.
Explain to the patient the test's purpose and procedure. The purpose of the test is to determine whether the enzyme lipase is elevated in the blood stream, which condition can occur in pancreatic disorders. The patient will be NPO for a specified time, except for water.
Record on the laboratory slip any narcotics the patient received within 24 hours prior to the test and any food eaten within 8 hours of the test.
Notify the physician when abdominal pain persists for several days. A serum lipase determination may be ordered, since it is an effective test for latent diagnosis of acute pancreatitis. Lipase levels may remain elevated in the blood for 2 weeks.

LIPOPROTEINS, LIPOPROTEIN ELECTROPHORESIS, LIPIDS (Serum)

NORMAL RANGE
Adult: *Total:* 400–800 mg/dl, 4–8 g/L (SI units) (differs in various laboratories). *Cholesterol:* 150–250 mg/dl (see Cholesterol). *Triglycerides:* 10–190 mg/dl (see Triglycerides). *Phospholipids:* 150–380 mg/dl.
Child: similar to adult.

DESCRIPTION
Lipoproteins are lipids bound to protein, and the three main lipoproteins are cholesterol, triglycerides, and phospholipids. There are two major classes or fractions of lipoproteins, alpha and beta, which can be separated by the method of electrophoresis. The alpha fraction is the high-density lipoprotein (HDL) and is predominantly composed of protein with small amounts of cholesterol, triglycerides, and phospholipids. The beta fraction is the low-density lipoprotein, which is predominantly

LIPOPROTEIN CLASSIFICATION*

Subgroup Classes of Lipoproteins	Protein Composition	Cholesterol	Triglycerides	Phospholipids
Chylomicrons	2%	3%	90%	5%
Very Low-density (VLDL, pre-beta)	10%	10%	70%	10%
Low-density (LDL, beta)	25%	45%	10%	20%
High-density (HDL, alpha)	50%	20%	Trace	30%

Adapted from Henry, J.B. Todd-Sanford–Davidsohn Clinical Diagnosis and Management. Philadelphia: Saunders, 1979.

composed of varying amounts of cholesterol, triglycerides, and phospholipids and small amounts of protein. The beta class is subgrouped into chylomicrons, very low-density lipoprotein (VLDL), known as pre-beta), and low-density lipoprotein (LDL, known as beta-lipoprotein). The beta groups are the largest contributors to atherosclerosis and coronary artery disease.

Increased lipoproteins (hyperlipidemia or hyperlipoproteinemia) can be phenotyped into five major types (I, IIA and IIB, III, IV, V). Cholesterol and triglycerides are the two lipids in each type found in varying amounts. With Type II, the cholesterol is highly elevated and the triglycerides are slightly increased; with Type IV, the triglycerides are highly elevated and the cholesterol is slightly increased. Types II and IV are the most common phenotypes and are the most prevalent in atherosclerosis and coronary artery disease.

Lipoprotein electrophoresis is a valuable tool used to assign the "risk factor" in cardiovascular disease. It is frequently used for screening, preventive, and diagnostic purposes. It is also a useful test for determining genetic disorders of lipoprotein metabolism (phenotyping).[8,9,11,14,27,30,31,34,36]

CLINICAL PROBLEMS

Decreased level *(↓ 400 mg/dl [adult, total])*: beta-lipoproteins—A-betalipoproteinemia, Tangier disease, chronic obstructive lung disease. *Drug influence:* see Cholesterol and Triglycerides.

Elevated level *(↑ 800 mg/dl [adult, total])*: beta-lipoproteins—hyperlipoproteinemia (especially Type II); acute myocardial infarction; hypothyroidism; diabetes mellitus; nephrotic syndrome; eclampsia; Laennec's cirrhosis; multiple myeloma; diet (high in saturated fats). *Drug influence:* see Cholesterol and Triglycerides.

PROCEDURE

Keep the patient NPO except for water for 12 to 14 hours prior to the test. The patient should be on a normal (regular) diet for 3 to 7 days before the test. The laboratory policy concerning NPO differs among institutions.

Collect 10 ml of venous blood in a red-top tube.

FACTORS AFFECTING LABORATORY RESULTS

A diet high in saturated fats and sugar.

Drugs which increase or decrease serum lipoproteins (see *Clinical Problems, Drug Influence* for Cholesterol and Triglycerides).

NURSING IMPLICATIONS WITH RATIONALE

Elevated level (↑ 800 mg/dl)

Relate clinical problems to hyperlipoproteinemia and the serum lipoprotein level of the patient.

Recognize when lipoprotein electrophoresis is indicated. This test is used mainly for screening and preventive purposes, following several elevated cholesterol and/or triglyceride results. It also may be ordered to evaluate the cause of severe angina pectoris and after an acute myocardial infarction.

Explain to the patient the purpose of the test. Explanation could be brief, such as, "to determine the lipid content of the blood."

Explain to the patient that he should not eat or drink, except for water, for a specified time—i.e., for 12 hours before the test.

Teach the patient with hyperlipoproteinemia to avoid foods high in saturated fats and sugar—i.e., bacon, cream, butter, fatty meats, and candy.

Check the patient's serum cholesterol and serum triglyceride levels and compare with the lipoprotein electrophoresis results. This information is helpful for teaching purposes and in answering the patient's questions.
Ask the physician what he has told the patient.

LITHIUM (Serum)

NORMAL RANGE
Adult: *Normal:* negative. *Therapeutic:* 0.5–1.5 mEq/L. *Toxic:* > 2 mEq/L.
Child: not usually given to children.

DESCRIPTION
Lithium or lithium salt is used to treat manic–depressive psychosis. This agent is used to correct the mania in manic–depression and to prevent depression. If therapeutic levels become toxic, the dose should be decreased.
Lithium salt was first used in the 1940s as a salt substitute; this practice was abandoned in the late 1940s because of its high toxicity. It was not used in the United States until after 1965, and then was used for treatment of manic depression.[11,27,34]

CLINICAL PROBLEMS
Elevated level *(↑ 2 mEq/L): Toxicity:* lithium carbonate (Eskalith, Lithane, Lithonate) lithium bromide.

PROCEDURE
Collect 5 ml of venous blood in a red-top tube.
Lithium should not be taken for 8 to 12 hours before the test (the last lithium dose before the test differs among laboratories and physicians).
There is no food or drink restriction.
The lithium tolerance test may be ordered instead of the conventional blood sample. A base blood specimen is obtained, and then the lithium dose is given. Blood specimens are collected 1, 3, and 6 hours after the lithium dose.

FACTORS AFFECTING LABORATORY RESULTS
None reported.

NURSING IMPLICATIONS WITH RATIONALE

Explain to the patient that the test is to evaluate the lithium level in the blood.
Explain that lithium should be withheld for 8 to 12 hours (a definite time should be stated) before the test. Explain that food and drinks are not restricted.
Instruct the patient to take the prescribed lithium dosage daily and to keep his medical appointment. Periodic blood specimens will need to be drawn to determine lithium levels.
Suggest to the nursing mother taking lithium that the pediatrician should be notified before she breast-feeds the infant. Breast milk can contain high levels of lithium.
Encourage adequate fluid and sodium intake while the patient is maintained on lithium. Lithium inhibits anti-diuretic hormone (ADH) secretion, causing body water loss. Diuretics should be avoided.
Observe for signs and symptoms of lithium overdose—i.e., slurred speech, muscle spasm, confusion, and nystagmus. Lithium dosage should be lower in the older adult (over 65) than in the middle-aged adult. Lithium test results should always be reported to the physician because of the narrow range of the "therapeutic" dosage.

L/S (LECITHIN/SPHINGOMYELIN) RATIO (Amniotic Fluid)

NORMAL RANGE
Before 35 weeks of gestation: 1:1. *Lecithin (L):* 6–9 mg/dl. *Sphingomyelin (S):* 4–6 mg/dl.
After 35 weeks of gestation: 4:1. *Lecithin (L):* 15–21 mg/dl. *Sphingomyelin (S):* 4–6 mg/dl.

DESCRIPTION
The L/S ratio can be used to predict neonatal respiratory distress syndrome (also called hyaline membrane disease) before delivery. Lecithin (L), a phospholipid, is responsible mostly for the formation of alveolar surfactant. Surfactant lubricates the alveolar lining and inhibits alveoli collapse, thus preventing atelectasis. Sphingomyelin (S) is another phospholipid, the value of which remains the same throughout pregnancy. A marked rise in amniotic lecithin after 35 weeks (to a level three or four times higher than that of sphingomyelin) is considered normal, and so chances for having hyaline membrane disease are small. The L/S ratio is also used to determine fetal maturity in the event that the gestation period is uncertain. In this situation, the L/S ratio is determined at intervals of a period of several weeks.[27,31,35,36]

CLINICAL PROBLEMS
Decreased Ratio After 35 Weeks: (L/S ratio is 1:1): respiratory distress syndrome, hyaline membrane disease.

PROCEDURE
The physician obtains amniotic fluid by the method of amniocentesis. The specimen should be cooled immediately to prevent the destruction of lecithin by certain enzymes in the amniotic fluid. The specimen should be frozen if testing cannot be done at a specified time (check with the lab). The specimen should also be kept in the dark, since other tests (e.g., bilirubin) may be requested later on.
Care should be taken to prevent puncture of the mother's bladder. If urine in the specimen is suspected, then the specimen should be tested for urea and potassium, and if these two levels are higher than blood levels, the specimen could be urine and not amniotic fluid.
There is no food, drink, or drug restriction.

FACTORS AFFECTING LABORATORY RESULTS
Maternal vaginal secretions or a bloody tap into the amniotic fluid may cause a false increased reading for lecithin.
The amniotic fluid specimen should be tested immediately to prevent inaccurate results.

NURSING IMPLICATIONS WITH RATIONALE

Check the procedure for amniocentesis. Explain the procedure to the patient. Assist the physician in obtaining amniotic fluid.
Obtain a fetal history of problems occurring during gestation. Also ask for and report information on any previous children born with respiratory distress syndrome.
Be supportive of the mother and her family before, during, and after the test. Remain with the patient and answer her questions, if possible, or refer her questions to appropriate professional personnel.
Assess the newborn at delivery for respiratory complications—i.e., substernal retractions, increased respiratory rate, labored breathing, and expiratory grunts.

LYMPHOCYTES (Blood)
Part of the Differential White Blood Cell Count

NORMAL RANGE
Adult: 25–35 percent of the total leukocytes (WBC); mean, 34 percent or 1700–3400 mm^3.

Child: *Newborn:* 32 percent (mean). *2 Weeks old:* 41 percent. *4 Weeks old:* 56 percent. *6–12 Months old:* 61 percent. *4 Years old:* 50 percent. *6 Years old:* 42 percent. *12 Years old:* 38 percent.

DESCRIPTION
Lymphocytes are mononuclear agranulocytes. They comprise the second largest group of leukocytes (neutrophils are the largest group). Lymphocytosis (increased number of lymphocytes) frequently occurs in chronic and viral infections—e.g., infectious mononucleosis, hepatitis. Severe lymphocytosis is commonly caused by chronic lymphocytic leukemia.

Lymphocytes may be increased when the neutrophils are decreased or when the total white blood cell count is increased. Many consider lymphocytes to be under the influence of adrenocortical hormones, decreasing in number with excess hormone secretion or steroid therapy.

There have been continuous studies in the last 20 years of the role lymphocytes play in immunology. The B-lymphocytes (B-cells) and T-lymphocytes (T-cells) are parts of the immune response system, and the B-lymphocytes (humoral immunity) are necessary for the synthesis of immunoglobulins. T-lymphocytes are effective in destroying bacteria, viruses, and other foreign cells (e.g., cancer cells).[16,21,27,31,36]

CLINICAL PROBLEMS
Decreased level *(↓ 25 percent):* cancer—esophagus, stomach, brain, melanoma; myelocytic leukemia; adrenal cortical hyperfunction; agranulocytosis; aplastic anemia; neurologic disorders—myasthenia gravis, multiple sclerosis, Guillain–Barré syndrome; renal failure; nephrotic syndrome; systemic lupus erythematosus. *Drug influence:* steroids—cortisone, ACTH; chemotherapeutic cancer agents.

Elevated level *(↑ 35 percent):* chronic lymphocytic leukemia; viral infections—infectious mononucleosis, hepatitis, mumps, pertussis, rubella, viral pneumonia; Hodgkin's disease; multiple myeloma; adrenal cortical hypofunction; anterior pituitary hypofunction; chronic infections.

PROCEDURE
See White Blood Cell and Differential Count.

FACTORS AFFECTING LABORATORY RESULTS
The age of the individual—infants and children have twice as many lymphocytes as adults.

Steroids decrease the lymphocyte count.

NURSING IMPLICATIONS WITH RATIONALE

Explain to the patient the purpose of the blood test. Explanation could be brief, such as, "to determine the number of lymphocytes." A more detailed explanation may be needed.

Instruct the patient that food and drinks are not restricted.

Decreased level (↓ 25 percent—lymphocytopenia)

Relate the decrease in lymphocytes to clinical problems and drugs. With a decrease in T-lymphocytes (for cellular immunity), cancer cells grow, and neurologic and collagen diseases progress.

Recognize that continued use of steroids (e.g., cortisone) could decrease the number of lymphocytes. Steroids may be ordered for lymphocytosis or for inflammatory conditions. Regardless of the purpose, the immune system is inhibited.

Check the total WBC and differential count.

Elevated level (↑ 35 percent—lymphocytosis)

Relate an elevated lymphocyte count to clinical problems.

Note the age of the patient. Children normally have an increased number of lymphocytes; the number is especially high before the age of 6. The ratio of neutrophils to lymphocytes in the first few years of life is 1:2, whereas with adults, the ratio is 2:1. Childhood diseases (e.g., mumps, German measles) can cause lymphocytosis.

Check the total WBC and differential count. With neutropenia, lymphocytosis could be present, and the WBC could be normal or slightly to moderately increased.

M

MAGNESIUM (Mg) (Serum)

NORMAL RANGE
Adult: 1.5–2.5 mEq/L, or 1.2–2.6 mEq (wide range to cover various institutions).
Newborn: 1.4–2.9 mEq/L.
Child: 1.6–2.6 mEq/L.

DESCRIPTION
Magnesium is most plentiful in the cells (intracellular fluid). One-third of the magnesium ingested is absorbed through the small intestine, and the remaining unabsorbed magnesium is excreted in the stools. The absorbed magnesium is eventually excreted through the kidneys.

As with potassium, sodium, and calcium, magnesium is needed for neuromuscular activity. Magnesium influences utilization of potassium, calcium, and protein, and when there is a magnesium deficit, there is frequently a potassium and calcium deficit. Magnesium is also responsible for the transport of sodium and potassium across the cell membranes. Another function of magnesium is its activation of enzymes for carbohydrate and protein metabolism.

Magnesium is found in most foods, so it would be difficult for a person who maintains a normal diet to have a magnesium deficiency. The daily required magnesium intake for an adult is 200 to 300 mg, or 0.2 to 0.3 g.

A serum magnesium deficit is known as hypomagnesemia, and a serum magnesium excess is called hypermagnesemia.[5,6,8,9,11,17,22,24,30]

CLINICAL PROBLEMS
Decreased level (↓ 1.5 mEq/L [adult]): protein malnutrition, malabsorption, cirrhosis of the liver, alcoholism, hypoparathyroidism, hyperaldosteronism, hypokalemia (↓ K), IV solutions without Mg, chronic diarrhea, bowel resection complications, dehydration. *Drug influence:* diuretics—mercurial, ethacrynic acid (Edecrin); calcium gluconate; amphotericin B; neomycin; insulin.

Elevated level (↑ 2.5 mEq/L [adult]): severe dehydration, renal failure, leukemia (lymphocytic and myelocytic), diabetes mellitus (early phase). *Drug influence:* antacids—Maalox, Mylanta, Aludrox, DiGel; laxatives—epsom salts ($MgSO_4$), milk of magnesium, magnesium citrate.

PROCEDURE
Collect 5 to 10 ml of venous blood in a red-top tube.
There is no food or drink restriction.
Prevent hemolysis.

FACTORS AFFECTING LABORATORY RESULTS
Hypokalemia and hypocalcemia.
Drugs—laxatives and antacids containing magnesium can cause hypermagnesemia, and diuretics, calcium gluconate, and insulin can cause hypomagnesemia. Insulin moves magnesium back into the cells, causing a serum Mg deficit.

NURSING IMPLICATIONS WITH RATIONALE

Decreased level (↓ 1.5 mEq/L [adult])

Recognize clinical problems and drugs related to hypomagnesemia. Malabsorption, continuously administered IV solutions without magnesium, and selected disease entities cause most serum magnesium deficits.

Explain to the patient the purpose of the blood test. Explanation could be brief, such as, "to determine if there is a magnesium (electrolyte) loss."

Observe for signs and symptoms of hypomagnesemia—i.e., tetany symptoms (twitching and tremors, carpopedal spasm, generalized spasticity), restlessness, confusion, and arrhythmia. Neuromuscular irritability can be mistakenly attributed to hypocalcemia.

Check serum potassium, sodium, calcium, and magnesium levels. Electrolyte deficits may accompany a magnesium deficit. If hypokalemia and hypomagnesemia are present, potassium supplements will not completely correct the potassium deficit until the magnesium deficit is corrected.

Check for a positive Chvostek sign by tapping the facial nerve in front of ear and observing for spasm of the cheek and twitching at the corner of the lip.

Teach the patient to eat foods rich in magnesium—i.e., fish, seafood, meats, green vegetables, whole grain, and nuts.

Report to the physician if the patient has been NPO and receiving IV fluids without magnesium salts for weeks. Hyperalimentation solutions should contain magnesium.

Check patients receiving digitalis preparations for digitalis intoxication (anorexia, nausea, vomiting, bradycardia). A magnesium deficit enhances the action of digitalis, causing digitalis toxicity.

Assess renal function when the patient is receiving magnesium supplements. Excess magnesium is excreted by the kidneys.

Assess ECG changes. A flat or inverted T-wave can be indicative of hypomagnesemia. It can also indicate hypokalemia.

Administer IV magnesium sulfate in solution slowly to prevent a hot or flushed feeling.

Have IV calcium gluconate available to reverse hypermagnesemia due to overcorrection. Calcium antagonizes the sedative effect of magnesium.

Elevated level (↑ 2.5 mEq/L [adult])

Recognize clinical problems and drugs related to hypermagnesemia—i.e., dehydration, renal failure, and laxatives and antacids containing magnesium.

Observe signs and symptoms of hypermagnesemia—i.e., flushing, a feeling of warmth, increased perspiration (with the Mg level at 3 to 4 mEq/L); muscular weakness, diminished reflex, respiratory distress, hypotension, a sedative effect (with the Mg level at 9 to 10 mEq/L).

Monitor urinary output. Effective urinary output (>750 ml daily) will decrease the serum magnesium level.

Assess the patient's level of sensorium and muscle activity.

Assess ECG changes. A peaked T-wave and wide QRS complex can indicate hyperkalemia (↑ K) and hypermagnesemia, so the serum potassium and magnesium levels should be checked.

Teach patients to avoid constant use of laxatives and antacids containing magnesium. Suggest to patients that they check drug labels.

Provide adequate fluids to improve kidney function and restore body fluids. Dehydration can cause hemoconcentration and, as a result, magnesium excess.

Check for digitalis intoxication if the patient is receiving calcium gluconate for hypermagnesemia. Calcium excess enhances the action of digitalis.

MALARIA SMEAR (Blood)

NORMAL RANGE
   Adult: negative.
   Child: negative.

DESCRIPTION
   Malaria is caused by malarial parasites transmitted by mosquitos. The parasites rupture the red blood cells (hemolysis), causing the patient to have chills and fever.
   Malarial parasites can be detected by blood smears (venous or capillary blood). Blood samples are usually taken in the presence of chills and fever daily for 3 days or at specified times—every 6 or 12 hours.[27,31,36]

CLINICAL PROBLEMS
   Positive: malaria (Plasmodium species).

PROCEDURE
   Venous or capillary blood can be used for the malarial smear.
   Collect 5 ml in a lavender-top tube.
   There is no food or drink restriction.

FACTORS AFFECTING LABORATORY RESULTS
   None known.

NURSING IMPLICATIONS WITH RATIONALE

Explain to the patient the purpose of the blood test. Explanation could be brief, such as, "to identify the organism which is causing the symptoms."

Explain the procedure to the patient. The patient should inform the nurse when he or she is having chills and fever, since a blood sample is usually requested at that time. The blood sample may also be requested daily for 3 days or at specified times during the day.

Monitor the patient's temperature every 4 hours or as ordered. Record temperature changes.

Report chills and fever to the physician.

MONOCYTES (Blood)
Part of the Differential White Blood Cell Count

NORMAL RANGE
   Adult: 4–6 percent (200–600 mm^3) of total WBC (leukocytes).
   Child: similar to adult.

DESCRIPTION

Monocytes are mononuclear agranulocytes, which comprise only a small percentage of the total white blood cells (leukocytes). Monocytes are the second line of defense against bacterial infections and foreign substances. They are slower to react to infections and inflammatory diseases, but once they do, they are stronger than neutrophils, ingesting larger particles of debris.

Monocytes act as powerful macrophages and respond late to acute infections, but they continue to function (by phagocytosis) during the chronic phase. They are scavengers, ingesting dead bacteria, dead neutrophils, and protein debris, preparing the damaged tissues for the healing process.[8,9,16,21,36]

CLINICAL PROBLEMS

Decreased level (↓ *4 percent):* lymphocytic leukemia, aplastic anemia.

Elevated level (↑ *6 percent):* viral diseases—infectious mononucleosis, mumps, herpes zoster; infections and parasitic diseases—tuberculosis, malaria, brucellosis, toxoplasmosis, Rocky Mountain spotted fever, trypanosomiasis, bacterial endocarditis, osteomyelitis; monocytic leukemia and other leukemias; cancer—esophagus, stomach, colon, liver, bone, prostate, uterus, brain, bladder, pancreas; multiple myeloma; collagen diseases—rheumatoid arthritis, systemic lupus erythematosus; ulcerative colitis; anemias—sickle cell, hemolytic.

PROCEDURE

Same as for Differential White Blood Cell Count.

FACTORS AFFECTING LABORATORY RESULTS

None known.

NURSING IMPLICATIONS WITH RATIONALE

Explain to the patient the purpose of the blood test. Explanation could be brief, such as, "to determine the number of monocytes." A more detailed explanation may be needed.

Inform the patient that food and drinks are not restricted.

Elevated level (↑ 6 percent)

Relate an increased monocyte count to clinical problems. Recognize that monocytes occur late during the acute stage and throughout the chronic stage of infections.

Check the differential WBC count for monocytes. An elevated percentage is indicative of an acute and chronic infectious process. Note if there are increases in other leukocytes.

Assess for signs and symptoms of infectious mononucleosis. These include malaise, sore throat, enlarged lymph nodes, headache, increased nasal secretions, a positive heterophil agglutination test, an elevated monocyte level, and an elevated total WBC count.

N

NEUTROPHILS (SEGS OR POLYS) (Blood)
Part of the Differential White Blood Cell Count

NORMAL RANGE
Adult: *Total Neutrophils:* 50-70 percent (2500-7000 mm^3) of WBC (leukocytes). *Neutrophils, Segments:* 50-65 percent (2500-6500 mm^3). *Neutrophils, Bands:* 0-5 percent (0-500 mm^3).
Child: *Newborn:* Total neutrophils: 61 percent (5490-18,300 mm^3). *1 Year Old:* Total neutrophils: 32 percent (1920-5600 mm^3). *Older Child:* Total neutrophils: similar to adult.

DESCRIPTION
Neutrophils are the most numerous circulating white blood cells (leukocytes), and they respond more rapidly in large numbers to the inflammatory and tissue injury sites than other leukocytes. During an acute infection, the body's first line of defense is the neutrophils. Their major function is phagocytosis (engulfing and digesting bacteria or foreign substances). Usually neutrophils live from 14 hours to several days, unless an acute inflammatory process or infection has occurred. They attack the invaders with so much force that they only live for 1 or 2 hours before dying.

The neutrophils undergo three stages of development before they are mature. The myeloblasts are the earliest immature neutrophils and are found mostly in the bone marrow. The metamyelocytes are fairly young neutrophils; the bands are early mature neutrophils; and the segments are the mature neutrophils. In most acute illnesses, the total neutrophil count increases in the blood, as does the count of the immature neutrophils.[8,9,11,16,21,27,36]

CLINICAL PROBLEMS
Decreased level *(↓ 50 percent [adult, total]):* viral diseases—chicken pox, measles, rubella; leukemias—lymphocytic, monocytic; systemic lupus erythematosus; agranulocytosis; anemias—aplastic, folic acid deficiency, iron deficiency. *Drug influence:* antiobiotic therapy, immunosuppressive drugs, steroids (differs among individuals).

Elevated level *(↑ 70 percent [adult, total]):* acute infections—localized and systemic; inflammatory diseases—acute rheumatic fever, rheumatoid arthritis, gout, bacterial endocarditis; pneumonia and influenza; chronic obstructive lung disease; tissue damage—acute myocardial infarction, burns, acute and chronic renal failure, crushed injury; cancer—stomach, lung, and pancreas; leukemia (myelocytic); Hodgkin's disease; acquired hemolytic anemia; acute cholecystitis; peritonitis; acute appendicitis; acute pancreatitis; hemolytic disease of newborns; diabetes mellitus. *Drug Influence:* epinephrine (Adrenalin), digitalis, heparin, sulfonamides, lithium, steroids (cortisone, ACTH).

PROCEDURE
See Differential White Blood Cell Count.

FACTORS AFFECTING LABORATORY RESULTS
Drugs that may increase the neutrophil count (see *Drug Influence* above).

NURSING IMPLICATIONS WITH RATIONALE

Explain to the patient the purpose of the blood test. Explanation could be brief, such as, "to check the number of white blood cells." A more detailed explanation may be needed.

Inform the patient that food and drinks are not restricted.

Decreased level (↓ 50 percent)

Relate a decreased number of neutrophils to clinical problems. Note that neutrophils are decreased in lymphocytic and monocytic leukemias, but are increased in myelocytic leukemia.

Elevated level (↑ 70 percent)

Relate an increased number of neutrophils to clinical problems and drugs. Recognize that neutrophils are the first line of defense and respond immediately to acute infections and inflammatory disease.

Check the WBC count and, if it is increased, check the neutrophils. If the neutrophils comprise more than 70 percent of the total, an acute inflammatory process may be occurring due to infection or disease. The neutrophils can also increase following surgery due to trauma.

Assess the patient for signs and symptoms of an infection—i.e., elevated temperature, increased pulse rate, edema, redness, and exudate (wound drainage).

O

OCCULT BLOOD (Feces)

NORMAL RANGE
Adult: negative.
Child: negative.
Note: with a diet rich in meats, poultry, and fish, the occult blood test could be positive.

DESCRIPTION
Blood in the feces (stools) usually indicates gastrointestinal (GI) bleeding. If the blood is bright red, it can be indicative of bleeding in the lower large intestine or could indicate hemorrhoids. With upper gastrointestinal bleeding, blood may not be visible in the stools and an occult blood test on the feces is necessary to detect small quantities of GI bleeding. If more than 50 ml of blood is lost in the upper GI tract, the stools will appear dark and may be referred to as tarry stools, depending on the amount of bleeding.

Occult blood (nonvisible) in the feces may be present days or several weeks after a single bleeding episode. False positive occult blood test results may be due to ingestion of meats, poultry, and fish which contain heme compounds.[4,8,9,11,30]

CLINICAL PROBLEMS
Negative results: *Drug influence:* ascorbic acid (large amounts of vitamin C).
Positive results: peptic ulcer, gastritis, gastric carcinoma, bleeding esophageal varices, colitis, intestinal carcinoma, diverticulitis. *Drug influence:* boric acid, bromides, colchicine, iron preparations, iodine, indomethacin (Indocin), reserpine, potassium preparations, salicylates (aspirin), steroids (cortisone preparations), thiazide diuretics.

PROCEDURE
There are a variety of blood test reagents which may be used to test for occult blood. Some are more sensitive than others, and so the laboratory should indicate which test method was used. Orthotoluidine (Occultest) is considered the most sensitive test, more sensitive than the guaiac (least sensitive).

The patient should avoid meats, poultry, and fish for 3 days prior to obtaining the stool specimen, especially if orthotoluidine or benzidine tests are used.

Obtain a single random stool specimen and send it to the laboratory. Only a small amount of fecal material is needed. Stool may be obtained from a rectal examination. Many times the stool test is done on the nursing floor using a commercial kit.

The stool specimen does not need to be kept warm or examined immediately.

FACTORS AFFECTING LABORATORY RESULTS
Drugs (see *Drug Influence* above).
Foods; meats; poultry; fish; and green, leafy vegetables can cause a false positive test result.
Urine and soap solution in the feces may affect the test result.

NURSING IMPLICATIONS WITH RATIONALE

Explain to the patient that the purpose of the test is to determine whether hidden blood is present in the stools.

Instruct the patient not to eat meats, poultry, or fish for 3 days prior to the test. Green, leafy vegetables, if eaten in abundance, could cause a false positive test.

Instruct the patient not to take drugs which could cause false positive results for 3 days before the test, if possible.

Positive Result for Occult Blood

Relate clinical problems and drugs to a positive test for occult blood (see *Clinical Problems* above).

Obtain a history of recent or past bleeding episodes. Inform the physician of a history of GI bleeding.

Inform the physician if the patient is receiving medication which could cause a false positive test result (see *Drug Influence* above).

Encourage the patient to report abnormal-colored stools (e.g., tarry stools). Oral iron preparations can cause the stools to be black.

Determine whether the patient has had epigastric pain between meals. This type of pain could be indicative of a peptic ulcer.

Be sure the stool is not contaminated with menstrual discharge.

OSMOLALITY (Serum)

NORMAL RANGE

Adult: 280–300 mOsm/kg/H_2O.
Child: 270–290 mOsm/kg/H_2O.

DESCRIPTION

Serum osmolality is an indicator of serum concentration. It measures the number of dissolved particles (electrolytes, urea, sugar) in the serum and is helpful in the diagnosis of fluid and electrolyte imbalances. Sodium contributes 85 to 90 percent of the serum osmolality; changes in osmolality are usually due to changes in the serum sodium concentration. Doubling the serum sodium can give a rough estimate of the serum osmolality.

The hydration status of the patient is usually determined by the serum osmolality. An increased value (>300 mOsm/kg) can indicate dehydration, and a decreased value (<280 mOsm/kg) can indicate overhydration, or water excess. An osmometer is used in laboratories to determine serum osmolality; however, if the serum sodium, urea, and sugar are known, the serum osmolality can be calculated by the nurse, as follows.[11,12,16,30,36]

$$\text{Serum osmolality} = 2 \times \text{Serum sodium} + \frac{\text{BUN}}{3} + \frac{\text{Sugar}}{5}$$

CLINICAL PROBLEMS

Decreased level *(↓ 280 mOsm/kg H_2O [adult]):* excessive fluid intake, cancer of the bronchus and lung, adrenal cortical hypofunction.

Elevated level *(↑ 300 mOsm/kg H_2O [adult]):* diabetes insipidus, dehydration, hypernatremia, hyperglycemia, uremia.

PROCEDURE
Collect 5 to 10 ml of venous blood in a red-top tube. Prevent hemolysis.
There is no food or drink restriction.

FACTORS AFFECTING LABORATORY RESULTS
Hyperglycemia increases the serum osmolality.

NURSING IMPLICATIONS WITH RATIONALE

Explain to the patient the purpose of the test. Explanation could be brief, such as, "to
determine the hydration status of the body."
Explain to the patient that food and drinks are not restricted.

Decreased level ($\downarrow$ 280 mOsm/kg H_2O [adult])
Associate a decreased serum osmolality with serum dilution due to excessive fluid
intake (overhydration).
Observe for signs and symptoms of overhydration—i.e., a constant, irritated cough;
dyspnea; neck and hand vein engorgement; and chest rales.
Instruct the patient to decrease fluid intake.
Observe for signs and symptoms of water intoxication—i.e., headaches, confusion, irritability. Excessive amounts of hyposmolar solutions can "super-dilute" the intravascular fluid.

Elevated level ($\uparrow$ 300 mOsm/kg H_2O [adult])
Associate elevated serum osmolality with fluid volume deficit (hypovolemia or
dehydration), sodium overload, or hyperglycemia.
Assess for signs and symptoms of dehydration—i.e., thirst, dry mucous membranes,
poor skin turgor, and shock-like symptoms.
Encourage the patient to increase fluid intake.
Check for glycosuria. Increased sugar in the urine could indicate the presence of hyperglycemia.
Check the serum sodium, urea, and glucose for increased values. Calculate the serum
osmolality by either doubling the serum sodium or using the formula given in the
description.

OSMOLALITY (Urine)

NORMAL RANGE
Adult: 50–1200 mOsm/kg/H_2O, average 200–800 mOsm/kg H_2O.
Newborn: 100–600 mOsm/kg/H_2O.
Child: same as adult.

DESCRIPTION
The urine osmolality test is more accurate than the specific gravity in determining the
urine concentration, since its value reflects the number of particles, ions, and molecules and is not unduly influenced by large molecules. Specific gravity measures the
quantity and nature of the particles—i.e., sugar, protein, and intravenous dyes (these
elevate specific gravity but have little affect on osmolality).
The urine osmolality fluctuates in the same way that the specific gravity of urine does,
and it can be low or high according to the patient's state of hydration. A dehydrated

patient with normal kidney function could have a urine osmolality of 1000 mOsm/kg H_2O or more. When hemoconcentration occurs as a result of acidosis, shock, or hyperglycemia, the serum osmolality is elevated, and so should the urine osmolality be elevated.

If serum hyposmolality and hyponatremia occur with urine hyperosmolality, the problem is most likely the syndrome of inappropriate antidiuretic hormone (SIADH). ADH causes water reabsorption from the kidney, thus diluting the serum.[9,11,30,36]

CLINICAL PROBLEMS

Decreased level *(↓ 200 mOsm/kg H_2O [adult, average])*: excessive water intake, continuous IV 5 percent dextrose/water, diabetes insipidus, glomerulonephritis, acute renal failure, sickle cell anemia, multiple myeloma. *Drug influence:* diuretics.

Elevated level *(↑ 800 mOsm/kg H_2O [adult, average])*: high-protein diet, SIADH, Addison's disease (adrenal gland insufficiency), dehydration, hyperglycemia with glycosuria.

PROCEDURE

Give a high-protein diet for 3 days prior to the urine osmolality test.

Restrict fluids for 8 to 12 hours before the test.

Collect a random urine specimen, preferably in the morning. Label the specimen as a single random urine collection. Urine osmolality should be high in the morning, and if it is not, kidney dysfunction should be considered.

Send the urine specimen to the laboratory.

FACTORS AFFECTING LABORATORY RESULTS

Diuretics can cause urine hyposmolality.

A high-protein diet can cause urine hyperosmolality.

NURSING IMPLICATIONS WITH RATIONALE

Explain to the patient that the purpose of the test is to determine the kidney's ability to concentrate urine, or give a similar response.

Explain the procedure of the test if it requires more than a random urine sample for urine osmolality. A high-protein diet is taken for 3 days before the test, and oral fluids are restricted the night before. The first urine specimen of the morning is discarded, and the second specimen, taken an hour or two later, is sent to the laboratory.

Decreased level (↓ 200 mOsm/kg H_2O [adult, average])

Determine whether the decreased urine osmolality could be due to excessive intake of water (>2 quarts daily) or continuous IV administration of dextrose in water. A urine osmolality that remains less than 200 mOsm/kg after fluids are restricted could be indicative of early kidney impairment.

Explain to the patient the need to decrease excessive water intake.

Report to the physician when the patient is receiving 5 percent dextrose in water (D/W) continuously without any other solutes, such as saline (NaC1). The 5 percent D/W not only dilutes the urine, it can decrease the serum osmolality and cause water intoxication.

Observe for signs and symptoms of water intoxication—i.e., headaches, confusion, irritability, weight gain, and, later, cerebral edema (if severe).

Elevated level (↑ 800 mOsm/kg H_2O [adult, average])

Relate the elevated urine osmolality to clinical problems.

Instruct patients on high-protein diets to increase water intake.

Determine the hydration status of the patient. Dehydration will cause an elevated urine osmolality as well as elevated serum osmolality. A urine osmolality of 1000 mOsm/kg is not abnormal if the patient has a decreased fluid intake.

Check the serum osmolality. If the serum is hyposmolar and the urine is hyperosmolar, the problem could be due to SIADH. SIADH (continuous secretion of ADH) frequently occurs following surgery, trauma, or pain and will correct itself in a day or two. The function of ADH is to promote water reabsorption from the kidney tubules. The serum is diluted and the decreased urine is concentrated.

Keep an acurate intake and output record. The fluid intake should be comparative to the urine output.

OXYGEN SATURATION (So$_2$) (Arterial Blood)

NORMAL RANGE

Adult: arterial blood saturation (So$_2$) >95 percent, venous blood saturation (Svo$_2$) 70–80 percent.

Child: same as adult.

DESCRIPTION

The oxygen saturation is the percentage of oxygen in the blood that is combined with hemoglobin compared to the maximum amount of oxygen that the hemoglobin is capable of holding. The combination of oxygen saturation (So$_2$), partial pressure of oxygen (Po$_2$), and hemoglobin (Hgb or Hb) can indicate tissue oxygenation.

The oxygen saturation test is done during cardiac catheterization and respiratory function tests for diagnostic purposes and after open-heart surgery.[4,8,14,27,31]

CLINICAL PROBLEMS

Decreased level: lung diseases—asthma, emphysema, cancer of the lung, tuberculosis, cystic fibrosis (lung); cor pulmonale; pulmonary embolism; acute myocardial infarction; pulmonary edema; myasthenia gravis; sickle cell anemia; congenital heart defects.

Elevated level: O$_2$ administration.

PROCEDURE

Blood oxygen saturation is usually measured by spectrophotometry. It can be obtained from blood gas studies (see Arterial Blood Gases).

FACTORS AFFECTING LABORATORY RESULTS

Improper procedure and equipment.

NURSING IMPLICATIONS WITH RATIONALE

Explain to the patient the purpose and procedure of the test. Explain that the blood sample will be taken from an artery and that afterwards pressure will be applied for 5 minutes at the needle site.

Assess for signs of respiratory distress—i.e., pallor, apprehension, and dyspnea.

Be supportive to the patient and family. Respiratory disorders can cause apprehension and anxiety which can intensify breathing difficulty.

P

PARASITES AND OVA (Feces)

NORMAL RANGE
  Adult: negative.
  Child: negative.

DESCRIPTION
  Parasites may be present in various forms in the intestine, including the ova (eggs), larvae (immature form), cysts (inactive stage), and trophozoites (motile form) of protozoa. It is vitally important to detect parasites so that proper treatment can be ordered. Some of the organisms identified are amoeba, flagellates, tapeworms, hookworms, and roundworms. A history of recent travel outside of the United States should be reported to the laboratory, since it may help in identifying the parasite.[4,8,9,11,27,30]

CLINICAL PROBLEMS
  Positive result: protozoa—*Balantidium coli, Chilomastix mesnili, Entamoeba histolytica, Giardia lamblia, Trichomonas hominis;* helminths (adults)—*Ascaris lumbricoides* (roundworm), *Diphyllobothrium latum* (fish tapeworm), *Enterobius vermicularis* (pinworm), *Necatar americanus* (American hookworm), *Strongyloides stercoralis* (threadworm), *Taenia saginata* (beef tapeworm), *Taenia solium* (pork tapeworm).

PROCEDURE
  Usually, three stool specimens are collected, daily for 3 days or every other day (three specimens in 6 days). Stool specimens should be taken immediately to the laboratory.
  Mark the laboratory slip if the patient has been outside the United States in the last 1 to 3 years. Laboratories may require different information concerning the number of years spent outside the United States.
  A loose or liquid stool is more likely to indicate that trophozoites are present, and so the liquid stool should be kept warm and taken to the laboratory within 30 minutes. If the stool is semiformed or well-formed, it does not need to be kept warm, but should be taken to the laboratory at once.
  If the stool is tested for tapeworm, the entire stool should be sent to the laboratory so that the head (scolex) of the tapeworm can be identified. The tapeworm will continue to grow as long as the head is lodged in the intestine.
  Anal swabs are used to check for pinworm eggs, and the swabbing should be done in the morning before defecation or the morning bath.
  The stool specimen should be collected in a sterile bedpan and transferred to a sterile container, using a sterile tongue blade.
  Some laboratories may recommend that formalin be added to the specimen to preserve the ova and parasites.

FACTORS AFFECTING LABORATORY RESULTS
  Urine, toilet paper, soap, disinfectants, antibiotics, antacids, barium, harsh laxatives, and hypertonic saline enemas (Fleets) may affect the result of the test.

NURSING IMPLICATIONS WITH RATIONALE

Explain to the patient the procedure for collecting the stool specimen. The stool should be collected in the morning, preferably before a bath. Explain to the patient that he should not use soap or a Fleets enema, for this may destroy the parasite. The stool specimen should be obtained before treatment is initiated.

Administer a mild laxative or normal saline enema, with the physician's approval, to obtain the stool specimen, if necessary.

Take the fresh stool specimen to the laboratory immediately.

Report to the physician if the patient is taking antacids and/or antibiotics or has received barium in the last 7 days. These agents can alter the stool examination for parasites and ova.

Tell the patient not to put urine or toilet paper in the sterile bedpan. Disinfectants should not be used, for they can cause the ova to deteriorate.

Obtain a history from the patient concerning recent travel. Certain parasites are common to certain countries, and the physician and laboratory should be notified of this information.

Handle the stool specimen with care to prevent parasitic contamination of yourself and other patients.

Instruct the patient to wash his hands thoroughly after urinating and defecating.

PARTIAL THROMBOPLASTIN TIME (PTT), ACTIVATED PARTIAL THROMBOPLASTIN TIME (APTT) (Plasma)

NORMAL RANGE

Adult: Results vary in accordance with equipment and laboratory values. *PTT:* 60–70 seconds. APTT: 30–45 seconds (>50 seconds is abnormal).

Child: same as adult.

DESCRIPTION

The partial thromboplastin time (PTT) is a screening test used to detect deficiencies in all clotting factors except VII and XIII and to detect platelet variations. This test determines defects in the intrinsic coagulation system, bypassing the extrinsic system (factor VII cannot be detected with the PTT). It is more sensitive than the prothrombin time (PT) in detecting minor deficiencies, but is not as sensitive as the APTT.

The PTT is useful for monitoring heparin therapy. Heparin doses are adjusted according to the PTT test.

The activated partial thromboplastin time (APTT) is more sensitive in detecting clotting factor defects than the PTT, since the activator added in vitro shortens the clotting time. By shortening the clotting time, minor clotting defects can be detected.

The APTT is similar to the PTT, except that the thromboplastin reagent used in the APTT test contains an activator (kaolin, celite, or ellagic acid) for identification of deficient factors. This test is commonly used to monitor heparin therapy.[4,8,9,11,20,27,30,31,36]

CLINICAL PROBLEMS

Decreased level *(<30 seconds):* extensive cancer.

Increased level *(>70 seconds [PTT], >45 seconds [APTT]):* factor deficiency—factors V, VIII (hemophilia), IX (Christmas disease), X, XI, XII, cirrhosis of the liver; vitamin K deficiency; hypofibrinogenemia; prothrombin deficiency; von Willebrand disease (vascular hemophilia); disseminated intravascular coagulation (DIC) effects of fibrin degradation products (FDP); leukemias—myelocytic, monocytic; malaria. *Drug influence:* heparin, salicylates.

PROCEDURE

The test (collection) tube should contain the anticoagulant sodium citrate.

Collect 7 to 10 ml of venous blood in a blue-top tube. The tube should be filled to its capacity. The blood sample should be packed in ice and taken to the laboratory immediately.

An activated thromboplastin mixture (thromboplastin reagent and an activator, such as kaolin) is added to the patient's plasma sample and the control sample. When a small amount of calcium solution is added, the stopwatch is started; it is stopped when fibrin strands are noted. The tests are usually duplicated and should agree to within 1 to 1.5 seconds. The test can also be done using a "fibronmeter."

There is no food or drink restriction.

FACTORS AFFECTING LABORATORY RESULTS

A clotted blood sample.

A test (collection) tube without an anticoagulant.

NURSING IMPLICATIONS WITH RATIONALE

Explain to the patient the purpose of the test. Explanation could be brief, such as, "to determine whether there is a clotting problem or deficiency" *or* "to check on the effectiveness of heparin" *or* "to monitor the heparin dosage."

Check the APTT or PTT and report the results to the physician. The heparin dosage may need to be adjusted. The APTT range for heparin therapy is 1.5 to 3 times the normal value.

Assess the patient for signs and symptoms of bleeding—e.g., purpura (skin), hematuria, and nosebleeds.

Administer heparin subcutaneously or intravenously through a heparin lock. Do not aspirate when giving heparin subcutaneously, for a hematoma (blood tumor) could occur at the injection site.

Pco₂ (PARTIAL PRESSURE OF CARBON DIOXIDE) (Arterial Blood)

NORMAL RANGE

Adult: 35–45 mmHg (arterial), 35–50 mmHg (venous).
Child: similar to adult.

DESCRIPTION

The partial pressure of carbon dioxide (Pco_2) is the pressure exerted by CO_2 in the blood, and it reflects the ability of the lungs to exhale carbon dioxide. Carbon dioxide diffuses across the alveolar surfaces of the lung faster than oxygen. When there is alveolar (air sac) damage, CO_2 cannot escape, and the partial pressure of carbon dioxide builds up in the blood. Carbon dioxide (in the blood) combines with water (H_2O) to form carbonic acid ($H_2CO_3 \rightleftharpoons H^+ + HCO_3^-$), causing an acidotic state.

When the Pco_2 is elevated, hypoventilation occurs and respiratory acidosis results. Chronic obstructive lung disease (COLD) is a major cause of respiratory acidosis. With a decrease in Pco_2, hyperventilation (blowing off CO_2) occurs and respiratory alkalosis results.[8,9,17,27,30,36]

CLINICAL PROBLEMS

Decreased level *(↓ 35 mmHg [arterial]):* anxiety, hysteria; salicylate toxicity; tetany; hypoxia; fever; swimming, running; pregnancy; hyperthyroidism; delirium tremens; hepatic encephalopathy.

Elevated level *(↑ 45 mmHg [arterial]):* chronic obstructive lung disease (COLD)—emphysema, chronic bronchitis, bronchiectasis; severe asthmatic attack; pneumonia; anesthesia; cerebral trauma; flail chest—crush injury; obesity hypoventilation; kyphoscoliosis; neuromuscular disorders—Guillain-Barré, myasthenia gravis. *Drug influence:* narcotics—meperidine (Demerol), morphine; sedatives—barbituates.

PROCEDURE

Same as for Arterial Blood Gases and pH.

FACTORS AFFECTING LABORATORY RESULTS

See Arterial Blood Gases or pH.

Note: If venous blood is drawn, be sure this is noted on the report, since the respective normal values for arterial and venous blood vary greatly.

NURSING IMPLICATIONS WITH RATIONALE

Explain to the patient the purpose of the blood test. Explanation may be brief, such as, "to determine the lungs' ability to excrete (exhale) carbon dioxide."

Explain to the patient the procedure for the arterial blood gases (ABGs) test. Explanation could include: "Blood will be taken from an artery in the arm or groin; hand pressure will be applied to the puncture site to control bleeding."

Instruct the patient that he may eat and drink before the test.

Decreased level (↓ 35 mmHg [arterial])

Relate a low Pco_2 to clinical problems and respiratory alkalosis. Anxiety, hysteria, nervousness, and strenuous physical exertion can cause tachypnea (overbreathing). With rapid breathing, an excess of CO_2 is lost.

Check the results of the ABGs test. If the bicarbonate or base excess is decreased (metabolic acidosis), the lungs could be compensating (respiratory compensation) by hyperventilating to blow off CO_2, thus decreasing the acidotic state of the body fluids.

Assess for signs and symptoms of respiratory alkalosis, such as dizziness, rapid breathing, tetany spasms, and a Pco_2 lower than 35 mmHg.

Elevated level (↑ 45 mmHg [arterial])

Relate an elevated Pco_2 level to clinical problems, drugs, and/or respiratory acidosis. Emphysema, acute respiratory distress syndrome, and use of narcotics are the major causes of CO_2 retention.

Teach the patient breathing exercises to enhance CO_2 excretion from the lungs.

Perform chest clapping to break up bronchial and alveolar secretions. Carbon dioxide can be trapped in the lungs due to excess secretions and mucous plugs.

Encourage the patient to use the Intermittent Positive Pressure Breathing (IPPB) machine, if ordered, and make sure that it is being used properly. Intermittent positive pressure breathing improves ventilation and exchanges of gases in the lungs.

Demonstrate the postural drainage procedure, if not contraindicated, by lowering the head of the bed or having the patient lie over the side of the bed. Secretions are excreted by gravity.

Assess for signs and symptoms of respiratory acidosis, such as dyspnea (difficulty in breathing), disorientation, confusion, and an increased Pco_2 (> 45 mmHg).

pH (Arterial Blood)

NORMAL RANGE
 Adult: 7.35–7.45 (arterial), 7.34–7.42 (venous).
 Newborn: 7.27–7.47.
 Child: 7.36–7.44.

DESCRIPTION
 The pH is the negative logarithm of the hydrogen ion concentration, determining the acidity and alkalinity of body fluids. A low pH (<7.35) indicates an acid state of acidosis, either respiratory or metabolic, and a high pH (>7.45) indicates an alkaline state or alkalosis, either respiratory or metabolic. To determine whether the acidosis is due to respiratory or metabolic causes, the PCO_2 (respiratory) and bicarbonate level (HCO_3, metabolic) need to be known.
 A pH within the range of 6.8 to 7.8 is compatible with life.[8,9,17,27,30,36]

CLINICAL PROBLEMS
 Decreased level (↓ *7.35 [adult, arterial]): Metabolic acidosis:* diabetic ketoacidosis, severe diarrhea, starvation/malnutrition, kidney failure, burns, shock, acute myocardial infarction, acute alcoholic intoxication, adrenal cortical hypofunction. *Respiratory acidosis:* chronic obstructive lung disease (COLD)—emphysema; chronic bronchitis; severe asthma; Guillain–Barré syndrome; respiratory distress syndrome; pneumonia; anesthesia. *Drug influence:* narcotics—meperidine (Demerol), morphine; sedatives—barbiturates; acetazolamide (Diamox); ammonium chloride; paraldehyde.
 Elevated level (↑ *7.45 [adult, arterial]): Metabolic alkalosis:* severe vomiting, gastric suction, peptic ulcer, potassium loss (hypokalemia), excess administration of $NaHCO_3$, adrenal cortical hyperfunction, cystic fibrosis, hepatic failure. *Respiratory alkalosis:* salicylate toxicity (early phase); anxiety, hysteria; tetany; strenuous exercise (swimming, running); fever; hyperthyroidism; delirium tremens; pulmonary embolism. *Drug influence:* sodium bicarbonate, sodium oxalate, potassium oxalate.

PROCEDURE
 See Arterial Blood Gases.
 Collect 1 to 5 ml of arterial blood in a heparinized needle and syringe, remove the needle, and apply an airtight cap over the tip of the syringe.
 Place the syringe with arterial blood in an ice bag or container with some water and deliver it immediately to the laboratory. A gas analyzer machine is used for analyzing the ABGs.
 Indicate on the ABGs (arterial blood gases) slip if the patient is receiving oxygen, and give the rate of flow.
 Apply pressure to the puncture site for 2 to 5 minutes.
 There is no food or drink restriction.

FACTORS AFFECTING LABORATORY RESULTS
 Hemolysis of the blood sample.
 Improper handling of the blood sample (e.g., no ice around the blood or exposure to air.
 Drugs that can increase and decrease pH levels (see *Drug Influence* above).

NURSING IMPLICATIONS WITH RATIONALE

Explain to the patient the purpose of the arterial blood test. Explanation could be brief, such as, "to determine the acid–base status of the body fluids."
Explain to the patient the procedure for the ABGs test. Explanation could include:

"Blood will be taken from an artery in the arm or groin, hand pressure will be applied to the puncture site for 2 to 5 minutes to control bleeding."
Instruct the patient that he may eat and drink before the test.

Decreased level (↓ 7.35 [adult, arterial])
Relate a low pH (<7.35) to clinical problems associated with acidosis. This could be metabolic acidosis or respiratory acidosis.
Assess for signs and symptoms of metabolic acidosis, such as rapid, vigorous breathing (Kussmaul breathing); flushing of the skin; restlessness; and decreased HCO_3 and serum CO_2 levels.
Assess for signs and symptoms of respiratory acidosis, such as dyspnea (difficulty in breathing), disorientation, and an increased PCO_2.

Elevated level (↑ 7.45 [adult, arterial])
Relate a high pH (>7.45) to clinical problems associated with alkalosis. This could be metabolic alkalosis or respiratory alkalosis.
Assess for signs and symptoms of metabolic alkalosis, such as shallow breathing, vomiting, and increased HCO_3 and serum CO_2 levels.
Assess for signs and symptoms of respiratory alkalosis, such as overbreathing (hyperventilation), dizziness (vertigo), tetany spasms, and a decreased PCO_2.

PHENYLKETONURIA (PKU) (Urine), GUTHRIE TEST FOR PKU (Blood)

NORMAL RANGE
Adult: PKU and Guthrie test not usually done.
Child: *Phenylalanine:* 0.5–2.0 mg/dl. *PKU:* negative—positive when the serum phenylalanine is 12–15 mg/dl. *Guthrie:* negative—positive when the serum phenylalanine is 4 mg/dl.

DESCRIPTION
The urine phenylketonuria (PKU) and Guthrie (blood) tests are two screening tests used for detecting a hepatic enzyme deficiency (phenylalanine hydroxylase) which prevents the conversion of phenylalanine (amino acid) to tyrosine in the infant. Phenylalanine from milk and other protein products accumulates in the blood and tissues and can lead to brain damage and mental retardation. When the accumulation of phenylalanine is approximately 12 to 15 mg/dl, it converts to phenylpyruvic acid and is excreted in the urine.
At birth, the newborn's serum phenylalanine level is less than 2 mg/dl because of the mother's enzyme activity. After the third day of life or after 48 hours of milk ingestion, the serum level increases if phenylalanine is not metabolized.
The Guthrie procedure is the test of choice, since a positive test result occurs when the serum phenylalanine reaches 4 mg/dl (at 3 to 5 days of life), when the infant may still be in the hospital. A positive Guthrie test does not always indicate PKU, but, if it is positive, a specific blood phenylalanine test should be performed. The PKU urine test is done after the infant is 3 weeks old and should be repeated a week or two later. Significant brain damage usually occurs when the serum level is 15 mg/dl. If either the Guthrie test or the urine PKU is positive, the infant should be maintained on a low phenylalanine diet for 6 to 8 years.[8,11,27,30,35,36]

CLINICAL PROBLEMS
Elevated level *(↑ 4 mg/dl [child, Guthrie]):* phenylketonuria (PKU), low birth weight infants, hepatic encephalopathy, septicemia, galactosemia. *Drug influence:* aspirin and salicylate compounds, chlorpromazine (Thorazine), ketone bodies.

PROCEDURE

Guthrie test/Guthrie inhibition test: This is a bacterial inhibition procedure. Phenylalanine promotes bacterial growth (bacillus subtilis) when the serum level is greater than 4 mg/dl.

Cleanse the infant's heel and prick it with a sterile lancet. Obtain several drops of blood on the filter paper. The surface of the filter paper is streaked with bacillus subtilis, and if the bacillus grows, the test is positive. Check the procedure outlined by your institution.

The test should not be done before 2 to 4 days of milk intake (cow's milk or breast milk), and should preferably be done on the fourth day.

The date of birth and the date the first milk was ingested should be written on the laboratory slip.

Urine PKU: There are several urine tests for detecting phenylpyruvic acid. All utilize the reagent ferric chloride, which causes the urine specimen to turn green, when positive. The Phenistix (Ames Co.) is a dipstick with ferric salt in the filter paper; it is dipped in fresh urine or pressed against a wet diaper. The dipstick will turn green, if positive.

The urine PKU test should be done 3 to 4 weeks after birth. It is usually not positive for PKU until the serum phenylalanine levels are between 10 and 15 mg/dl.

The infant should be receiving milk for accurate Guthrie and urine PKU test results.

FACTORS AFFECTING LABORATORY RESULTS

Urine that is not fresh.

Vomiting and/or decreased milk intake—this may cause a normal serum phenylalanine level in the infant with PKU.

Aspirins and salicylate compounds can cause a false positive result.

Early PKU testing before the infant is 3 days old (Guthrie) or 2 weeks old (Phenistix).

NURSING IMPLICATIONS WITH RATIONALE

Elevated level (↑ 4 mg/dl)

Relate positive Guthrie and urine PKU test results to the clinical problem, phenylketonuria.

Explain to the mother the purpose of the Guthrie test for her infant. Explanation could be brief, such as, "to determine if an enzyme deficiency is present." A more detailed explanation may be needed, including information concerning the effects of the amino acid phenylalanine when it is not metabolized.

Explain to the mother the screening tests used to detect PKU. The Guthrie test is normally done while the mother and infant are in the hospital. Many pediatricians want the urine PKU done at home by the parent or in the doctor's office 3 to 4 weeks after birth as a follow-up test.

Teach the mother how to perform a urine PKU test accurately. A fresh, wet diaper or a fresh urine specimen should be used.

Instruct the mother that the baby should not receive aspirin or salicylate compounds for 24 hours before testing the urine. A false positive test could result. Tylenol should be given instead of aspirin.

Determine whether the infant has been taking adequate feedings (cow's milk or breast milk) before performing the Guthrie test. Vomiting and/or refusing to eat are common problems of PKU infants. This may cause a normal serum phenylalaline level.

Tell the mother which foods the baby should and should not have. The preferred milk substitute is Lofenalac (Mead Johnson and Co.), an enzymic casein hydrolysate with vitamins and minerals. It provides a balanced nutritional formula. Other low-phenylalanine foods are fruits, fruit juices, vegetables, cereals, and breads. High-protein foods should be avoided (such as milk shakes, ice cream, and cheese).

It is thought that after the age of 6 to 8 years, 90 percent of the brain growth has occurred, and the diet does not need to be as restrictive.

PHOSPHORUS (P)—INORGANIC (Serum)
Phosphate (PO$_4$)

NORMAL RANGE
Adult: 1.7–2.6 mEq/L or 2.5–4.5 mg/dl.
Newborn: 3.5–8.6 mg/dl.
Infant: 4.5–6.7 mg/dl.
Child: 4.5–5.5 mg/dl.

DESCRIPTION
Phosphorus is the principal intracellular anion, and most of phosphorus exists in the blood as phosphate. From 80 to 85 percent of the total phosphates in the body are combined with calcium in the teeth and bones.

Phosphorus is the lab term used, since phosphates are converted into inorganic phosphorus for the test. The many functions of phosphorus include metabolism of carbohydrates and fats, maintenance of the acid–base balance, utilization of B vitamins, promotion of nerve and muscle activity, and transmission of hereditary traits.

Phosphorus (P) metabolism and homeostasis are associated with calcium (Ca) metabolism. Both ions need vitamin D for their absorption from the GI tract. Phosphorus and calcium concentrations are controlled by the parathyroid hormone. Usually there is a reciprocal relationship between Ca and P—i.e., when serum phosphorus levels increase, serum calcium levels decrease, and when serum phosphorus levels decrease, serum calcium levels increase. In certain neoplastic bone diseases, this relationship is no longer true, since both Ca and P are increased.

A high serum phosphorus (serum phosphate) level is called hyperphosphatemia, which is usually associated with kidney dysfunction (poor urinary output). Hypophosphatemia means a low serum phosphorus or serum phosphate level.[4,5,8,9,11,30]

CLINICAL PROBLEMS
Decreased level (↓ *1.7 mEq/L [adult]):* starvation, malabsorption syndrome, hyperparathyroidism, hypercalcemia, hypomagnesemia, chronic alcoholism, vitamin D deficiency, diabetic acidosis, myxedema, continuous IV fluids with glucose. *Drug influence:* antacids—aluminum hydroxide (Amphojel); epinephrine (adrenalin); insulin; Mannitol.

Elevated level (↑ *2.6 mEq/L [adult]):* renal insufficiency, renal failure, hypoparathyroidism, hypocalcemia, hypervitaminosis D, bone tumors, acromegaly, fractures (healing). *Drug influence:* antibiotics—methicillin, tetracyclines; diphenylhydantoin (Dilantin); heparin; Lipomol; laxatives with phosphate.

PROCEDURE
Collect 5 ml of venous blood in a red-top tube.

The patient should be NPO (nothing by mouth) except for water for 8 hours before the test. Some laboratories will require NPO for 4 hours. Carbohydrate lowers serum phosphorus levels, because phosphate goes into the cells with glucose.

The blood sample should be taken to the laboratory within 30 minutes. The serum should be separated from the red blood cells quickly.

Prevent hemolysis of the blood sample. Do not shake the tube.

FACTORS AFFECTING LABORATORY RESULTS

A high-carbohydrate diet and IV fluids with glucose can lower the serum phosphorus level; hence a fasting specimen is needed.

Hemolysis of the blood sample can increase the serum phosphorus level. When red blood cells rupture, they release intracellular phosphate into the serum.

Late delivery of the blood sample (longer than 30 minutes) may cause the release of phosphorus from the blood cells into the serum. The serum should be separated from the blood clot within 30 minutes.

Drugs (see *Drug Influence* above). Amphojel can lower the serum phosphorus level.

NURSING IMPLICATIONS WITH RATIONALE

Explain to the patient the purpose of the test. Explanation could be brief, such as, "to determine the concentration of an ion (phosphorus) in the blood."

Tell the patient that food and beverages are restricted, except for water, after midnight until the blood is drawn. Call the dietary department to release the patient's breakfast tray after the blood sample is taken.

Hold medications in the morning until the blood sample is taken.

Hold intravenous fluid with glucose for 4 to 8 hours before the blood test, if possible. Glucose can lower the serum phosphorus level by promoting the shift of phosphate back into the cells.

Decreased level (↓ 1.7 mEq/L [adult])

Recognize clinical problems and drugs which can cause a phosphorus deficit—e.g., malnutrition, malabsorption syndrome, hypercalcemia, and vitamin D deficiency.

Teach the patient to eat foods rich in phosphorus (i.e., meats (beef, pork, turkey), milk, whole grain cereals, and almonds) if the decrease is due to malnutrition. Most carbonated drinks are high in phosphates.

Instruct the patient not to take antacids which contain aluminum hydroxide (Amphojel). Phosphorus binds with aluminum hydroxide; a low serum phosphorus level results.

Check the serum phosphorus, calcium, and magnesium levels and report changes to the physician if the serum levels are unknown. An elevated calcium level causes a decreased phosphorus level.

Monitor oral and intravenous phosphorus replacements. Some of the oral phosphate salts (Neutrophos) come in capsules, which are indicated if nausea is present. Administer IV phosphate (KH_2PO_4) slowly to prevent hyperphosphatemia.

Observe for signs and symptoms of hypophosphatemia—i.e., anorexia and pain in the muscles and bone. Relate symptoms to the patient's clinical condition or problem.

Observe for signs and symptoms of hypocalcemia (tetany) while the patient is receiving phosphate supplements.

Elevated level (↑ 2.6 mEq/L [adult])

Recognize clinical problems and drugs which can increase the serum phosphorus level—e.g., poor urinary output, hypocalcemia, and hypervitaminosis D.

Teach the patient to eat foods that are low in phosphorus—i.e., vegetables. Instruct the patient to avoid drinking carbonated sodas which contain phosphates.

Check the serum phosphorus, calcium, and magnesium levels. Observe for signs and symptoms of hypocalcemia (tetany); with an increased phosphorus level, calcium is usually low.

Monitor urinary output. A decreased urine output (<25 ml/hour or <600 ml/day) can increase the serum phosphorus level. Notify the physician of changes in urinary status.

PLATELET COUNT (Blood—Thrombocytes)

NORMAL RANGE
    Adult: 150,000–400,000 mm³ (mean, 250,000 mm³), 0.15–0.4 × 10¹²/L (SI units)
    Premature: 100,000–300,000 mm³.
    Newborn: 150,000–300,000 mm³.
    Infant: 200,000–475,000 mm³.

DESCRIPTION
    Platelets (thrombocytes) are fragments of cytoplasm from megakaryocyte in the bone marrow. Platelets are much smaller than erythrocytes. However, they are needed for blood coagulation (clotting), in which they clump and stick to rough surfaces and injured sites. A decrease in circulating platelets (less than 50 percent of the normal value) will cause bleeding, and if the decrease is severe, hemorrhaging may occur.
    Thrombocytopenia is the term for platelet deficiency or a low platelet count. It is commonly associated with leukemias, aplastic anemia, and idiopathic thrombocytopenic purpura. Increased platelet counts (thrombocytosis) occur in polycythemia, and fractures and after splenectomy. During chemotherapy, the platelet count (along with the WBC count) is extremely important in monitoring the effective dosage.[4,8,9,11,27,30,36]

CLINICAL PROBLEMS
    Decreased level *(<100,000 mm³ [adult]):* idiopathic thrombocytopenic purpura; multiple myeloma; cancer—bone, GI, brain; leukemias—lymphocytic, myelocytic, monocytic; anemias—aplastic, iron deficiency, pernicious, folic acid deficiency, sickle cell; liver disease—cirrhosis, chronic active hepatitis; systemic lupus erythematosus; disseminated intravascular coagulopathy (DIC); kidney diseases; eclampsia; acute rheumatic fever. *Drug influence:* antibiotics—chloromycetin, streptomycin; sulfonamides; aspirin (salicylates); quinidine; quinine; acetazolamide (Diamox); amidopyrine; thiazide diuretics; meprobamate (Equanil); phenylbutazone (Butazolidin); tolbutamide (Orinase); vaccine injections; chemotherapeutic agents.
    Elevated level *(>400,000 mm³ [adult]):* polycythemia vera; trauma—surgery, fractures; postsplenectomy; acute blood loss (peaks in 7 to 10 days); metastatic carcinoma; pulmonary embolism; high altitudes; tuberculosis; reticulocytosis; severe exercise. *Drug influence:* epinephrine (adrenalin).

PROCEDURE
    Venous blood: Collect 5 ml of venous blood in a lavender-top tube.
    Capillary blood: After bleeding occurs, discard the first few drops. Collect a drop of blood from a finger puncture and dilute the blood immediately with the appropriate diluting solution.
    There is no food or drink restriction.

FACTORS AFFECTING LABORATORY RESULTS
    Chemotherapy and X-ray therapy can cause a decreased platelet count.
    Drugs (see *Drug Influence* above).

NURSING IMPLICATIONS WITH RATIONALE

Explain to the patient that the purpose of the blood test is to determine the platelet count, or give a similar response.
Check the platelet count and report abnormal levels to the physician (if they are not known by the physician).

Decreased level (<100,000 mm³ [adult])

Recognize clinical problems and drugs related to platelet deficiency.

Observe for signs and symptoms of bleeding—skin (purpura, petechiae) or gastro-intestinal (hematemesis, rectal bleeding). Record findings on the chart and report them to the physician.

Inform the patient to avoid injury to himself, if possible. Mild injury could cause bleeding.

Monitor the platelet count, especially when the patient is receiving chemotherapy or radiation therapy for cancer.

Elevated level (>400,000 mm³ [adult])

Recognize clinical problems related to an elevated platelet level.

Po₂ (PARTIAL PRESSURE OF OXYGEN) (Arterial Blood)

NORMAL RANGE

Adult: 75–100 mmHg (arterial).

Child: similar to adult.

DESCRIPTION

The Po_2 measures the pressure of the oxygen dissolved in plasma. The Po_2 determines the amount of oxygen that can bind with hemoglobin. The pH affects the combining power of oxygen and hemoglobin, and with a low pH, there will be less oxygen in the hemoglobin.

The Po_2 indicates the ability of the lung to oxygenate the blood. There is a decrease in Po_2 in respiratory diseases, such as emphysema, pneumonia, and pulmonary edema.[8,9,14,31,36]

CLINICAL PROBLEMS

Decreased level (↓ 75 mmHg): chronic obstructive lung disease (COLD)—emphysema; cancer of the bronchus and lung; sickle cell anemia; cystic fibrosis; anemias; chronic bronchitis; cor pulmonale; acute myocardial infarction; pulmonary edema; respiratory distress syndrome; atelectasis; pulmonary embolism; myasthenia gravis.

Elevated level (↑ 100 mmHg): polycythemia.

PROCEDURE

See Arterial Blood Gases and pH.

FACTORS AFFECTING LABORATORY RESULTS

See Arterial Blood Gases or pH.

NURSING IMPLICATIONS WITH RATIONALE

Decreased level (↓ 75 mmHg)

Relate a low Po_2 value to clinical problems.

Explain to the patient the purpose of Po_2 test results—e.g., to determine the oxygen content in the blood, or to determine the ability of the lungs to oxygenate the blood.

Check the arterial blood gas reports for Po_2 levels.

Assess for signs and symptoms of oxygen deficit, such as dyspnea (difficulty in breathing), increased pulse rate, and cyanosis.

Administer oxygen at a low concentration (2 to 3 liters) when emphysema is present and at 6 liters for acute myocardial infarction, anemias, and myasthenia gravis.

PORPHOBILINOGEN (Urine)

NORMAL RANGE
Adult: *Random (qualitative):* Negative. *24 Hour (quantitative):* 0–1 mg/24 hours.
Child: same as adult.

DESCRIPTION
Porphobilinogen is one of the precursors of porphyrins, and large amounts are excreted during an acute attack of porphyria. Between attacks, there may not be an appreciable amount of porphobilinogen present. The test should be conducted during the acute phase.

The urine porphobilinogen test is ordered to detect the presence of porphyrias. Porphyrias are inherent metabolic disorders which affect the synthesis of heme of hemoglobin. Congenital porphyria (erythropoietic porphyria) is characterized by pinkish brown-stained teeth, pinkish yellow to reddish black urine, and skin photosensitivity. Uroporphyrin and coproporphyrin I are excreted.

Hereditary hepatic porphyria can be divided into three types: acute intermittent porphyria, porphyria variegate, and herditary coproporphyria. During an acute attack of porphyria, the urine becomes deep red and there are mental disturbances and severe abdominal pain. These attacks mimic various diseases (such as appendicitis and pancreatitis), and the leukocyte (WBC) count becomes elevated. Barbiturates, alcohol, and estrogen can precipitate an acute attack of porphyria.[8,9,11,14,20,27,30,36]

CLINICAL PROBLEMS
Elevated level *(>1 mg/24 hours):* acute intermittent porphyria, porphyria variegata, secondary malignant neoplasm, Hodgkin's disease, cirrhosis of the liver (occasionally).
Drug influence: antibiotics—penicillin, tetracyclines; antiseptics—ethoxazene (Diaphenyl), phenazopyridine (Pyridium); barbiturates, hypnotics; phenothiazines—chlorpromazine (Thorazine); procaine; sulfonamides.

PROCEDURE
Qualitative *(screening test):* Collect a random 30 ml or more of fresh urine during or immediately after an acute attack of porphyria. The patient will have acute abdominal pain. Protect the specimen from light.

Quantitative *(24 hour):* Collect the urine in a dark container. If it is collected in a clear container, protect it from light and refrigerate. The container should have an acidic preservative (hydrochloric acid, or HC1). Delta amino levulinic acid (ALA), which forms porphobilinogen, is not stable unless the urine is acidic. Urine should be collected immediately after the patient has an acute attack. Have the patient void, discard the urine, and then save all urine for 24 hours. Label the specimen with the date and the exact time the test started and ended.

Encourage the patient to take fluids. There is no food restriction.

FACTORS AFFECTING LABORATORY RESULTS
Exposure of the urine sample to light.
Drugs (see *Drug Influence* above).
Contamination of the urine with toilet paper or feces.

NURSING IMPLICATIONS WITH RATIONALE

Explain the procedure to the patient and family and tell them not to throw away any urine. Tell them that urine should not be exposed to light and should be refrigerated.

Post a sign on the patient's bed or door and in the Kardex saying that all urine should be saved for 24 hours and placed in a container in the refrigerator.

Inform the patient that he should not contaminate the urine with toilet paper or stools.

Elevated level (>1.0 mg/24 hours)

Recognize that this test is usually done during an acute attack (acute abdominal pain) to detect porphyria.

Observe and report urine color prior to an acute attack. The urine color could be amber to burgundy.

Observe for signs and symptoms of an acute porphyria attack—i.e., severe abdominal pain (colicky), mental disturbances, and neuropathy. Respiratory distress could occur.

Instruct the patient with porphyria to stay away from bright sunlight. Skin photosensitivity is a common problem, and skin lesions could result. Suggest that the patient use sun screen on exposed skin areas and wear protective clothing.

Emphasize that the patient should not take barbiturates, alcohol, or estrogens without the physician's permission. These agents can precipitate an acute attack of porphyria.

PORPHYRINS—COPROPORPHYRINS, UROPORPHYRINS (Urine)

NORMAL RANGE

Coproporphyrins: *Adult:* Random: 3–20 µg/dl (mcg/dl), 50–160 µg/24 hours. *Child:* 0–80 µg/24 hours.

Uroporphyrins: *Adult:* Random: negative. *Child:* 10–30 µg/24 hours.

DESCRIPTION

Porphyrins are utilized in the synthesis of hemoglobin and of any hemoproteins that are carriers of oxygen. The porphyrins are eliminated from the body in feces and urine, mainly as coproporphyrin I and III and as uroporphyrins. Normal excretion of coproporphyrins is minimal, but the amount excreted rises during liver damage, lead poisoning, and congenital porphyria (an inherent error of metabolism).

There is an increase in urine porphobilinogen with disorders of porphyrin metabolism. Porphobilinogen is one of the precursors of porphyrins (formed in the liver).[8,9,11,14,20,27,30,36]

CLINICAL PROBLEMS

Elevated level *(>160 µg/24 hours [adult, coproporphyrins]):* lead toxicity, cirrhosis of the liver, acute intermittent porphyria, viral hepatitis, infectious mononucleosis, porphyria variegata, porphyria cutanea tarda, acquired hemolytic anemia (autoimmune). *Drug influence:* antibiotic—tetracyclines, penicillin; antiseptics—ethoxazene (Diaphenyl), phenazopyridine (Pyridium); sulfonamides—sulfamethoxazole (Gantanol); barbiturates and hypnotics; phenothiazines—chlorpromazine (Thorazine); procaine.

PROCEDURE
Collect urine in a dark container containing the preservative sodium carbonate. If a large, clear container is used, protect it from light and refrigerate it.
Have the patient void, discard the urine, and then save all urine for 24 hours.
Label the specimen with the exact date and time the test started and ended (e.g., 7/24/84, 7:00 A.M. to 7/25/84, 7:01 A.M.).
There is no food or drink restriction.

FACTORS AFFECTING LABORATORY RESULTS
Exposure of the urine to light.
Drugs (see *Drug Influence* above).
Contamination of the urine with toilet paper and feces.

NURSING IMPLICATIONS WITH RATIONALE

Explain the procedure to the patient. Inform the patient and family that all urine must be saved for 24 hours. Have the patient participate in the urine collection if he or she is able. Emphasize that the urine should *not* be exposed to light.
Inform the patient not to contaminate the urine with toilet paper or feces.
Post a sign on the patient's bed or door and in the Kardex saying that all urine should be saved for 24 hours.

Elevated level (>160 μg/24 hours [adult, coproporphyrins])
Recognize clinical problems and drugs related to elevated prophyrin levels. Liver disease and lead poisoning cause an excessive amount of coproporphyrin III to be excreted.
Observe the color of a urine specimen exposed to light. A pinkish or red color should be reported.

POTASSIUM (Serum)

NORMAL RANGE
Adult: 3.5–5.0 mEq/L.
Infant: 3.6–5.8 mEq/L.
Child: 3.5–5.5 mEq/L.

DESCRIPTION
Potassium is the electrolyte found most abundantly in intracellular fluids (cells), with a cellular potassium level of 150 mEq/L. The serum potassium level is the measurable body potassium, and death could occur if serum levels are less than 2.5 mEq/L or greater than 7.0 mEq/L persist.
Eighty to ninety percent of the body potassium is excreted by the kidneys. When there is tissue breakdown, potassium leaves the cells and enters the extracellular fluid (interstitial and intravascular fluids). With adequate kidney functions, the potassium in the intravascular fluid (plasma/blood vessels) will be excreted, and with excessive excretion, a serum potassium deficit (hypokalemia) occurs. However, if the kidneys are excreting less than 600 ml/24 hours, potassium will accumulate in the intravascular fluid and serum potassium excess (hyperkalemia) can occur.
The body does not conserve potassium, and the kidneys excrete an average of 40 mEq/L daily (the range is 25 to 120 mEq/L/24 hours), even with a low dietary potas-

sium intake. The daily potassium requirement is 3 to 4 g, or 40 to 60 mEq/L.[8,11,17,27,30,31,34,36]

CLINICAL PROBLEMS

Decreased level *(↓ 3.5 mEq/L):* vomiting/diarrhea; dehydration; malnutrition/starvation; crash diet; stress; trauma, injury, or surgery; gastric suction; intestinal fistulas; diabetic acidosis; burns; renal tubular disorders; hyperaldosteronism; excessive ingestion of licorice; excessive ingestion of glucose; alkalosis (metabolic). *Drug influence:* potassium-wasting diuretics—i.e., furosemide (Lasix), thiazides (Hydrodiuril), ethacrynic acid (Edecrin); steroids—i.e., cortisone, estrogen; antibiotics—i.e., gentamicin, amphotericin, polymyxin B; bicarbonate; insulin; laxatives; lithium carbonate; sodium polystyrene sulfonate (Kayexalate); salicylates (aspirin).

Increased level *(↑ 5.0 mEq/L):* oliguria and anuria, acute renal failure, IV potassium in fluids, Addison's disease (adrenocortical hormone), crushed injury and burns (with kidney shutdown), acidosis (metabolic or lactic). *Drug influence:* potassium-sparing diuretics—i.e., spironolactone (Aldactone), triamterene (Dyrenium); antibiotics—i.e., penicillin G potassium, cephaloridine (Loridin); heparin; epinephrine; histamine (IV); marijuana; isoniazid.

PROCEDURE

Collect 5 to 10 ml of venous blood in a red-top tube.

Remove 5 to 10 ml of venous blood without the use of a tourniquet. Using a tourniquet can increase the serum potassium level by 5 to 20 percent. If a tourniquet is needed to obtain the specimen, then it should be released 1 to 2 minutes before the blood is drawn.

Prevent hemolysis of the blood specimen to avoid false high results.

Food, fluid, and drug restrictions are not necessary.

FACTORS AFFECTING LABORATORY RESULTS

The hydration status of the patient can cause false potassium test values. Overhydration can cause a false serum potassium deficit through hemodilution. Dehydration can cause a serum potassium excess through hemoconcentration. After the patient is hydrated, his or her serum potassium level may be normal or slightly low.

The use of a tourniquet can cause an increase in the serum potassium level.

Hemolysis of the specimen (blood) can result in high serum potassium level.

Drugs (see *Drug Influence* above).

NURSING IMPLICATIONS WITH RATIONALE

Explain to the patient that the test is to measure the potassium (electrolyte) level in the blood.

Explain the procedure involving use of the tourniquet.

Instruct the patient that he may eat and drink before the test.

Decreased level *(↓ 3.5 mEq/L)*

Recognize the clinical problems and drugs related to hypokalemia.

Observe for signs and symptoms of hypokalemia (serum potassium deficit)—i.e., vertigo (dizziness), hypotension, arrhythmias, nausea, vomiting, diarrhea, abdominal distention, decreased peristalsis, muscle weakness, and leg cramps.

Record intake and output. Polyuria can cause an excessive loss of potassium. Potassium is not conserved well in the body, and the kidney excretes potassium regardless of potassium intake.

Report serum potassium levels below 3.5 mEq/L. If the potassium (K) level is 3.0 to 3.5 mEq/L, it will take 100 to 200 mEq/L of potassium chloride (KCl) to raise the K level 1 mEq/L. If the K level is 2.9 mEq/L or less, it will take 200 to 400 mEq/L of KCl to raise the level 1 mEq/L.

Determine the patient's hydration status when hypokalemia is present. Overhydration can dilute the serum potassium level.

Recognize behavioral changes as a sign of hypokalemia. Low potassium levels can cause confusion, irritability, and mental depression. The serum potassium level should be checked in the present of any behavioral changes.

Teach the patient and family to eat foods high in potassium—i.e., fruits, dry fruits, vegetables, meats, nuts, coffee, tea, cocoa, and Coca Cola. The daily potassium requirements is 3 to 4 g, or 40 to 60 mEq/L.

Report ECG (EKG) changes. A prolonged and depressed ST segment and a flat or inverted T-wave is indicative of hypokalemia.

Dilute oral potassium supplements in at least 4 ounces of water or juice. Potassium is a corrosive agent and is most irritating to the gastric mucosa.

Monitor the serum potassium level in patients receiving potassium-wasting diuretics and steroids. Examples of potassium-wasting diuretics are Hydrodiuril, Lasix, and Edecrin. Cortisone steroids (such as prednisone) cause sodium retention and potassium excretion.

Assess for signs and symptoms of digitalis toxicity when the patient is receiving a digitalis preparation and a potassium-wasting diuretic or steroid. A lower serum potassium level enhances the action of digitalis. Signs and symptoms of digitalis toxicity are nausea and vomiting, anorexia, bradycardia, arrhythmia, and visual disturbances.

Teach patients to eat foods rich in potassium when they are taking drugs and foods (i.e., cortisone, potassium-wasting diuretics, laxatives, lithium carbonate, salicylates, insulin, glucose, and licorice) that decrease body potassium.

Monitor serum chloride, serum magnesium, and serum protein test results when hypokalemia is present. Correcting a potassium deficit with potassium only is not effective if chloride, magnesium, and protein levels are also low.

Administer intravenous potassium chloride (KCl) in a liter of parenteral fluids. Never give a bolus or IV push of KCl intravenously, for cardiac arrest can occur. Parenteral potassium chloride can only be administered intravenously when it is diluted (20 to 40 mEq/L per liter) and should never be given subcutaneously or intramuscularly. Concentrated IV KCl is irritating to the heart muscle and to the veins, causing phlebitis.

Check the intravenous site when the patient is receiving KCl in IV fluids. Infiltrated potassium is most irritating to the subcutaneous tissues (fatty tissues) and can cause tissue sloughing.

Measure gastrointestinal fluid loss from suctioning, vomiting, or diarrhea for appropriate potassium and other electrolyte replacement. Potassium, sodium, hydrogen, and chloride are most plentiful in the GI tract.

Irrigate gastrointestinal tubes with normal saline solution to prevent electrolyte loss.

Increased level (↑ 5.0 mEq/L)

Recognize clinical problems and drugs related to hyperkalemia.

Observe for signs and symptoms of hyperkalemia (serum potassium excess)—i.e., slow pulse rate (bradycardia), abdominal cramps, oliguria or anuria, tingling, and twitching or numbness of the extremities.

Assess urine output to determine renal function. Urine output should be at least 25 ml/hour, or 600 ml daily, and a urine output of less than 600 ml/day could cause hyperkalemia.

Report serum potassium levels greater than 5.0 mEq/L. High serum potassium levels can cause cardiac arrest.

Regulate the rate of IV fluids so that no more than 10 mEq KCl/L are administered per hour. Rapid administration of KC1 intravenously can result in hyperkalemia.

Check the age of whole blood before administering it to a patient with hyperkalemia. Blood 2 weeks old or older has an elevated serum potassium level.

Assess the patient's serum potassium level every 6 to 8 hours when it is elevated (↑ 7.0 mEq/L) and during treatment for hyperkalemia. The serum potassium level can change frequently during treatment.

Monitor the ECG (EKG) for QRS spread and peaked T-waves (signs of hyperkalemia). The pulse may be rapid, but if hyperkalemia persists, bradycardia or slow pulse can occur.

Restrict potassium intake when the serum potassium level is greater than 6.0 mEq/L.

Monitor patients receiving various medical treatments for hyperkalemia for signs and symptoms of continuous hyperkalemia or developing hypokalemia. The various medical treatments are as follows: (1) IV sodium bicarbonate increases the pH, causing potassium to shift back into the cells; (2) IV glucose and insulin can also cause potassium to shift back into the cells and are usually effective for 6 hours; (3) calcium gluconate decreases the myocardial irritability resulting from hyperkalemia but does not decrease the serum potassium level; (4) kayexalate (sodium polystyrene sulfonate) is a drug used as ion (resin) exchange, sodium for potassium. It can be administered orally or rectally and is considered the most effective method for treating hyperkalemia.

Notify the physician if the patient is receiving a digitalis preparation when calcium gluconate is given. An elevated serum calcium level enhances the action of digitalis, causing digitalis toxicity.

Observe for signs and symptoms of hypokalemia when adminstering Kayexalate for a prolonged period of time (two or more days).

POTASSIUM (Urine)

NORMAL RANGE
Adult: *Broad range:* 25–120 mEq/24 hours. *Average range:* 40–80 mEq/24 hours, 40–80 mmol/24 hours (SI units).

DESCRIPTION
Eighty to ninety percent of the body's potassium is excreted in the urine. A 24 hour urine potassium level is a valuable indicator of serum potassium status. A decrease in urinary potassium can indicate hyperkalemia (elevated serum potassium), and an increase in urinary potassium can indicate hypokalemia (low serum potassium) or may result from an increased potassium intake. If the kidneys are not functioning properly and there is decreased urine output (oliguria), the potassium excreted in the urine will be decreased and the serum potassium level will be elevated.[8,11,27,30,36]

CLINICAL PROBLEMS
Decreased level *(↓ 25 mEq/24 hours):* elevated serum potassium level, acute renal failure, diarrhea. *Drug influence:* potassium-sparing diuretics (e.g., Aldactone.)
Elevated level *(↑ 120 mEq/24 hours):* decreased serum potassium level, dehydration/starvation, chronic renal failure, diabetic acidosis, vomiting and gastric suction,

↑ adrenal cortical hormone or Cushing's disease, salicylate toxicity. *Drug influence:* potassium-wasting diuretics (e.g., Hydrodiuril, Lasix), prednisone.

PROCEDURE

The 24 hour urine specimen should be kept on ice or refrigerated.

Food and fluid do not need to be restricted.

Potassium supplements given as salt replacement should be eliminated for 48 hours.

FACTORS AFFECTING LABORATORY RESULTS

Failure to refrigerate the urine container.

Fecal material and toilet paper contamination.

Vomiting or gastric suctioning can cause hypokalemia due to potassium loss from the GI tract, and the accompanying metabolic alkalosis can cause an increase in urinary potassium loss. With a high urinary potassium excretion, the hypokalemic state could become more severe.

NURSING IMPLICATIONS AND RATIONALE

Decreased level (↓ 24 mEq/24 hours)

List the clinical problems attributing to a low urinary potassium excretion.

Explain to the patient that the purpose of the test is to determine whether his kidneys are excreting an adequate amount of potassium or whether the body is retaining it.

Instruct the patient to save all of his urine for 24 hours and place it in the container, which should be on ice or refrigerated.

Observe for signs and symptoms of hyperkalemia. When urinary potassium excretion is decreased, the serum potassium level may be increased. Signs and symptoms of hyperkalemia are oliguria, abdominal cramps, bradycardia, and tingling, twitching, or numbness in the extremities.

Check the arterial pH or the serum CO_2 levels. If metabolic acidosis is present (decreased pH and serum CO_2), the serum potassium may be elevated and the urinary potassium may be decreased. Potassium is frequently retained in the body during metabolic acidosis.

Metabolic acidosis: ↓ pH, ↓ serum CO_2 → ↑ Serum K, ↓ urinary K.

Elevated level (↑ 120 mEq/24 hours)

List clinical problems contributing to a high urine potassium excretion.

Explain to the patient that an increase in potassium intake or the use of diuretics (potassium-wasting) will result in an excess urinary potassium excretion.

Observe for signs and symptoms of hypokalemia. When urinary potassium excretion is increased, the serum potassium level is frequently decreased. Signs and symptoms of hypokalemia are vertigo (dizziness), hypotension, arrhythmia, muscle weakness, and decreased peristalsis.

Determine arterial pH or serum CO_2 levels. If metabolic alkalosis is present (elevated pH and serum CO_2), the serum potassium level may be low and the urine potassium may be increased. Hydrogen and potassium are excreted together in the urine and alkalosis results. Vomiting and gastric suction can cause metabolic alkalosis.

Metabolic alkalosis: ↑ pH, ↑ serum CO_2 → ↓ Serum K, ↑ urinary K.

PREGNANEDIOL (Urine)

NORMAL RANGE
Adult: *Women:* 0.5-1.5 mg/24 hours (proliferative phase), 2-7 mg/24 hours (luteal phase), 0.1-1.0 mg/24 hours (postmenopausal). *Men:* 0.1-1.5 mg/24 hours.
Child: 0.4-1.0 mg/24 hours.

DESCRIPTION
Pregnanediol is the major metabolite of progesterone produced by the ovary during the secretary phase of the menstrual cycle (second half) and by the placenta. Progesterone is responsible for uterine changes after ovulation and for maintaining pregnancy after fertilization. A steady rise in urinary pregnanediol levels occurs during pregnancy, and a decrease in these levels indicates placental dysfunction (not fetal) and the possibility of an abortion. Progesterone therapy would most likely be indicated in such a case.

Urinary pregnanediol levels may be used to determine menstrual disturbances and are used to verify ovulation in those who haven't been able to become pregnant. The pregnanediol levels rise rapidly after ovulation, and they can be used as an indicator of ovulation time. This test should not be mistaken for the pregnanetriol test.[4,8,27,30,36]

CLINICAL PROBLEMS
Decreased level *(↓ 0.5 mg/24 hours):* amenorrhea (menstrual disorders), ovarian hypofunction, threatened abortion, pregnancy complicated by intrauterine death, benign neoplasms of the ovary and breast, lutein cell tumor of the ovary, preeclampsia.
Elevated levels *(↑ 7 mg/24 hours):* pregnancy, ovarian cyst, choriocarcinoma of the ovary, adrenal cortex hyperplasia.

PROCEDURE
Collect urine over a 24 hour period in a large container/bottle and keep it refrigerated. Label the bottle with the patient's name and the dates and exact times of collection (e.g., 4/10/83, 8:00 A.M. to 4/11/83, 8:00 A.M.).
The container usually contains a preservative (boric acid).
Record on the laboratory slip the date of the last menstrual period.
Take the urine bottle to the laboratory immediately after the urine collection has been completed.
There is no food or drink restriction.
The urine may also be used to determine estradiol (E_3) levels in conjunction with the pregnanediol levels.

FACTORS AFFECTING LABORATORY RESULTS
Toilet paper and feces in the urine.
An unrefrigerated urine collection which has not been analyzed for several days.

NURSING IMPLICATIONS WITH RATIONALE

Explain to the patient the purpose of the urine test. A brief explanation could be "to determine the amount of a hormone in the urine." A more detailed explanation may be needed, such as, "to determine whether there is a decreased amount of hormone (progesterone) which is causing the menstrual disorder" *or* "to determine whether there is an increased amount of hormone in the urine, which usually indicates normal pregnancy."

Explain to the patient the procedure for collecting urine. Explain that all urine should be saved and placed in the labelled container in the refrigerator.

Instruct the patient not to put toilet paper or feces in the urine.

Post on the patient's door or bed and in the Kardex the date and time of urine collection.

Decreased level (↓ 0.5 mg/24 hours)

Recognize clinical problems that may cause a decreased pregnanediol level—i.e., menstrual disorder (amenorrhea), threatened abortion, and complicated pregnancy.

Obtain a history of menstrual changes (menstruation patterns—frequency, length of period, flow, and discomfort).

Obtain a history of pregnancy complications or problems. Record when the patient had her last menstrual period and whether bleeding is present (how long has it occurred, how much bleeding, and is it continuous?).

Give support to the patient and family by listening, spending time with them, and answering questions, if possible. Supportive care can reduce anxiety.

Monitor the urine pregnanediol levels if several tests have been ordered over a period of days or weeks. The levels can indicate progesterone production and whether progesterone therapy is needed.

Elevated level (↑ 7 mg/24 hours)

Recognize clinical problems that can cause an elevated pregnanediol level, such as pregnancy and an ovarian cyst. Pregnanediol level should increase during pregnancy. After 18 to 24 weeks, the level should be 13 to 22 mg/24 hours, and after 28 to 32 weeks, the level should be 27 to 47 mg/24 hours. In the last 2 weeks of pregnancy, the urine pregnanediol level decreases.

Ask when the patient had her last period; this should be recorded on the laboratory slip.

PREGNANETRIOL (Urine)

NORMAL RANGE

Adult: Male: 0.4–2.4 mg/24 hours. *Female:* 0.5–2.0 mg/24 hours.
Infant: 0–0.2 mg/24 hours.
Child: 0–1.0 mg/24 hours.

DESCRIPTION

Pregnanetriol (17-hydroxyprogestone) comes from adrenal corticoid synthesis. It should not be mistaken for pregnanediol, because it is not a derivative of progesterone. The pregnanetriol test is useful in diagnosing congenital adrenal cortical hyperplasia.[2,8,36]

CLINICAL PROBLEMS

Decreased level *(↓ 0.4 mg/24 hours):* anterior pituitary hypofunction.
Elevated level *(↑ 2.4 mg/24 hours):* congenital adrenal cortical hyperplasia, adrenal cortical hyperfunction, malignant neoplasm of the adrenal gland.

PROCEDURE

Collect urine for 24 hours in a large bottle and keep the urine refrigerated. No preservative is needed.

Label the bottle with the patient's name and the dates and exact times of collection (e.g., 2/3/84, 8:00 A.M. to 2/4/84, 8:02 A.M.).

There is no food or drink restriction.

FACTORS AFFECTING LABORATORY RESULTS
None known.

NURSING IMPLICATIONS WITH RATIONALE

Explain to the patient that the purpose of the test is to determine the amount of a substance which comes from the adrenal gland and is excreted in the urine.

Instruct the patient and family to save all urine for 24 hours and to keep the urine refrigerated.

Tell the patient not to put toilet paper or feces in the urine.

Explain to the patient that food and drink before and during the test are permitted.

Post on the patient's door or bed and in the Kardex instructions for the 24 hour urine collection—i.e., the date and time of urine collection, and that all urine be refrigerated.

PROTEIN (TOTAL) (Serum)

NORMAL RANGE
   Adult: 6.0–8.0 g/dl.
   Premature: 4.2–7.6 g/dl.
   Newborn: 4.6–7.4 g/dl.
   Infant: 6.0–6.7 g/dl.
   Child: 6.2–8.0 g/dl.

DESCRIPTION

The total protein is composed mostly of albumin and globulins (see Protein Electrophoresis). The use of the total serum protein test is limited unless the serum albumin, A/G ratio, or protein electrophoresis tests are also performed.

The protein level needs to be known to determine the significance of its components. With certain disease entities (i.e., collagen diseases, cancer, and infections), the total serum protein levels may be normal when the protein fractions are abnormal (decreased or elevated).[4,9,11,30,35]

CLINICAL PROBLEMS

Decreased level *(↓ 6 g/dl [adult]):* prolonged malnutrition, starvation, low-protein diet, diet, malabsorption syndrome, cancer of the GI tract, ulcerative colitis, Hodgkin's disease, severe liver disease, chronic renal failure, severe burns, water intoxication.

Elevated level *(↑ 8 g/dl [adult]):* dehydration (hemoconcentration), vomiting, diarrhea, rhea, multiple myeloma, respiratory distress syndrome, sarcoidosis.

PROCEDURE

Collect 5 to 10 ml of venous blood in a red-top tube.

Prevent hemolysis of the blood sample.

The patient should be NPO (food) for 8 hours before blood is drawn. There are no restrictions on water and medications. A high-fat diet should not be given for 24 hours before the test.

FACTORS AFFECTING LABORATORY RESULTS

Hemolysis of the blood sample.

A high-fat diet before the test.

The bromsulphalein (BSP) test for liver function can cause a false serum protein elevation and should not be performed for 48 hours before the total protein test.

NURSING IMPLICATIONS WITH RATIONALE

Explain the purpose of the test to the patient. Explanation may be brief, such as, "to determine the protein level in the blood."

Instruct the patient to avoid eating foods high in fat content for 24 hours before the test. Explain to the patient that he or she will be NPO (nothing by mouth) after the dinner meal or after midnight, except for water and medications.

Decreased level (↓ 6 g/dl)

Recognize clinical problems associated with a serum protein deficit—i.e. malabsorption, malnutrition, prolonged inadequate protein intake, and others (see *Clinical Problems* above).

Assess the patient's dietary intake. If the deficit is due to poor nutrition, encourage the patient to increase protein intake (eggs, cheese, meats, beans).

Plan a well-balanced diet with the patient. Collaborate with the dietitian and/or have the dietitian see the patient.

Elevated level (↑ 8 g/dl)

Recognize clinical problems associated with a serum protein excess. Hemoconcentration caused by dehydration is a frequent cause of total serum protein excess.

Assess the patient for signs and symptoms of dehydration—i.e., extreme thirst, poor skin turgor, dry mucous membranes, tachycardia, and increased respirations.

Check urinary output. The serum protein level may be increased (it also could be decreased) with kidney dysfunction. If kidney dysfunction is due to dehydration, vomiting, or diarrhea, the serum protein level will most likely be elevated.

Monitor fluid replacement (IV or orally). The serum protein level should return to normal when the patient is adequately hydrated. Care should be taken to prevent overhydration when forcing fluids.

PROTEIN ELECTROPHORESIS (Serum)

NORMAL RANGE
Adult:

	Weight (g/dl)	% of Total Protein
Albumin	3.5–5.0	52–68
Globulin	1.5–3.5	32–48
Alpha-1 (α1)	0.1–0.4	2–5
Alpha-2 (α2)	0.4–1.0	7–13
Beta (β)	0.5–1.1	8–14
Gamma (γ)	0.5–1.7	12–22

Child:

	Albumin (g/dl)	Globulins (g/dl)			
		α1	α2	β	γ
Premature	3.0–4.2	0.1–0.5	0.3–0.7	0.3–1.2	0.3–1.4
Newborn	3.5–5.4	0.1–0.3	0.3–0.5	0.2–0.6	0.2–1.2
Infant	4.4–5.4	0.2–0.4	0.5–0.8	0.5–0.9	0.3–0.8
Child	4.0–5.8	0.1–0.4	0.4–1.0	0.5–1.0	0.3–1.0

DESCRIPTION

Serum proteins are made up of albumin and globulins. Albumin is the smallest of the protein molecules, but it makes up the largest percentage of the total protein value. Changes in the albumin level will affect the total protein value. Albumin plays an important role in maintaining serum colloid osmotic pressure. The globulin molecules are about 2.5 times as large as albumin molecules, but they are not as effective in maintaining serum osmotic pressure as albumin molecules are.

Serum protein electrophoresis is a process which separates various protein fractions into albumin, alpha-1-globulin, alpha-2-globulin, beta-globulin, and gamma-globulin. The gamma-globulins are the body's antibodies, which contribute to immunity.[4,8,9,11,27,30,35,36]

CLINICAL PROBLEMS

Protein Fraction	Decreased Level	Elevated Level
Albumin	Chronic liver disease	Dehydration
	Malnutrition	Exercise
	Starvation	
	Malabsorption syndrome	
	Advanced malignancy	
	Leukemia	
	Congestive heart failure	
	Toxemia of pregnancy	
	Nephrotic syndrome	
	Chronic renal failure	
	Burns	
	Systemic lupus erythematosus	
Globulin		
$\alpha 1$	Emphysemia due to	Pregnancy
	α1-antitrypsin deficiency	Neoplasm
		Acute infection
		Tissue necrosis
$\alpha 2$	Hemolytic anemia	Acute infection
	Severe liver disease	Injury, trauma
		Burns
		Extensive neoplasma
		Rheumatic fever
		Rheumatoid arthritis
		Acute myocardial infarction
		Nephrotic syndrome
β	Hypocholesterolemia	Hypothyroidism
		Biliary cirrhosis
		Kidney nephrosis
		Diabetes mellitus
		Cushing's disease
		Malignant hypertension
γ	Nephrotic syndrome	Collagen disease
	Lymphocytic leukemia	Rheumatoid arthritis
	Lymphosarcoma	Lupus erythematosis
		Hodgkin's disease

Protein Fraction	Decreased Level	Elevated Level
	Hypogammaglobulinemia or agammaglobulinemia	Malignant lymphoma Chronic lymphocytic leukemia Multiple myeloma Liver disease
Electrophoretic patterns:		
Pattern I	↓ albumin ↑ α2-globulin	Acute stressful situation Acute infections Myocardial infarction Severe burns Surgery
Pattern II	↓ (slightly) albumin ↑ (slightly) 2-globulin ↑ (slightly) gamma globulin	Chronic infection and inflammatory Cirrhosis Collagen disease (rheumatoid)
Pattern III	↓ (moderately) albumin ↑ gamma globulin ↑ or normal beta	Collagen disease (lupus) Subacute bacterial endocarditis Sarcoidosis

PROCEDURE

Collect 5 to 10 ml of venous blood in a red-top tube.
There is no food or drink restriction.

FACTORS AFFECTING LABORATORY RESULTS

The Bromsulphalein (BSP) test could cause a false elevation; however, this test is no longer performed.

NURSING IMPLICATIONS WITH RATIONALE

Explain to the patient that the purpose of the test is to determine the increases and decreases of the protein components in the blood. A more detailed explanation may be needed.

Explain to the patient that food and drink are not restricted.

Check the albumin level from the protein electrophoresis results. Many clinical problems are the result of a serum albumin deficit.

Assess for peripheral edema in the lower extremities when the albumin level is decreased. Albumin is the major protein compound responsible for plasma colloid osmotic pressure. With a decreased albumin level, fluid seeps out of the blood vessels into the tissue spaces. Cirrhosis of the liver and congestive heart failure are clinical problems which can cause an albumin deficit and edema.

Encourage the patient to increase protein intake. Malnutrition and cirrhosis of the liver are associated with a poor-protein diet. Suggest foods high in protein—i.e., beans, eggs, meats, and milk.

Check electrophoretic patterns and associate abnormal protein fractions with clinical problems (see *Clinical Problems* above).

Assess urinary output. Renal and collagen (lupus) diseases occur with abnormal protein fractions. Urine output should be 25 ml/hour or 600 ml/24 hours. Check for albumin in the urine.

PROTHROMBIN TIME (PT) (Plasma)
Pro-time

NORMAL RANGE
Adult: 11–15 seconds (depending on the method and reagents used) *or* 70–100 percent. *For anticoagulant therapy:* 2–2.5 times the control in seconds *or* 20–30 percent.
Child: same as adult.

DESCRIPTION
Prothrombin (factor II of the coagulation factors) is produced by the liver and requires vitamin K for its synthesis (see Factor Assay). Prothrombin is converted to thrombin by the action of thromboplastin, which is needed to form a blood clot.

The prothrombin time (PT) is one of the tests usually performed to test clot formation. The prothrombin time measures the clotting ability of factors I (fibrinogen), II (prothrombin), V, VII, and X. Alterations of factors V and VII will prolong the PT for about 2 seconds, or 10 percent of normal. In liver disease, the PT is usually prolonged, since the liver cells cannot synthesize prothrombin.

The major use of the PT test is to monitor oral anticoagulant therapy—i.e., with bishydroxycoumarin (Dicumarol) and warfarin sodium (Coumadin).[4,8,9,11,20,30,31,36]

CLINICAL PROBLEMS
Decreased level *(<11 seconds):* thrombophlebitis, myocardial infarction, pulmonary embolism. *Drug influence:* barbiturates, digitalis preparations, diuretics, diphenhydramine (Benadryl), oral contraceptives, rifampin, metaproterenol (Metaprel) vitamin K.

Increased level *(>15 seconds):* liver diseases—cirrhosis of the liver, hepatitis, liver abscess, cancer of the liver; afibrinogenemia; factor II deficiency; factor V deficiency; factor VII deficiency; factor X deficiency; fibrin degradation product (FDP); leukemias; congestive heart failure; erythroblastosis fetalis (hemolytic disease of the newborn). *Drug influence:* antibiotics—penicillin, streptomycin, carbenicillin, chloramphenicol (Chloromycetin), kanamycin (Kantrex), neomycin, tetracyclines; anticoagulants, oral (Dicumarol, Coumadin); chlorpromazine (Thorazine); chlordiazepoxide (Librium); diphenylhydantoin (Dilantin); heparin; methyldopa (Aldomet); mithramycin; reserpine (Serpasil); phenylbutazone (Butazolidin); quinidine; salicylates (aspirin); sulfonamides.

PROCEDURE
The test (collection) tube should contain an anticoagulant, either sodium oxalate or sodium citrate.

Collect 7 to 10 ml of venous blood in a black-top tube (sodium oxalate). The blood must be tested within 1 hour after the blood has been drawn. The tube should be filled to its capacity. Some black-top tubes contain sodium citrate, so check with the laboratory.
OR
Collect 7 to 10 ml of venous blood in a blue-top tube (sodium citrate). The blood should be tested within 4 hours to prevent inactivation of some of the factors. The tube should be filled to its capacity.

Deliver the blood sample to the lab packed in ice. If the blood clots before testing, a new blood sample should be taken.

The blood sample is mixed with the reagents calcium chloride and thromboplastin. Blood testing is run in duplicate or triplicate. Agreement between the tests should be within 1 second for duplicates. If it is not, a third test must be run (PT values from 1 to 30 seconds).

Control values are given with the patient's PT values. Control values may change from day to day; this is an indication of the minor variables in the testing conditions.

There is no food or drink restriction.

FACTORS AFFECTING LABORATORY RESULTS
A clotted blood sample will cause an inaccurate result.
A high-fat diet (decreased PT) and alcohol (increased PT) may cause an endogenous change of PT production.
Leaving a blood sample at room temperature for several hours (1 to 4 hours).

NURSING IMPLICATIONS WITH RATIONALE

Explain to the patient the purpose of the test. Explanation may be brief, such as, "to determine how fast the blood clots." If the purpose of the test is to monitor anticoagulant therapy, inform the patient that blood will be drawn daily or at specified times.

Explain to the patient that food and drinks are not restricted.

Hold medications (if possible) that may affect the PT test results. If such medications *are* given, list the names of the drugs on the lab slip and in the Kardex or the patient's chart.

Take the blood sample immediately to the laboratory for testing. There should be an anticoagulant in the tube and the blood should fill the tube.

Increased level (>15 seconds)

Monitor the prothrombin time when the patient is receiving anticoagulant therapy. The desired PT with anticoagulant therapy is 2 to 2.5 times the control PT in seconds. The PT may be slightly lower when treating cardiac patients—18 to 24 seconds in patients with a thrombus. The desired PT range is 26 to 40 seconds. When the PT is above 40 seconds, bleeding may occur.

Inform the physician of the patient's PT daily or as ordered. The physician may want the anticoagulant held (drug adjustment) until the current PT has been received. The results are usually called to the floor by the laboratory personnel.

Observe the patient for signs and symptoms of bleeding—purpura (skin), hematuria (hemastix test), hematemesis, nosebleeds, etc. Report observations to the physician and record them in the patient's chart.

Administer vitamin K intramuscularly (IM) *as ordered* when the PT is over 40 seconds or when there is bleeding. IM injections can cause hematomas at the injection site when anticoagulants are used.

Instruct the patient not to self-medicate when receiving anticoagulant therapy. Over-the-counter drugs may either increase or decrease the effects of the anticoagulants (drug interaction) and the results of the PT test.

Instruct the patient to take the prescribed anticoagulants as ordered by the physician. Missed doses could affect the PT test.

Assess the alcohol consumption. Constant alcohol intake over a period of time can affect liver function, which in turn can cause a prolonged prothrombin time.

See Partial Thromboplastin Time, Activated Partial Thromboplastin Time.

R

RED BLOOD CELL INDICES (MCV, MCH, MCHC) (Blood)
Erythrocyte Indices

NORMAL RANGE

	Adult	Newborn	Child
RBC count (million/mm^3 $\times$ 10^{12}/L [SI units])	Male: 4.6–6.0 Female: 4.0–5.0 4.6–6.0 $\times$ 10^{12}L	4.8–7.2 4.8–7.2 $\times$ 10^{12}L	3.8–5.5 3.8–5.5$\times$ 10^{12}L
MCV (cuμ, [conventional]) or fl [SI units])	80–98	96–108	82–92
MCH (pg [conventional and SI units])	27–31	32–34	27–31
MCHC (% or g/dl [conventional] or SI units)	32–36% 0.32–0.36	32–33% 0.32–0.33	32–36% 0.32–0.36

DESCRIPTION

Red blood cells (RBC) contain hemoglobin, which is needed to carry oxygen to body cells. The red blood cell count is usually given in SI units (number of RBC per liter) of blood; hemoglobin is given in grams per deciliter (g/dl); and hematocrit is expressed as the percentage of the cells in a unit volume of blood. The values for the total number of RBC, hemoglobin, and hematocrit have to be known to calculate the red blood cell indices: MCV (mean corpuscular volume), MCH (mean corpuscular hemoglobin), and MCHC (mean corpuscular hemoglobin concentration). Other names for red blood cell indices are *erythrocyte indices* and *corpuscular indices.*

To identify the types of anemias, the physician depends on RBC indices (MCV, MCH, MCHC), which give the size, hemoglobin content, and hemoglobin concentration of the red blood cells.

MCV: This is the mean volume of red blood cells, measured as cubic microns (cuμ or $\pounds$) or femtoliters (fl). The value indicates the size of the red blood cells—microcytic, normocytic, or macrocytic. If the cells are microcytic, the MCV would be less than 80 fl, and if they are macrocytic, the MCV would be greater than 98 fl. Iron deficiency anemia is associated with microcytic cells, and pernicious anemia is associated with macrocytic cells. The red blood cells are normocytic when the MCV value is in the normal range.

MCH: This is the weight of hemoglobin in red blood cells, regardless of their size. In macrocytic anemias, the MCH is elevated, and it is decreased in hypochromic anemia. The MCH is derived by dividing the RBC count into ten times the hemoglobin (Hb) value:

$$\text{MCH} = \frac{\text{Hb} \times 10}{\text{RBC count}}.$$

The new Coulter Counter gives very accurate results.

MCHC: This is the hemoglobin concentration per unit volume of red blood cells. The MCHC can be calculated from the MCH and MCV, as follows:

$$\text{MCHC} = \frac{\text{MCH}}{\text{MCV}} \times 100 \ or \ \text{MCHC} = \frac{\text{Hb}}{\text{HCT}} \times 100.$$

A decreased MCHC can indicate hypochromic anemias.[4,8,20,27,36]

CLINICAL PROBLEMS

Indices	Decreased level	Elevated level
RBC count	Hemorrhage (blood loss)	Polycythemia vera
	Anemias	Hemoconcentration/dehydration
	Chronic infections	High altitude
	Leukemias	Cor pulmonale
	Multiple myeloma	Cardiovascular disease
	Excessive IV fluids	
	Chronic renal failure	
	Pregnancy	
	Overhydration	
MCV	Microcytic anemia:	Macrocytic anemia
	Iron deficiency	Aplastic, hemolytic,
	Malignancy	Pernicious
	Rheumatoid arthritis	Chronic liver disease
	Hemoglobinopathies	Hypothyroidism (myxedema)
	Thalassemia	*Drug influence*
	Sickle cell anemia	Vitamin B_{12} deficiency
	Hemoglobin C	Anticonvulsants
	Lead poisoning	Antimetabolics
	Radiation	
MCH	Microcytic, hypochromic anemia	Macrocytic anemias
MCHC	Hypochromic anemia	
	Iron deficiency anemia	
	Thalassemia	

PROCEDURE

Collect 7 to 10 ml of venous blood in a lavender-top tube.

There is no food or drink restriction.

Usually a particle counter is used which will provide all complete blood count (CBC) results along with all the indices.

FACTORS AFFECTING LABORATORY RESULTS

Drugs (see *Clinical Problems* above).

NURSING IMPLICATIONS WITH RATIONALE

Explain to the patient that the purpose of the test is to determine red blood cell count and composition.

Decreased levels

Relate a decreased RBC count, MCV, MCH, and MCHC to clinical problems.

Assess for the cause(s) of a decreased RBC count. Check for blood loss and obtain a history of anemias, renal insufficiency, chronic infection, or leukemia. Determine whether the patient is overhydrated.

Observe for signs and symptoms of advanced iron deficiency anemia—i.e., fatigue, pallor, dyspnea on exertion, tachycardia, and headache. Chronic symptoms include cracked corners of the mouth, smooth tongue, dysphagia, and numbness and tingling of the extremities. With mild iron deficiency, the patient is usually asymptomatic.

Instruct the patient to follow the physican's orders (medical regime)—e.g., iron supplement therapy and a diet rich in iron.

Instruct the patient to eat foods rich in iron—i.e., liver, red meats, green vegetables, iron-fortified bread, and milk.

Explain to the patient who is taking iron supplements that the stools usually appear dark in color (tarry appearance). Tell the patient to take an iron medication with meals. Milk and antacids can interfere with iron absorption.

Elevated levels

Relate an elevated RBC count, MCV, MCH, and MCHC to clinical problems and drugs.

Assess for signs and symptoms of hemoconcentration. Dehydration, shock, and severe diarrhea are some of the causes of hemoconcentration which can elevate the RBC count.

RENIN (Plasma)

NORMAL RANGE

Adult: 0.4–4.5 ng/ml/hour (upright, normal salt intake).
Child: not usually done.

DESCRIPTION

Renin is an enzyme secreted by the kidneys. This enzyme activates the renin–angiotension system, which causes vasoconstriction and the release of aldosterone (a hormone from the adrenal medulla that causes sodium and water retention). Vasoconstriction and aldosterone can cause hypertension.

Increased plasma renin levels can occur as a result of hypovolemia and kidney disorders. In addition, postural change (from a recumbent to an upright position) and a decreased sodium (salt) intake will stimulate renin secretion. Plasma renin levels are usually higher from 8:00 A.M. to noon and lower from noon to 6:00 P.M.

This test can be complicated, for plasma renin cannot be measured directly but is estimated indirectly. Since renin is an unstable enzyme, plasma renin samples are usually frozen and sent to a special laboratory.[2,27,30]

CLINICAL PROBLEMS

Decreased level *(<0.4 ng/ml/hour):* adrenal cortical hyperfunction, diabetes mellitus, hypothyroidism, high-sodium diet. *Drug influence:* antihypertensives—methyldopa (Aldomet), guanethidine (Ismelin); propranolol (Inderal); L-dopa.

Elevated level *(>4.5 ng/ml/hour):* hypertension—essential renal, malignant; hyperaldosteronism; cancer of the kidney; acute renal failure; adrenal cortical hypofunction; chronic obstructive lung disease (COLD); acute alcoholic intoxication; manic depressive disorder; pregnancy (first trimester); pre-eclampsia and eclampsia; hyperthyroidism; hypokalemia; low-sodium diet. *Drug influence:* estrogens; diuretics; antihypertensives—hydralazine (Apresoline), diazoxide (Hyperstat), nitroprusside.

PROCEDURE

Check with the laboratory and physician to determine whether the plasma renin test is to include urine aldosterone and/or urine sodium tests.

Plasma renin: Keep the tube and/or syringe cold in an ice bath before collection.
The tourniquet should be released before the blood is drawn.
The patient should be in an upright position since the "normal" is established for this position.
A normal or low-salt diet may be indicated.
Collect 5 to 7 ml of venous blood in a lavender-top tube.
The blood sample should be placed in an ice bath; after centrifugation, the plasma is separated, frozen immediately to preserve renin activity, and sent to a special laboratory.
Protocol for plasma renin and urine aldosterone: This protocol can be modified:

1. A diet high in sodium (9 g) and with normal potassium is ordered for 4 days. Medications should be withheld for 4 days.
2. Obtain a blood sample to determine the plasma renin on the morning of the fourth day. The patient should remain in a lying-down position.
3. A 24 hour urine sample to determine aldosterone and sodium should be collected on the fourth day.
4. A low-sodium diet (0.5 g) and normal potassium intake should be continued for 3 days.
5. A blood sample for plasma renin should be drawn on the fourth day in the morning after the patient has been NPO and remained upright for 2 hours.[9]

FACTORS AFFECTING LABORATORY RESULTS
Drugs (see *Drug Influence* above).

NURSING IMPLICATIONS WITH RATIONALE

Explain the procedure for the test as well as the purpose, which is to determine the enzyme (renin) level. For the explanation of procedure, see *Procedure* above. Check with the laboratory on procedural changes or modifications.

Elevated level (>4.5 ng/ml/hour)
Recognize clinical problems and drugs associated with an elevated plasma renin level (see *Clinical Problems* above).
Monitor the patient's blood pressure every 4 to 6 hours or as ordered.
Assess kidney function by recording urinary output. If urinary output is less than 25 ml/hour or 600 ml/day, renal insufficiency should be suspected.

RETICULOCYTE COUNT (Blood)

NORMAL RANGE
Adult: 0.5–1.5 percent of all red blood cells (RBC), 25,000–75,000 mm³ (absolute count).
Newborn: 2.5–6.5 percent of all RBC.
Infant: 0.5–3.5 percent of all RBC.
Child: 0.5–2.0 percent of all RBC.

DESCRIPTION
The reticulocyte count is an indicator of bone marrow activity. Reticulocytes are immature, nonnucleated red blood cells which are formed in the bone marrow and passed into circulation. Normally, there is a small number of reticulocytes in circulation; however, an increased number (count) indicates an erythropoietic (red blood cell

production) acceleration. An increased count could be due to hemorrhage or hemolysis, or treatment of iron deficiency, vitamin B12 deficiency, or folic acid deficiency anemia. This test is also done to check on persons working with radioactive material or receiving radiotherapy. A persistently low count could be suggestive of bone marrow hypofunction or aplastic anemia.

Giving a percentage is not always the most accurate way of reporting the reticulocyte count, especially when the total red blood cell (RBC or erythrocyte) count is *not* within normal range. For example, say the RBC count is 7,000,000 and the reticulocyte count is reported as 1.5. Looking at the reticulocyte count as a percentage makes it appear normal; however, the absolute count of reticulocytes is increased (7,000,000 × 0.015 = 105,000 mm^3). Both the red blood cell count and the reticulocyte count should be reported.[4,8,9,11,30]

CLINICAL PROBLEMS

Decreased level *(↓ 0.5 percent, or ↓ 25,000 mm^3 [adult]):* anemias—pernicious, folic acid deficiency, aplastic (absolute count reduced); radiation therapy; effects of x-ray irradiation; adrenal cortical hypofunction (absolute count is decreased); anterior pituitary hypofunction (absolute count is decreased); cirrhosis of the liver (alcohol suppresses reticulocytes).

Elevated level *(↑ 1.5 percent, or ↑ 75,000 mm^3 [adult]):* anemias—hemolytic, sickle cell; thalassemia major; chronic hemorrhage; posthemorrhage (3 to 4 days); treatment for anemias: iron deficiency, vitamin B12, folic acid; leukemias; erythroblastosis fetalis (hemolytic disease of the newborn); hemoglobin C and D diseases; pregnancy.

PROCEDURE

Venous or capillary blood could be used for the reticulocyte count test.

Venous blood: Collect 5 to 7 ml of venous blood in a lavender-top tube.

Capillary blood: Cleanse the finger and puncture the skin with a sterile lancet. Wipe the first drop of blood away. Collect the blood by using a micropipette. The blood is mixed in equal proportions with methylene blue solution. The reticulocytes stain blue. There is no food or drink restriction.

FACTORS AFFECTING LABORATORY RESULTS

The use of the wrong colored-top tube for venous blood. The tube should contain anticoagulant (EDTA).

NURSING IMPLICATIONS WITH RATIONALE

Explain to the patient the purpose of the test. Explanation may be brief, such as, "a test which helps to determine bone marrow function" *or* "to determine whether there is an excess or decreased number of premature red blood cells."

Explain to the patient that food, drink, and medication are not restricted.

Decreased level (↓ 0.5 percent, or 25,000 mm^3 [adult])

Recognize clinical problems related to a decreased reticulocyte count.

Obtain a history regarding radiation exposure—x-ray and others.

Check the reticulocyte count and the red blood cell count. If the reticulocyte count is given as a percentage, convert the percentage to the absolute count (see *Description* above).

Elevated level (↑ 1.5 percent, or 75,000 mm^3 [adult])

Recognize clinical problems related to an elevated reticulocyte count.

Monitor the reticulocyte count when the patient is being treated for pernicious anemia or folic acid anemia. There is usually an increase in reticulocytes.

Rh TYPING (Blood)

NORMAL RANGE
Adult: Rh + (positive), Rh − (negative).
Child: same as adult

DESCRIPTION
Rh typing is one of the major procedures used for cross-matching blood for transfusion services and typing donors' and maternal blood for screening and prevention of blood incompatibility.

Rh factor (also known as Rh antigen) was first discovered by Landsteiner and Weiner in 1941; it was named "Rh" because of the use of rhesus monkeys in the research. Most people have Rh-positive factor—only a small percentage of the population does not have the factor, and these persons are considered to have Rh-negative blood. Persons usually do not have anti-Rh agglutinins (antibodies) unless they have been sensitized by Rh incompatability as a result of a blood transfusion or pregnancy.

If an Rh-negative woman is carrying a fetus with an Rh-positive blood group, the Rh-positive antigens (from the fetus) may seep into the mother's blood, causing Rh antibody formation. Usually the first-born child is not affected; however, when the second child has Rh-positive blood, the mother frequently develops a high anti-Rh antibody titer and the child can be born with a condition called erythroblastosis fetalis (hemolysis of the red blood cells). This is due to the infant's Rh-positive antigen reacting to the mother's Rh antibodies. To prevent this condition, the Rh-negative woman is given Rho (D) immune globulin (RhoGAM) within 3 days after delivery or after a miscarriage/abortion to neutralize any anti-Rh antibodies.[4,8,9,11]

CLINICAL PROBLEMS
Elevated anti-Rh agglutinins titer: *Infant:* erythroblastosis fetalis.

PROCEDURE
Collect 5 ml of venous blood in a red-top tube.
There is no food or drink restriction.
Blood testing for Rh factor (antigen) should be done with care to avoid false positive and false negative results.

FACTORS AFFECTING LABORATORY RESULTS
None known.

NURSING IMPLICATIONS WITH RATIONALE

Explain to the patient that the blood sample is being drawn to determine his or her Rh factor. The blood sample is usually drawn to determine blood type and Rh factor.

Obtain a history of previous blood transfusions the patient has received. If the patient/client is a pregnant woman, determine whether she has been pregnant before and whether the child (children) was (were) born jaundiced.

Ask the patients if they know their Rh factor. Compare the tested Rh factor with the patient's stated Rh factor. This could prevent administering incorrect blood.

Inform the pregnant woman with Rh-negative factor that her blood will be tested at intervals during her pregnancy to find out whether antibodies are produced. The pregnant woman usually receives RhoGAM (Rh immune globulin) after delivery to prevent production of anti-Rh antibodies.

RHEUMATOID FACTOR (RF), RHEUMATOID ARTHRITIS (RA) FACTOR, RA LATEX FIXATION (Serum)

NORMAL RANGE
Adult: <1:20 titer; 1:20–1:80 positive for rheumatoid arthritis and other conditions; >1:80 positive for rheumatoid arthritis.
Child: not usually done.

DESCRIPTION
The rheumatoid factor (RF) or rheumatoid arthritis (RA) factor test is a screening test used to detect antibodies, considered autoantibodies, which are believed to be a mixture of IgM particles in the serum of many patients with rheumatoid arthritis. The antibodies will agglutinate the red blood cells of sheep, bacteria, or latex particles coated with an IgG fraction. The most common agglutination test is the latex fixation for RA. RF occurs in 53 to 94 percent (average 76 percent) of patients with rheumatoid arthritis. Of all the tests, latex fixation is the most specific, since it gives the lowest percentage of positives in normal adults (1 percent). The Rose–Waaler test, using sensitized red blood cells of sheep, is the second most common RF test, giving 58 to 78 percent (average 64 percent) positive results in RA patients. In normal adults, it can give positive results in 5.6 percent of patients. The Hyland RA slide test gives positive results in 78 to 98 percent (average 82 percent) of RA patients, but it also gives the largest percentage of false positives (8 to 10 percent) in normal adults.

The rheumatoid factor tests can be positive in many of the collagen diseases. However, the latex fixation test has the lowest percentage of positives in collagen diseases—i.e., systemic lupus erythematosus and scleroderma.

The RF tests should not be used for monitoring follow-up or treatment stages of RA, since RF tests often remain positive when clinical remissions have been achieved. It also takes approximately 6 months for a significant elevation of titer. For diagnosing and evaluating rheumatoid arthritis, the C-reactive protein agglutination test is frequently used.[8,9,11,27,30,31,34,36]

CLINICAL PROBLEMS
Elevated level *(↑ 1:20 liter):* rheumatoid arthritis, lupus erythematosus, dermatomyositis, scleroderma, infectious mononucleosis, tuberculosis, leukemia, sarcoidosis, cirrhosis of the liver, hepatitis, syphilis, chronic infections, old age persons.

PROCEDURE
Collect 5 to 10 ml of venous blood in a red-top tube.
There is no food or drink restriction.

FACTORS AFFECTING LABORATORY RESULTS
A positive RF test result frequently remains positive regardless of clinical improvement.

The RF test result can be positive in various clinical problems—i.e., collagen diseases, cancer, and liver cirrhosis.

The older adult may have an increased RF titer without the disease.

Due to the variability in the sensitivity and specificity of these screening tests, positive results must be interpreted in corroboration with the patient's clinical status.

NURSING IMPLICATIONS WITH RATIONALE

Elevated level (>1:20 titer)
Relate an increased RF titer to clinical problems. A titer greater than 1:80 is most

likely due to rheumatoid arthritis. Titers between 1:20 and 1:80 could be due to lupus, scleroderma, or liver cirrhosis.

Consider the age of the patient when the RF is slightly increased. There can be a slight titer increase in the older adult without there being clinical symptoms of RA. With juvenile rheumatoid arthritis, only 10 percent of the children have a positive RF titer.

Explain to the patient the purpose of the test. Explanation could be brief, such as "This is one of the tests used to detect antibodies in the body." A more detailed explanation may be needed.

Tell the patient that food and drinks are not restricted.

Assess for pain in the small joints of the hands and feet (especially the proximal interphalangeal), which could be indicative of an early stage of rheumatoid arthritis.

RPR (RAPID PLASMA REAGIN) (Serum)

NORMAL RANGE
Adult: nonreactive.
Child: nonreactive.

DESCRIPTION
See *Description* for VDRL.
The rapid plasma reagin (RPR) test is a rapid screening test for syphilis. A nontreponemal antibody test like VDRL, the RPR test detects reagin antibodies in the serum and is more sensitive but less specific than VDRL. As with other nonspecific reagin tests, false positives can occur as the result of acute and chronic diseases. A positive RPR should be verified by VDRL and/or FTA-ABS tests.
The RPR test is carried out with a commercial kit prepared by Hynson, Westcott, and Dunning, Inc.[8,11,27]

CLINICAL PROBLEMS
Reactive (positive): syphilis. *False positive:* See *Clinical Problems* for VDRL.

PROCEDURE
Follow the directions on the RPR kit.

FACTORS AFFECTING LABORATORY RESULTS
False positive results due to acute and chronic diseases (see *Clinical Problems* for VDRL).

NURSING IMPLICATIONS WITH RATIONALE

Explain to the patient that the purpose of the test is to check for syphilis.

Reactive (Positive)
Explain to the patient that further testing will be done to verify test results.
See VDRL for nursing implications for reactive test results.

RUBELLA ANTIBODY DETECTION (Serum)
Hemagglutination Inhibition Test (HI or HAI) for Rubella (German Measles)

NORMAL RANGE
   Adult: titer <1.8, susceptibility to rubella; titer 1.8–1.32, past rubella exposure; titer 1.32–1.64, immunity; titer 1.64 and greater, definite immunity.

DESCRIPTION
   Rubella (German Measles) is a mild viral disease of short duration causing a fever and a transient rash. If it occurs in a woman in early pregnancy who is not immune from previous rubella infection and has not received rubella vaccination, the disease can produce serious deformities in her unborn child. Women should be made immune to rubella (vaccinated) before marriage and definitely before pregnancy.
   The rubella virus produces antibodies (natural immunity) against future rubella infections, but the exact antibody titer in the blood is unknown. Hemagglutination inhibition (HI or HAI) measures rubella antibody titers and is considered sensitive and reliable and is easy to perform. To test for antibodies, the patient's serum is mixed with a viral preparation, and if the mixture does not agglutinate added red blood cells, then the serum has rubella antibodies. If the antibody titer is 1.64 or higher, protection against rubella infection is assured.
   Clinical indications for the HAI antibody (screening) test are:

1. To determine the person's rubella antibody titer if she has previously had the rubella infection. She will need the rubella vaccine if her titer is less than 1.8 (some physicians state less than 1.20, others 1.32 or less).
2. To determine the rubella antibody titer at the first antepartum visit.
3. To check pregnant women (during their first trimester of pregnancy) at the time of rubella exposure and again in 3 to 4 weeks.
4. To check personnel who work in obstetrics in the hospital, clinic or physician's office.
5. To diagnose a recent rubella infection in pregnant women (first trimester of pregnancy). The HAI test is done 3 days following the onset of the rash and is repeated 2 to 3 weeks later. A four-fold increase with the second HAI test usually indicates that the rash was due to rubella. A therapeutic abortion may be indicated.[8,9,11,30,36]

CLINICAL PROBLEMS
   Decreased level *(<1.8):* susceptible to rubella (German measles).
   Elevated level *(>1.64):* definite immunity (resistance) to rubella.

PROCEDURE
   Collect 3 to 5 ml of venous blood in a red-top tube.
   There is no food or drink restriction.

FACTORS AFFECTING LABORATORY RESULTS
   None known.

NURSING IMPLICATIONS WITH RATIONALE

Explain to the patient the HAI antibody titer for rubella susceptibility (<1.8) and for rubella immunity (1.64 and greater). The antibody titer to protect the unborn child differs among experts and physicians. Some of them feel 1.20 gives adequate immunity, while others think it should be greater than 1.32. All agree that a 1.64 or higher dilution is a definite immunity titer.

Explain to the patient that the purpose of the test is to determine whether she would be susceptible to German measles or to check the rubella antibody for protection against German measles.

Teach young female adults and families about the need to have their blood checked for rubella immunity (against German measles). This test should be done before pregnancy, and if the titer is less than 1.8, they should receive the rubella vaccine. Some States require a rubella test before a marriage license is issued.

Instruct the pregnant women who are suspectible to German measles to avoid exposure to the disease if at all possible. If they have been exposed to German measles or develop a rash, they should notify the obstetrician immediately so that HAI antibody titer testing can be done. Exposure to German measles does not mean that the person will develop the disease, but it does mean that the antibody titer must be monitored. Emphasize the importance of calling the physician when exposed to German measles.

Explain to interested persons some of the fetal abnormalities (congenital heart disease, deafness, mental retardation) which can occur if the woman develops German measles during the first 3 months of pregnancy.

S

SALICYLATE (Serum)

NORMAL RANGE
Adult: *Normal:* negative. *Therapeutic:* 15–30 mg/dl, 1.44–1.80 mmol/L (SI units).
>30 mg/dl.
Child: *Toxic:* >25 mg/dl.

DESCRIPTION
Salicylate levels are measured to check the therapeutic level, as in the treatment of rheumatic fever, and to check the levels due to an accidental or deliberate overdose. Blood salicylate reaches its peak in 2 to 3 hours, and the blood level can be elevated for as long as 18 hours.

Excessive salicylate increases metabolism, resulting in greater oxygen needs. Respiratory alkalosis will first occur, and as excess salicylates interfere with normal carbohydrate and fat metabolism, metabolic acidosis will result from accumulation of ketones (fatty acids) and organic acids. Prolonged use of salicylates (aspirins) can cause bleeding tendencies, since it inhibits platelet and prothrombin productions.[8,11,30,35]

CLINICAL PROBLEMS
Elevated level *(>30 mg/dl):* acetylsalicylic acid (aspirin; ASA), drugs containing aspirin.

PROCEDURE
Collect 5 ml of venous blood in a green-top tube.
There is no food or drink restriction.
A urine test may also be done as a screening test.

FACTORS AFFECTING LABORATORY RESULTS
None reported.

NURSING IMPLICATIONS WITH RATIONALE

Explain to the patient and/or parent the reason for the test, which is to evaluate the salicylate (aspirin) level in the blood.

Explain that food and drinks are not restricted.

Observe for signs and symptoms of early aspirin overdose—i.e., hyperventilation, flushed skin, and ringing in the ears.

Obtain a history from the child or parent concerning the approximate number of aspirins taken. A toxic dose for a small child is 3.33 grains/kg, or 200 mg/kg. For a child weighing 15 kg (33 lb), the toxic dose would be 10 adult aspirins (5 grains each).

Instruct the patient who takes aspirins constantly that before any surgery he should inform the surgeon of the number of aspirins he takes daily. He should be informed that aspirins will prolong bleeding time.

Recognize that acid–base imbalance is common with salicylate toxicity. Respiratory alkalosis usually occurs first, followed by metabolic acidosis. Symptoms of toxicity usually occur 6 hours following aspirin ingestion. Most of the aspirin has already been absorbed by that time.

SEMEN EXAMINATION

NORMAL RANGE
  Male adult: *Count:* 60–150 million/ml (20 million/ml—low normal). *Volume:* 1.5–5.0 ml.
  Morphology: >75 percent mature spermatozoa. *Motility:* >60 percent actively mobile
  spermatozoa.
  Child: not usually done.

DESCRIPTION
  Semen examination is used as one of the tests to determine the cause of infertility. The
  sperm count, volume of fluid, percent of normal mature spermatozoa (sperms), and percent of actively mobile spermatozoa are studied when analyzing the semen content.
  The normal pH of the semen fluid is 7.0 to 8.0, and the fresh opaque semen should
  liquify and become translucent in approximately 30 minutes. Conception has been
  reported even when the sperm count has been as low as 10 million/ml.
  Sperm count is frequently used to monitor the effectiveness of sterilization after a
  vasectomy (severing of the vas deferens). The sperm count is checked periodically.
  The three methods used to collect semen are masturbation, coitus interruptus, and
  intercourse using a condom. Sexual abstinence is usually required for 3 days before the
  test. Masturbation is the usual method for obtaining a semen specimen; however, for
  religious reasons, intercourse with a condom is sometimes preferred. With coitus interruptus, only a partial semen specimen may be obtained.
  A semen specimen may be collected at home or in the physician's office. In cases of
  rape, a forensic or medicolegal analysis is done to detect semen in vaginal secretions or
  on clothes.[9,30,36]

CLINICAL PROBLEMS
  Decreased level *(<60 million/ml; <20 million/ml—low normal):* infertility; surgery on the
  vas deferens (vasectomy) 0–2 million/ml.

PROCEDURE
  Abstinence from intercourse for 3 days before collecting semen.
  Collect semen by:

  1. Masturbation—collect in a clean container.
  2. Coitus interruptus—collect in a clean glass container.
  3. Intercourse with a clean, washed condom—place the condom in a clean con-
     tainer.

  Keep the semen specimen from chilling and take it immediately to the laboratory. It
  should be tested within 2 hours after collection—the sooner, the better.
  Alcoholic beverages should be avoided for several days (at least 24 hours) before the
  test. There is no other drink or food restriction.

FACTORS AFFECTING LABORATORY RESULTS
  Recent intercourse (within 3 days) could have an effect on the sperm count.

NURSING IMPLICATIONS WITH RATIONALE

  Explain to the patient the purpose of the test. He will most likely know the reason for
      semen collection and examination, which is either to determine the cause of in-
      fertility or to determine the effectiveness of sterilization following vasectomy.
  Check with the physician on what he has told the patient. Be able to supplement the
      physician's explanation to the patient, with the physician's approval.

Be available to discuss methods of semen collection with the patient and his spouse—i.e., masturbation, coitus interruptus, and intercourse with a condom. This can be most embarassing for the man and woman. Some persons prefer to discuss the test in detail with the nurse rather than with the physician. Religious beliefs need to be considered.

Be supportiive of the patient and his spouse. Be a good listener and give them time to express their concerns.

Answer their questions and, if you are unable to respond, refer the question to the appropriate person—i.e., the physician, a clergyman, etc.

Avoid giving your moral convictions about the test or the surgical procedure (vasectomy).

SGOT (SERUM GLUTAMIC OXALOACETIC TRANSAMINASE)

See Aspartate Aminotransferase.

SGPT (SERUM GLUTAMIC PYRUVIC TRANSAMINASE)

See Alanine Aminotransferase.

SICKLE CELL (SCREENING) TEST (Blood)

NORMAL RANGE
   Adult: 0.
   Child: 0.

DESCRIPTION
   See Hemoglobin Electrophoresis.
   Hemoglobin S (sickle cell), an abnormal hemoglobin, causes red blood cells (erythrocytes) to form a cresent or sickle shape when deprived of oxygen. With adequate oxygen, the red cells with hemoglobin S will maintain a normal shape.
   Sickle cell screening tests, such as Sickledex, are useful for determining the presence of hemoglobin S. A positive test does not differentiate between sickle cell anemia caused by hemoglobin S/S and sickle cell trait caused by hemoglobin A/S. If the Sickledex is positive, hemoglobin electrophoresis should be ordered to identify the abnormal hemoglobin combinations.[4,8,11,27,30]

CLINICAL PROBLEMS
   Positive results: sickle cell anemia, sickle cell trait.

PROCEDURE
   Collect 5 to 7 ml of venous blood in a lavender-top tube.
   If a commercial test kit (Sickledex) is used, follow the directions given on the kit.
   There is no food or drink restriction.

FACTORS AFFECTING LABORATORY RESULTS
   A blood transfusion given 3 to 4 months before the screening test may cause inaccurate results due to the donor's normal red blood cells.

If the patient's hemoglobin level is less than 10 g/dl or the hematocrit is less than 30 percent, test results could be falsely negative.

Reagents from the test kit may deteriorate and may no longer be active test agents.

The test result could be falsely negative in an infant less than 6 months old.

NURSING IMPLICATIONS WITH RATIONALE

Explain to the patient and/or family that the purpose of the test is to determine the presence of sickle cells (hemoglobin S).

Instruct the patient that food and drink are not restricted.

Positive test results

Observe for signs and symptoms of sickle cell anemia. Early symptoms are fatigue and weakness. Chronic symptoms are dyspnea on exertion, swollen joints, "aching bones," and chest pains.

Instruct the patient to avoid people with infections and colds. Persons with sickle cell anemia are susceptible to infections.

Encourage the patient to seek genetic counseling if he or she has sickle cell anemia or the sickle cell trait.

Instruct the patient with sickle cell anemia to minimize strenuous activity and avoid high altitudes and extreme cold. Encourage the patient to take rest periods.

SODIUM (Na) (Serum)

NORMAL RANGE
  Adult: 135–145 mEq/L, 135–145 mmol/L (SI units).
  Infant: 134–150 mEq/L.
  Child: 135–145 mEq/L.

DESCRIPTION

Sodium (Na) is the major cation in the extracellular fluid (ECF), and it has a water-retaining effect. When there is excess sodium in the ECF, more water will be reabsorbed from the kidneys.

Aldosterone, secreted from the adrenal cortex, promotes sodium reabsorption from the distal tubules of the kidneys. When there is a sodium deficit, more aldosterone is secreted and more sodium and water reabsorption occurs. With an increased serum sodium level, there is a decrease in aldosterone secretion, and excess sodium is excreted through the kidneys.

Sodium has many functions. It is responsible for conduction of neuromuscular impulses via the sodium pump (sodium shifts into cells as potassium shifts out for cellular activity), enzyme activity, the osmolality of intravascular fluid (doubling the sodium valve gives the approximate serum osmolality), and regulation of acid–base balance (combining with chloride or bicarbonate ions).

The body needs approximately 2 to 4 g of sodium daily. The American people daily consume approximately 6 to 12 g (90 to 240 mEq/L) of sodium in the form of salt (NaCl). A teaspoon of salt contains 2.3 g of sodium.

The names for sodium imbalances are hyponatremia (serum sodium deficit) and hypernatremia (serum sodium excess). When the serum sodium level is 125 mEq/L, sodium replacement with normal saline (0.9 percent NaCl) should be considered, and if the serum sodium level is 115 mEq/L or lower, concentrated saline solutions (3 or 5 percent

NaCl) might be ordered. When rapidly replacing sodium loss, assessment for over-hydration is important.[7,8,13,16,17,19,22]

CLINICAL PROBLEMS

Decreased level *(↓ 135 mEq/L):* vomiting; diarrhea; gastric suction; excessive perspiration; continous IV 5 percent dextrose in water (D/W); SIADH (syndrome of inappropriate antidiuretic hormone; due to surgery, trauma, pain, narcotics); low-sodium diet; burns, inflammatory reactions, tissue injury (fluid and Na shift to the third space); psychogenic polydipsia; salt-wasting renal disease. *Drug influence:* potent diuretics (Lasix—furosemide; Edecrin—ethacrynic acid; thiazides; mannitol).

Elevated level *(↑ 145 mEq/L):* dehydration, severe vomiting and diarrhea (water loss is greater than sodium loss), congestive heart failure, hyperactivity of the adrenal gland (Cushing's disease), hepatic failure, high-sodium diet. *Drug influence:* cough medicines, cortisone preparations, antibiotics, laxatives, methyldopa (Aldomet), hydralazine (Apresoline), reserpine (Serpasil).

PROCEDURE

Collect 5 to 10 ml of venous blood in a red- or green-top tube.

There are no restrictions on food and drink. If the patient has eaten large quantities of foods high in salt content in the last 24 to 48 hours, this should be noted on the laboratory slip and the physician should be notified. Sodium is rarely requested alone, but is rather given as part of the serum electrolytes—i.e., Na, K, Cl, CO_2.

FACTORS AFFECTING LABORATORY RESULTS

A diet high in sodium.

Drugs—potent diuretics, cortisone preparations, various antihypertensive agents, cough medicines.

NURSING IMPLICATIONS WITH RATIONALE

Decreased level (↓ 135 mEq/L)

Recognize clinical problems and drugs related to hyponatremia—i.e., vomiting, diarrhea, continous use of electrolyte-free solutions (5 percent D/W), drinking copious amounts of plain water, a low-sodium diet, potent diuretics, and others.

Assess for signs and symptoms of hyponatremia—i.e., apprehension, anxiety, muscular twitching, muscular weakness, headaches, tachycardia, and hypotension.

Associate hyponatremia following surgery as the result of the syndrome of inappropriate ADH (SIADH). There is usually an excess secretion of ADH for several days after surgery which causes water reabsorption from the kidney and sodium dilution.

Encourage the patient to avoid drinking only plain water. Suggest fluids with solutes—i.e., broth and juices.

Report to the physician if the patient has received dextrose in water infusions for more than 2 days. Hyponatremia and water intoxication could occur. Intravenous fluids with dextrose and one-third or one-half normal saline solution (0.33 to 0.45 percent) are frequently ordered.

Monitor the medical regime for correcting hyponatremia—i.e., water restriction, normal saline (0.9 percent) solution to correct a serum sodium level of 120 to 130 mEq/L, and 3 or 5 percent saline to correct a serum sodium level of less than 115 mEq/L.

Observe for signs and symptoms of overhydration when the patient is receiving 3 or 5 percent saline intravenously. Symptoms of overhydration are a constant, irritated cough; dyspnea; neck and hand vein engorgement; and chest rales.

Check the specific gravity of urine. A specific gravity of less than 1.010 could indicate hyponatremia.

Check serum sodium and other laboratory results and report serum electrolyte changes. An extremely low serum sodium level requires that the test be repeated.

Irrigate nasogastric tubes and wound sites with normal saline instead of sterile water.

Take vital signs to determine cardiac status during hyponatremia.

Elevated level (↑ 145 mEq/L)

Recognize clinical problems and drugs related to hypernatremia—i.e., dehydration (hemoconcentration), severe vomiting and diarrhea, Cushing's syndrome, high salt intake, and cortisone agents.

Observe for signs and symptoms of hypernatremia—i.e., restlessness; thirst; flushed skin; dry, sticky mucous membranes; a rough, dry tongue; and tachycardia.

Encourage the patient to drink 8 to 10 glasses of water, unless this is contraindicated (for instance, with a history of congestive heart failure [CHF]).

Instruct the patient to avoid foods which are high in sodium—i.e., corned beef, bacon, ham, tuna fish, cheese, celery, catsup, pickles, olives, potato chips, and Pepsi Cola.

Identify drugs which have a sodium-retaining effect on the body—i.e., steroids (cortisone), various antihypertensives (methyldopa—Aldomet; hydralazine—Apresoline; and reserpine—Serpasil). Diuretics are frequently prescribed with antihypertensive agents for decreasing sodium retention.

Check for body fluid loss by keeping an accurate intake and output record and weighing the patient daily. A liter of fluid will add on approximately 2.5 pounds of body weight.

Check the specific gravity of the urine. A specific gravity over 1.030 could indicate hypernatremia.

Teach the patient not to salt foods when cooking or use the salt shaker at mealtime.

Report to the physician if the patient is receiving intravenous fluids containing normal saline (0.9 percent NaCl). A liter of normal saline contains 155 mEq of sodium. The body needs 40 to 70 mEq/L of sodium daily, though the average daily intake for adults is 90 to 240 mEq/L. The maximum daily tolerance of sodium is 400 mEq/L, and if the patient receives 3 liters of normal saline, he will receive 465 mEq/L.

Explain to the patient the reason for drinking plain water, adding *no* salt to food, and avoiding foods that are high in sodium.

SODIUM (Na) (Urine)

NORMAL RANGE
  Adult: 40–220 mEq/L, 24 hours.
  Child: similar to adult.

DESCRIPTION

Sodium excretion varies according to the sodium intake, aldosterone secretion, urine volume, and disease entities—i.e., chronic renal failure, adrenal gland dysfunction (Addison's disease and Cushing's syndrome), cirrhosis of the liver, and congestive heart failure (CHF).

When the urine sodium level is less than 40 mEq/24 hours, the decreased sodium excretion could be due to sodium retention or decreased sodium intake. The body could be retaining sodium even with a low serum sodium level. Sodium could have shifted with water into tissue or cavity spaces (third space fluid) or into cells as potassium shifted out.

The urine sodium level should be monitored when edema is present and the serum sodium level is low or normal.[8,17,30,36]

CLINICAL PROBLEMS

Decreased level *(<40 mEq/24 hours):* hyperactive adrenal gland, congestive heart failure, hepatic failure, renal failure, COLD (chronic obstructive lung disease), low sodium (salt) intake. *Drug influence:* cortisone preparations.

Elevated level *(>220 mEq/24 hours):* hypoactive adrenal gland, dehydration, essential hypertension, diabetes mellitus, anterior pituitary hypofunction, high sodium intake. *Drug influence:* potent diuretics—i.e., Lasix, Edecrin.

PROCEDURE

Collect a 24 hour urine sample and place it in a large specimen container. Label the container with the exact times the urine collection started and ended. The patient should void first and this urine should be discarded.

The urine specimen should be refrigerated or placed in a container of ice.

There is no food or drink restriction.

Post a sign on the patient's door or by the bed and in the Kardex saying that a 24 hour urine specimen is being collected.

FACTORS AFFECTING LABORATORY RESULTS

A diet high or low in sodium content.

Drugs such as cortisone and potent diuretics.

Renal dysfunction.

Discarded urine.

NURSING IMPLICATIONS WITH RATIONALE

Explain to the patient that the purpose of the test is to determine whether sodium is excreted or retained in the body. Frequently, it is requested along with a urine osmolality test.

Explain the procedure for collecting the 24 hour urine. Inform the patient that all voidings (urine) should be placed in the large container. Have patients inform their families of the procedure. Tell the patient not to put toilet paper or feces in the urine.

Decreased level (<40 mEq/24 hours)

Recognize clinical problems and drugs associated with a decrease in sodium excretion.

Compare the serum sodium level with the urine sodium level. A low or normal serum sodium and a low urine sodium could indicate sodium retention or a decrease in sodium intake.

Elevated level (>220 mEq/24 hours)

Recognize clinical problems and drugs associated with an increase in sodium excretion.

Teach the patient to avoid eating foods high in sodium if the cause is due to high sodium intake.

Report to the physican if the patient is receiving several liters of normal saline solution intravenously (see Sodium [Serum]).

T

T₃ RESIN UPTAKE (TRIIODOTHYRONINE) (Serum)

NORMAL RANGE
Adult: 25–35 relative percentage uptake, 110–220 ng/dl.
Child: usually not done.

DESCRIPTION
Triiodothyronine (T_3), one of the thyroid hormones, is present in small amounts in the blood and is more short-acting and more potent than thyroxine (T_4). T_3 uptake is a useful test for determining thyroid function. The test can be performed when patients are receiving drugs containing iodine, diagnostic agents (x-ray contrast media), and foods. Usually, this test is not affected by inorganic or organic iodine, but it is affected by radioactive iodine, which interferes with the test reagents.[4,5,8,11,30,36]

CLINICAL PROBLEMS
Decreased level (↓ *25 percent*): hypothyroidism—cretinism, myxedema; pregnancy; menstruation; thyroiditis (Hashimoto); cirrhosis of the liver.* *Drug influence:* ACTH;* corticosteroids;* estrogen; oral contraceptives; antithyroid agents—methimazole, propylthiouracil; diuretics (thiazides); chlordiazepoxide (Librium); sulfonylureas (Orinase).

Elevated level (↑ *35 percent*): hyperthyroidism, protein malnutrition, malignancies (breast) and metastatic carcinoma, myasthenia gravis, liver disease,* nephrotic syndrome, uremia, threatened abortion. *Drug influence:* ACTH,* corticosteroids,* anticoagulant (oral), heparin, diphenylhydantoin (Dilantin), phenylbutazone (Butazolidin), salicylates (high doses of aspirin compounds), thyroid agents.

PROCEDURE
Radioimmunoassay technique is used to measure T_3 resin uptake. The patient's blood is mixed with radioactive T_3 and synthetic resin material in a test tube. The patient does *not* receive radioactive T_3, for this is an in vitro test.
Collect 5 ml of venous blood in a red-top tube.
There is no food or drink restriction.

FACTORS AFFECTING LABORATORY RESULTS
Drugs (see *Drug Influence* above).
Previous administration of radioactive iodine or other radioactive substances could cause inaccurate results.

NURSING IMPLICATIONS WITH RATIONALE

Explain to the patient the purpose and the procedure for the test. Explain that the test is to check the level of a (specific) thyroid hormone. Explain that the patient will not receive a radioactive substance.
Obtain a past and present history of the drugs the patient has taken or is taking, including any radioactive drugs.

---

* *May cause decreased or elevated T_3 uptake levels.*

Record in the patient's chart any drugs the patient is taking that could decrease or increase the T$_3$ uptake level, and report these drugs to the physician.

List on the laboratory slip any drugs the patient is taking that could cause a false negative or false positive result. Also note any radioactive substance the patient has taken.

Check results of the T$_4$ test.

Decreased level (↓ 25 percent)

Recognize clinical problems and drugs associated with a decreased T$_3$ uptake percentage.

Observe for signs and symptoms of hypothyroidism—i.e., fatigue, forgetfulness, weight gain, dry skin with poor turgor, dry and thin hair, bradycardia, decreased peripheral circulation, depressed libido, infertility, and constipation.

Elevated level (↑ 35 percent)

Recognize clinical problems and drugs associated with an elevated T$_3$ uptake percentage.

Observe for signs and symptoms of hyperthyroidism—i.e., nervousness, tremors, emotional instability, increased appetite, weight loss, palpitations, tachycardia, diarrhea, decreased fertility, and exophthalmos (eyeballs protruding).

Monitor the pulse rate. Tachycardia is common and, if severe, could cause heart failure and cardiac arrest.

T$_4$ (THYROXINE) (Serum)

NORMAL RANGE
Adult: *Reported as serum thyroxine:* T$_4$ by column: 4.5–11.5 µg/dl (mcg/dl). Murphy-Pattee: 6.0–11.8 µg/dl. T$_4$ radioimmunoassay (RIA): 5–12 µg/dl. Free T$_4$: 1.0–2.3 ng/dl. *Reported as thyroxine iodine:* T$_4$ by column: 3.2–7.2 µg/dl. Murphy-Pattee: 4.0–7.8 µg/dl.
Child: *Newborn:* 11–23 µg/dl. *1–4 Months old:* 7.5–16.5 µg/dl. *4–12 Months old:* 5.5–14.5 µg/dl. *1–6 Years old:* 5.5–13.5 µg/dl. *6–10 Years old:* 5–12.5 µg/dl.

DESCRIPTION
Thyroxine (T$_4$) is the major hormone secreted by the thyroid gland and is at least 25 times more concentrated than T$_3$ (triiodothyronine). The serum T$_4$ levels are commonly used to measure thyroid hormone concentration and the function of the thyroid gland. The use of protein-bound iodine (PBI) is considered obsolete, and this test is seldom performed.

In some institutions, the T$_4$ test is required for all newborns (as is the PKU test) to detect a decreased thyroxine secretion, which could lead to irreversible mental retardation.[4,8,11,14,30,36]

CLINICAL PROBLEMS
Decreased level *(↓ 4.5 µg/dl [adult, T$_4$ by column]):* hypothyroidism—cretinism, myxedema; protein malnutrition; anterior pituitary hypofunction; strenuous exercise. *Drug influence:* cortisone, chlorpromazine (Thorazine), diphenylhydantoin (Dilantin), heparin, lithium, sulfonamides, reserpine (Serpasil), testosterone, tolbutamide (Orinase).
Elevated level *(↑ 11.5 µg/dl [adult, T$_4$ by column]):* hyperthyroidism, acute thyroiditis, viral hepatitis, myasthenia gravis, pregnancy, pre-eclampsia. *Drug influence:* oral contraceptives, estrogens, clofibrate.

PROCEDURE

Various methods are used for measuring T_4. If the Murphy–Pattee method is used, the patient should not receive any radioisotopic substances prior to the test. Thyroid medication will interfere with the T_4 by column method.

Collect 5 ml of venous blood in a red-top tube.

There is no food or drink restriction.

FACTORS AFFECTING LABORATORY RESULTS

Drugs (see *Drug Influence* above).

Previously administered radioisotopes could affect test results (Murphy–Pattee procedure).

NURSING IMPLICATIONS WITH RATIONALE

Explain to the patient the purpose of the test. Explanation could be brief, such as, "to determine the thyroid hormone level in the blood."

Record in the patient's chart and on the laboratory slip the drugs the patient is taking which could affect the serum T_4 result, and report these drugs to the physician.

Inform the patient that food and drink are not restricted.

See the T_3 results.

Decreased level ($\downarrow$ 4.5 μg/dl [adult, T_4 by column])

Same as for T_3 Resin Uptake.

Elevated level ($\uparrow$ 11.5 μg/dl [adult, T_4 by column])

Same as for T_3 Resin Uptake.

TESTOSTERONE (Serum or Plasma)

NORMAL RANGE

Adult: *Male:* 0.3–1.0 μg/dl (mcg/dl), 300–1000 ng/dl. *Female:* 0.03–0.1 μg/dl, 30–100 ng/dl.

Child: *Male, 12–14 years:* >0.1 μg/dl, >100 ng/dl.

DESCRIPTION

Testosterone, a male sex hormone, is produced by the testes and adrenal glands in the male and by the ovaries and adrenal glands in the female. This hormone causes male sex characteristics, or masculinity.

In males, the highest serum testosterone levels occur in the morning. Serum testosterone is low in both primary and secondary hypogonadism.[27,30,34]

CLINICAL PROBLEMS

Decreased level *(<0.3 μg/dl [male], <0.03 μg/dl [female]):* testicular hypofunction, Klinefelter's syndrome (primary hypogonadism), alcoholism, anterior pituitary hypofunction, estrogen therapy, hypopituitarism.

Elevated level *(>1.0 μg/dl [male], >0.1 μg/dl [female]):* benign prostatic hypertrophy (BPH), neoplasm or hyperplasia of ovaries, adrenogenital syndrome in women, polycystic ovaries in females, adrenal hyperplasia or tumor.

PROCEDURE

Collect 10 ml of venous blood in a red- or green-top tube.

There is no food or drink restriction.

FACTORS AFFECTING LABORATORY RESULTS
None known.

NURSING IMPLICATIONS WITH RATIONALE

Explain to the patient that the purpose of the test is to determine the testosterone level in the blood *or* to determine whether there is a deficit or excess of a male hormone in the body.
Explain that food and drink are not restricted.

Decreased level (<0.3 μg/dl [male], <0.03 μg/dl [female])
Determine whether the patient is complying with medical treatment for testicular hypofunction or hypogonadism. Discuss the side-effects of testosterone.
Be supportive of the patient and his family concerning physical changes due to hormonal deficiency.

Elevated level (>1.0 μg/dl [male], >0.1 μg/dl [female])
Relate elevated testosterone levels to clinical problems.
Observe for signs and symptoms of excess testosterone secretion—i.e., hirsutism, masculine voice, and increased muscle mass (especially in women). Report findings to the physician and record on the chart.

THYROGLOBULIN ANTIBODIES

See Thyroid Antibodies.

THYROID ANTIBODIES (TA) (Serum)
Thyroglobulin Antibodies or Thyroid Hemagglutination Test

NORMAL RANGE
  Adult: negative to 1:20, tanned red cell (TRC) results under 100.
  Child: similar to adult, but usually not done.

DESCRIPTION
  A thyroid antoimmune disease usually produces thyroid antibodies (thyroglobulin antibodies). These autoantibodies (against the body's own tissue) combine with thyroglobulin from the thyroid gland and cause inflammatory lesions of the gland.
  A serum titer evaluation is ordered to detect the presence of thyroid antibodies. With Hasimoto's thyroiditis, the titer is high (1:5000); however, the titer can also be elevated with carcinoma of the thyroid, rheumatoid–collagen diseases, pernicious anemia, and thyrotoxicosis. A positive thyroid antibodies (TA) test does not always confirm the diagnosis of Hashimoto's thyroiditis, unless the titer is extremely high.[8,11,27,36]

CLINICAL PROBLEMS
  Elevated titer: Hashimoto's thyroiditis, carcinoma of the thyroid gland, pernicious anemia, lupus erythematosus, rheumatoid arthritis, thyrotoxicosis (Graves' disease).

PROCEDURE

Collect 5 ml of venous blood in a red-top tube.

The TA test uses the rapid latex agglutination slide test. A positive test result occurs when the patient's serum agglutinates the latex particles, which are coated with thyroglobulin antigen.

The tanned red cell (TRC) test is more sensitive for detecting thyroid autoimmune disease (such as Hasimoto's thyroiditis) than the TA test. It is useful for detecting microsomal antigen.

There is no food or drink restriction.

FACTORS AFFECTING LABORATORY RESULTS

Sex (thyroid disease is more common in women than in men).

NURSING IMPLICATIONS WITH RATIONALE

Explain to the patient that the purpose of the test is to detect thyroid antibodies in the blood which may be responsible for his or her symptoms.

Explain to the patient that food and drink are not restricted.

Elevated titer level

Check serum thyroglobin antibody titer results and relate them to clinical problems. The test is usually ordered to diagnose Hashimoto's thyroiditis; however, the titer level can be elevated in other clinical conditions (see *Clinical Problems* above).

Obtain a family history of thyroid disease. Determine whether the patient has had a viral infection in the last few weeks or months. It is believed that viral infections can trigger autoimmune disease.

THYROID-STIMULATING HORMONE (TSH) (Serum)

NORMAL RANGE

Adult: 2–5.4 µIU/ml, <10 µU/ml, <10^{-3} IU/L (SI units), <3 ng/ml.

Newborn: <25 µIU/ml by the third day.

DESCRIPTION

The anterior pituitary gland (anterior hypophysis) secretes thyroid-stimulating hormone (TSH) in response to thyroid-releasing hormone (TRH) from the hypothalamus. TSH stimulates the secretion of thyroxine (T_4) produced in the thyroid gland. The secretion of TSH is dependent on the negative feedback system—a decreased T_4 level promotes the release of TRH, which stimulates TSH secretion. An elevated thyroxine level suppresses TRH release, which suppresses TSH secretion.

TSH and T_4 levels are frequently measured to differentiate pituitary from thyroid dysfunctions. A decreased T_4 level and a normal or elevated TSH level can indicate a thyroid disorder. A decreased T_4 level with a decreased TSH level can indicate a pituitary disorder.[8,9,11,27]

CLINICAL PROBLEMS

Decreased level: secondary hypothyroidism (pituitary gland involvement), anterior pituitary hypofunction, Klinefelter's syndrome.

Elevated level: primary hypothyroidism (thyroid gland involvement with a decreased T_4); thyroiditis (Hashimoto's)—autoimmune disease; cirrhosis of the liver.

PROCEDURE

Collect 5 ml of venous blood in a red-top tube. The radioimmunoassay (RIA) procedure is usually used.

There is no food or drink restriction.

FACTORS AFFECTING LABORATORY RESULTS

None known.

NURSING IMPLICATIONS WITH RATIONALE

Explain to the patient the purpose of the test. Explanation may be brief, such as, "This is one of the tests used to determine thyroid function."

Recognize the cause of hypothyroidism by comparing the TSH level with the T_4 level. Decreased TSH and T_4 levels could be due to anterior pituitary dysfunction causing secondary hypothyroidism. A normal or elevated TSH and a decreased T_4 could be due to thyroid dysfunction.

Observe for signs and symptoms of myxedema (hypothyroidism)—i.e., anorexia; fatigue; weight gain; dry and flaky skin; puffy face, hands, and feet; abdominal distention; bradycardia; infertility; and ataxia.

Monitor vital signs before and during treatment for hypothyroidism. Report immediately if tachycardia occurs.

Refer to the patient's T_3, T_4, and thyroglobulin results to observe correlations with the TSH result.

TRIGLYCERIDES (Serum)

NORMAL RANGE

Adult: 10–190 mg/dl, 0.11–2.09 mmol/L (SI units).
Infant: 5–40 mg/dl.
Child: 10–140 mg/dl.

DESCRIPTION

Triglycerides are a blood lipid formed by esterification of glycerol and three fatty acids. They are carried by the serum lipoproteins. The intestine processes the triglycerides from dietary fatty acids (exogenous), and they are transported in the bloodstream as chlyomicrons (tiny fat droplets covered by protein), which gives the serum a milky or creamy appearance after a meal rich in fats. The liver is also responsible for manufacturing triglycerides, but these do not travel as chylomicrons. The majority of triglycerides is stored as lipids in the adipose tissue. A function of triglycerides is to provide energy to the heart and skeletal muscles.

Triglycerides are a major contributor to arterial diseases and are frequently compared with cholesterol by the lipoprotein electrophoresis. As the concentration of triglycerides increases, so will the "very low density lipoproteins" increase, leading to hyperlipoproteinemia.[8,9,14,34,36]

CLINICAL PROBLEMS

Decreased level (↓ 10 mg/dl [adult]): congenital a-β-lipoproteinemia, hyperthyroidism, hyperparathyroidism, protein malnutrition, chronic obstructive lung disease (COLD), exercise. *Drug influence:* ascorbic acid, clofibrate (Atromid-S), phenformin, metformin.

Elevated level *(↑ 190 mg/dl [adult]):* hyperlipoproteinemia (types I, IIB, III, IV, V), acute myocardial infarction, hypertension, cerebral thrombosis, hypothyroidism, nephrotic syndrome, arteriosclerosis, Laennec's or alcoholic cirrhosis, uncontrolled diabetes mellitus, pancreatitis, Down's syndrome, stress, high-carbohydrate diet, pregnancy. *Drug influence:* estrogen, oral contraceptives, cholestyramine resin (Questran).

PROCEDURE

Collect 5 ml of venous blood in a red-top tube.

The patient should be NPO (food, drink, medications) after 6 P.M. the night before the test, except for water. Medications should be held until after blood is drawn. The patient should be on a normal diet for several days to 2 weeks before the test.

FACTORS AFFECTING LABORATORY RESULTS

A high-carbohydrate diet can elevate the serum triglycerides level.

NURSING IMPLICATIONS WITH RATIONALE

Decreased level (↓ 10 mg/dl [adult])

Relate clinical problems and drugs to decreased serum triglycerides levels. The drugs that decrease the serum level are not all known.

Elevated level (↑ 190 mg/dl [adult])

Relate clinical problems and drugs to increased serum triglycerides levels. When triglycerides and/or cholesterol are elevated, a lipoprotein electrophoresis is frequently ordered.

Explain to the patient the purpose of the test. Explanation can be brief, such as, "to determine the triglycerides level in the blood." A more detailed explanation may be needed.

Instruct the patient that he is not to eat food or drink anything except water for 12 to 14 hours before the test. Medications may or may not be given during the NPO (nothing by mouth) period. The nurse should check with the physician and laboratory.

Teach the patient with a high serum triglycerides level to avoid eating excessive amounts of sugars and carbohydrates as well as dietary fats. The patient should be encouraged to eat fruit.

Check the serum cholesterol level. At times, only one of the body's lipids (cholesterol or triglycerides) will be elevated. If the cholesterol level is elevated, suggest which foods should be avoided (see Cholesterol). Consult with the dietetics department.

Check to see if a lipoprotein electrophoresis has been ordered. This is frequently done when the triglycerides are elevated.

U

URIC ACID (Serum)

NORMAL RANGE
 Adult: *Male:* 3.5–7.8 mg/dl. *Female:* 2.8–6.8 mg/dl (normal range may slightly differ among laboratories).
 Child: 2.5–5.5 mg/dl.

DESCRIPTION
 Uric acid is a byproduct of purine metabolism. When kidney excretory function is decreased, the serum uric acid will most likely be elevated. An elevated serum uric acid is called hyperuricemia. Serum uric acid is also elevated when there is marked cellular destruction, as in leukemia. The most common problem associated with hyperuricemia is gout. When uric acid is increased, it is important to know the clinical history in order to make a meaningful diagnosis.
 Patients/clients with elevated serum uric acid should avoid foods high in purine.[4,8,9,11,18,30,36]

CLINICAL PROBLEMS
 Decreased level (↓ *3.5 mg/dl [adult male]):* hepatolenticular degeneration, proximal renal tubular acidosis, anemia (folic acid deficiency), burn, pregnancy. *Drug influence:* acetohexamide (Dymelor), allopurinol, azathioprine (Imuran), coumarin, probenecid (Benemid), sulfinpyrazone (Anturan).
 Elevated level (↑ *7.8 mg/dl [adult male]):* gout; alcoholism; leukemias—lymphocytic, myelocytic, monocytic; metastatic cancer; multiple myeloma; severe eclampsia; hyperlipoproteinemia; diabetic mellitus (severe); congestive heart failure; glomerulonephritis; renal failure; stress; lead poisoning; x-ray exposure (excessive); exercise (prolonged); high-protein weight reduction diet. *Drug influence:* ascorbic acid; diuretics—acetazolamide (Diamox), thiazides (chlorothiazide), furosemide (Lasix); levodopa; methyldopa (Aldomet); 6-mercaptopurine; phenothiazines; salicylates (prolonged low dose); theophylline.

PROCEDURE
 Collect 5 to 10 ml of venous blood in a red-top tube.
 There is no food or drink restriction; however, in many cases, high purine foods, such as meats (liver, kidney, brain, heart, and sweetbreads), scallops, and sardines, are restricted for 24 hours before the test.

FACTORS AFFECTING LABORATORY RESULTS
 Excessive stress and fasting could cause an elevated serum uric acid level.
 Foods high in purine (see *Nursing Implications* below).
 Drugs (see *Drug Influence* above).

NURSING IMPLICATIONS WITH RATIONALE

Explain to the patient that the purpose of the test is to determine the cause of his or her symptoms *or* to determine the blood value for uric acid.
Check with the physician and/or laboratory to determine whether foods high in purine should be restricted.

Elevated level (↑ 7.8 mg/dl [adult male])
Recognize clinical problems and drugs related to hyperuricemia. Gout is a problem
   commonly associated with a high serum uric acid.
Teach the patient to avoid eating food that has moderate or high amounts of purines.
   Examples are as follows.

High (100–1000 mg purine nitrogen/ 100 g food)	Moderate (9–100 mg purine nitrogen/ 100 g food)
Brains	Meat
Heart	Poultry
Kidney	Fish
Liver	Shellfish
Sweetbreads	Asparagus
Roe	Beans
Sardines	Mushrooms
Scallops	Peas
Mackerel	Spinach
Anchovies	
Broth	
Consommé	
Mincemeat	

Ask the dietitian to visit the patient to talk about food preference and to plan a low-
   purine diet.
Instruct the patient to decrease alcoholic intake. Ethanol causes renal retention of
   urate.
Observe for signs and symptoms of gout—i.e., tophi of the ear lobe and joints, joint
   pain, and edema in the "big" toe. An elevated uric acid level leads to urate deposits
   in the tissues and in the synovial fluid of joints.
Monitor the pH of the urine and the amount of the urinary output. The urine pH
   should be kept alkaline to prevent the formation of uric acid stones in the kidney. A
   decreased urine output (< 600 ml/24 hours) with an elevated serum uric acid could
   indicate impaired renal function and/or kidney disease.
Check serum urea and serum creatinine levels if the serum uric acid level is elevated
   and the urinary output is decreased. If the serum urea, creatinine, and uric acid are
   elevated and the urine output is decreased, kidney dysfunction should definitely be
   suspected. It could be secondary to another clinical problem.

URIC ACID (Urine—24 Hour)

NORMAL RANGE
   Adult: 250–750 mg/24 hours (low-purine diet).
   Child: similar to adult.

DESCRIPTION
   See Uric Acid (Serum).
   Uric acid is the end-product of purine metabolism, which takes place in the bone
marrow, muscles, and liver. Excess quantities of uric acid are excreted in the urine,
unless there is renal dysfunction due to obstruction of renal flow.
   The main purpose of this 24 hour urine test is to detect and/or confirm the diagnoses of

gout or kidney disease. If severe kidney disease is due to obstruction, uric acid excretion will be decreased along with urea and phosphorus excretion and the urinary volume.[4,8,31]

CLINICAL PROBLEMS

Decreased level *(↓ 250 mg/24 hours):* renal diseases—glomerulonephritis (chronic), urinary obstruction, uremia; eclampsia (toxemia of pregnancy); lead toxicity. *Drug influence:* allopurinol, acetazolamide (Diamox), salicylates (prolonged low doses), triamterene.

Elevated level *(↑ 750 mg/24 hours):* gout, a diet high in purine and nucleic substances; leukemias—lymphocytic, myelocytic; polycythemia vera; Fanconi's syndrome; neurologic disorders—cerebral hemorrhage, cerebral thrombosis, brain infarction, cerebral embolism, encephalomyelitis; psychiatric disorders—manic-depressive, paranoid states, depressive neurosis; ulcerative colitis; viral hepatitis; x-ray therapy; febrile illnesses. *Drug influence:* bishydroxycoumarin, corticosteroids, cytotoxic agents (treatment for cancer), probenecid (Benemid), salicylates (high doses).

PROCEDURE

Collect a 24 hour urine sample in a large container with a preservative. (Some laboratories do not require a preservative.) If the urine is not tested immediately after collection, the urine container should be refrigerated. Check with the laboratory on the need for refrigeration.

Label the container with the patient's name and the dates and times of urine collection (e.g., 9/23/83, 7:11 A.M. to 9/24/83, 7:11 A.M.).

A diet low or high in purines may be ordered before and/or during the time of urine collection.

There is no drink restriction.

FACTORS AFFECTING LABORATORY RESULTS

Drugs (see *Drug Influence* above).

A high- or low-purine diet.

Excessive x-ray exposure.

Febrile illnesses.

NURSING IMPLICATIONS WITH RATIONALE

Explain to the patient the purpose of and procedure for the test. Explain to the patient and family that all urine should be saved for 24 hours. Tell the patient not to put feces or toilet paper in the urine.

Post a sign on the patient's door or bed and in the Kardex giving the dates and times of urine collection.

Tell the patient which foods to avoid before and during the test, as ordered by the physician.

Monitor urinary output. Poor urine output could indicate inadequate fluid intake or poor kidney function.

Compare the serum uric acid level with the urine acid level. An elevated serum uric acid level (hyperuricemia) and a decreased urine uric acid level can indicate kidney dysfunction. Increased serum and urine uric acid levels are frequently seen in gout, so it is important to obtain both the urine and serum values.

Check the urine pH, especially if a uric acid concentration is present. Uric acid stones can occur when the urine pH is low (acidic) and the serum and urine uric acid levels are elevated.

URINALYSIS (ROUTINE) (Color, Appearance, Odor, Foam, pH, Specific Gravity, Protein, Glucose, Ketones, RBC, WBC, and Casts)

NORMAL RANGE

	Adult	Newborn	Child
Color	Light straw to dark amber		Light straw to dark yellow
Appearance	Clear	Clear	Clear
Odor	Aromatic		Aromatic
Foam	White (small amount)		White (small amount)
pH	4.5–8 Average is 6	5–7	4.5–8
Specific Gravity (SG)	1.005–1.030 (1.015–1.024, normal fluid intake)	1.001–1.020	1.005–1.030
Protein	2–8 mg/100 ml— negative reagent strip test		
Glucose	Negative		Negative
Ketones	Negative		Negative
Microscopic examination			
RBC	1–2 per low power field		Rare
WBC	3–4		0–4
Casts	Occasional hyaline		Rare

DESCRIPTION

Urinalysis is a physical, chemical, and microscopic analysis of the urine. Routine urine tests were performed as early as 1821. Until recently, urine was manually tested for individual constituents, but now multiple-reagent strips are used for quick chemical screening.

Urinalysis is useful for diagnosing renal disease or urinary tract infection and for detecting metabolic disease not related to the kidneys. Many routine urinalyses are done in the physician's office as well as in the hospital or in a private laboratory. The color, appearance, odor, and foam of the urine are examined, and the pH, protein, glucose ketones, and bilirubin are tested with the reagent strips. Specific gravity is measured with a urinometer, and a microscopic examination of the urinary sediment is performed to detect red blood cells, white blood cells, casts, crystals, and bacteria.[3,4,8,11,20,27,30,31,36]

CLINICAL PROBLEMS

Property or Constituent	Clinical Conditions/Problems	Comments
Color		
Colorless (very pale)	Large fluid intake Diabetes insipidus Chronic kidney disease Alcohol ingestion Nervousness	A pale color usually indicates diluted urine and dark yellow or amber indicates concentrated urine.

Property or Constituent	Clinical Conditions/Problems	Comments

Red or red-brown	Hemoglobinuria
	Porphyrins
	Menstrual contamination
	Drug influence
	    Azo-gantrisin
	    Diphenylhydantoin
	    (Dilantin)
	    Cascara
	    Chlorpromazine
	    (Thorazine)
	    Doxidan
	    Ex-Lax (phenolphthalein)
	Foods
	    Beets
	    Rhubarb
	    Food color
		Drugs and foods will change the color of the urine.

Orange	Restricted fluid intake
	Concentrated urine
	Excess sweating
	Fever
	Drug influence
	    Amidopyrine
	    Furazolidone (Furoxone)
	    Nitrofurantoin
	    Phenazopyridine
	    (Pyridium)
	    Sulfonamides
	Foods and others
	    Carrots (carotene)
	    Rhubarb
	    Food color
	    Bilirubin	

Blue or green	Pseudomonas toxemia
	Drug influence
	    Amitriptyline (Elavil)
	    Methylene blue
	    Methocarbamol (Roboxin)
	    Vitamin B complex
	    Yeast concentrate	

Brown or black	Lysol poisoning
	Melanin
	Bilirubin
	Methemoglobin
	Porphyrin
	Drug influence
	    Cascara
	    Chloroquine (Aralen)
	    Iron injectable compounds
	    Phenylhydrazine	

Property or Constituent	Clinical Conditions/Problems	Comments
Appearance		
Hazy, cloudy	Bacteria	
	Pus, tissue	
	Red blood cells	
	White blood cells	
	Phosphates	
	Prostatic fluid	
	Spermatozoa	
	Urates, uric acid	
Milky	Fat	
	Pyuria	
Odor		
Ammonia	Urea breakdown by bacteria	
Foul or putrid	Bacteria (UTI)	
Mousey	Phenylketonuria	
Sweet or fruity	Diabetic acidosis (ketoacidosis)	
	Starvation	
Foam		
Yellow—large amounts	Severe cirrhosis of the liver	
	Bilirubin or bile pigment	
pH		
<4.5	Metabolic acidosis	
	Respiratory acidosis	
	Starvation	
	Diarrhea	
	Diet high in meat protein and/or cranberries	
	Drug influence	
	Ammonium chloride	
	Methenamine mandelate (mandelic acid)	
>8.0	Bacteriuria	
	Urinary tract infection due to Pseudomonas or Proteus	
	Drug influence	
	Antibiotics	
	Kanamycin	
	Neomycin	
	Streptomycin	
	Sulfonamides	
	Excess salicylates (aspirin)	
	Sodium bicarbonate	
	Acetazolamide (Diamox)	
	Potassium citrate	
	Diet	
	High in citrus fruits	
	High in vegetables	

Property or Constituent	Clinical Conditions/Problems	Comments
Specific gravity (SG)		
<1.005	Diabetes insipidus	Low fixed SG can indicate kidney disease due to inability to concentrate urine.
	Excess fluid intake	
	Overhydration	
	Renal disease	
	Glomerulonephritis	
	Pyelonephritis	
	Polycystic disease	
	Severe potassium deficit	
>1.026	Decreased fluid intake	
	Fever	
	Administration of IV	
	dextran, albumin	
	Diabetes mellitus	
	Vomiting, diarrhea	
	Dehydration	
	X-ray contrast media	
Protein		
>8 mg/dl or	Proteinuria	Proteinuria is a sensitive indicator of kidney dysfunction.
>80 mg/24 hrs	Mild, transitory	
	Protein	
	Exercise	
	Severe stress	
	Cold baths	
	Fever	
	Acute infectious diseases	
	Renal disease	
	Glomerulonephritis	
	Nephrotic syndrome	
	Polycystic kidney	
	Lupus Erythematosus	
	Leukemia	
	Multiple myeloma	
	Cardiac disease	
	Toxemia of pregnancy	
	Septicemia	
	Materials	
	Arsenic	
	Mercury	
	Lead	
	Carbon tetrachloride	
	Drug influence	
	Barbiturates	
	Neomycin	
	Massive doses of penicillin	
	Sulfonamides	
<2 mg/dl	Very diluted urine	
Glucose		
>15 mg/dl (random)	Diabetes mellitus	The renal threshold for blood glucose is 160–180 mg/dl.
	CNS disorders	
	Stroke (CVA)	

Property or Constituent	Clinical Conditions/Problems	Comments
	Meningitis	Tes-tape should be used in
	Cushing's syndrome	place of clinitest when the
	Anesthesia	patient is receiving drugs.
	Glucose infusions	
	Severe stress	
	Infections	
	Drug influence	
	(false positive results)	
	Ascorbic acid	
	Aspirin	
	Keflin	
	Streptomycin	
	Epinephrine	
Ketones	See Ketone Bodies, Acetone	Acetest or ketostix should be
Positive	Ketoacidosis	tested when clinitest
+1 to +3	Starvation	or tes-tape is tested.
	A diet high in protein and low in carbohydrates	

Microscopic examination of urinary sediment

Red blood cells (RBC) and RBC casts >2 per low power field	Trauma to the kidney Renal disease Pyelonephritis Glomerulonephritis Hydronephrosis Renal calculi Cystitis Lupus nephritis (collagen disease) Aspirins (excess) Anticoagulants Sulfonamides Menstrual contamination	
White blood cells (WBC) and WBC casts >4 per low power field	Urinary tract infection Fever Strenuous exercise Lupus nephritis Renal diseases	If WBC are present in the urine, a urine culture should be done.
Casts hyaline (most common form found in urine)	Fever Renal diseases Heart failure	

PROCEDURE

Collect a freshly voided urine specimen—approximately 50 ml or more—in a clean, dry container and take it to the laboratory within 30 minutes. An early morning urine specimen collected before breakfast is preferred. If the test is to check for glycosuria, collect the urine specimen 2 to 3 hours after eating.

The urine specimen could be refrigerated for 6 to 8 hours. The urine specimen could be obtained during working hours.

A clean-caught or midstream urine specimen could be requested if WBC are in the urine or if bacteria are suspected.

There is no food or drink restriction unless the urinalysis is to be done in the early morning.

FACTORS AFFECTING LABORATORY RESULTS

A urine specimen that has been sitting for an hour or longer without refrigeration.

Drugs and foods (see *Clinical Problems* above).

Feces or toilet paper in the urine.

NURSING IMPLICATIONS WITH RATIONALE

Explain to the patient the purpose of the test. Explanation could be brief, such as, "to do urinalysis" *or* "to check the substances in the urine."

Explain to the patient the procedure for collecting the urine. Inform the patient that an early morning urine specimen taken before breakfast is needed, unless the physician is checking for sugar in the urine (glycosuria), and then the specimen would be taken 2 to 3 hours after a meal. Instruct the patient that aproximately one-third or one-half of a small container of urine is needed. Have the patient void in a clean, dry container or a clean urinal or bedpan which can be poured into the container, and ask him or her to notify you immediately so that the urine can be taken to the laboratory within 30 minutes. Concentrated urine is desired when checking for protein and the content of urinary sediment.

Tell the patient not to put feces in the urine.

Teach the patient at home to place the fresh morning urine specimen in the refrigerator. The urine specimen, however, should be taken to the lab within an hour. Urine is an excellent medium for the growth of bacteria, and the bacterial growth begins approximately one-half hour after collection. Refrigeration may help to retard growth for a short period of time.

Explain to the patient the procedure for a clean-catch or midstream urine collection (see Cultures). This procedure may be requested when culture of the urine is needed as well as for urinalysis.

Assist the patient with the urine collection as needed.

Obtain a history of any drugs the patient is currently taking. Such drugs as cascara, Azo Gantrisin, nitrofurantoin, Thorazine, sulfonamides, Elavil, Ex-Lax, Pyridium, and others cause a discoloration of the urine.

Assess the fluid status of the patient. Urine should be concentrated if the urine specimen is obtained in the morning or if the patient has a decreased fluid intake or is dehydrated. An increase in fluid intake will dilute the urine contents.

Obtain a history of an excess amount of a certain food (e.g., carrots, rhubarb, beets) which can cause a change in the urine color or of foods (e.g., excess amounts of meat, cranberry juice) which could lower the urine pH (acidic).

UROBILINOGEN (Urine)

NORMAL RANGE
Adult: *Random:* 0.3–3.5 mg/dl. *2 hour specimen:* 0.3–1.0 Ehrlich units. *24 hour specimen:* 0.05–2.5 mg/24 hour, 0,5–4.0 Ehrlich units/24 hour, 0.09–4.23 μmol/24 hour (SI units).
Child: in Rh incompatibility, the infant's urine may be requested to check for a hemolytic problem; normal range similar to adult.

DESCRIPTION
Bile, which is formed mostly from conjugated bilirubin, reaches the duodenum, where the intestinal bacteria change the bilirubin to urobilinogen. Most of the urobilinogen is lost in the feces; a large amount goes back to the liver through the bloodstream, where it is reprocessed to bile; and approximately 1 percent is excreted by the kidneys in the urine.

The urobilinogen test is one of the most sensitive tests for determining liver damage, hemolytic disease, and severe infections. In early hepatitis, mild liver cell damage, or mild toxic injury, the urine urobilinogen level will increase despite an unchanged serum bilirubin level. The urobilinogen level will frequently decrease with severe liver damage, since less bile will be produced.[8,9,11,27,30,36]

CLINICAL PROBLEMS
Decreased level *(↓ 0.3 mg/dl [adult, random]):* biliary obstruction, severe liver disease, cancer of the pancreas, severe inflammatory disease, cholelithiasis, severe diarrhea. *Drug influence:* antibiotics (decreasing gut bacteria), ammonium chloride, ascorbic acid (vitamin C).

Elevated level *(↑ 3.5 mg/dl [adult, random]):* infectious hepatitis, toxic hepatitis, cirrhosis of the liver (early and recovery stages), hemolytic anemia, pernicious anemia, erythroblastosis fetalis, sickle cell anemia, infectious mononucleosis. *Drug influence:* sulfonamides—sulfisoxazole (Gantrisin); phenothiazines—chlorpromazine (Thorazine); acetazolamide (Diamox); cascara; phenazopyridine (Pyridium); mandalamine; paraminosalicylic acid (PAS); procaine; sodium bicarbonate.

PROCEDURE
There are three types for urobilinogen: the single or random specimen, the 2 hour urine specimen, and the 24 hour urine specimen.

The single urine specimen should be fresh (urine) and should be tested immediately. This may be done as part of the routine urinalysis. A reagent color dipstick is dipped in urine and is compared to a color chart, in Ehrlich units.

The 2 hour timed specimen is frequently taken between 1:00 and 3:00 P.M. or 2:00 and 4:00 P.M. The patient should first void and this urine should be discarded before beginning the test. The exact time of the urine collection should be posted and written on the bottle. The collecting bottle should be kept from light and refrigerated.

The 24 hour urine specimen should be kept from light and refrigerated. The urine container should have a preservative in it. The patient should first void and this urine should be discarded before beginning the test. The exact times of the urine collection should be posted and written on the bottle—e.g., 3/4/83, 8:01 A.M. to 3/5/83, 7:59 A.M. There is no food or drink restriction.

List any drugs the patient is receiving that could cause a false positive result. If possible and with the physician's permission, withhold the drugs for 24 hours before the test and during the test.

FACTORS AFFECTING LABORATORY RESULTS

Bananas.

Antibiotics which decrease the bacterial flora in the intestine.

Certain drugs increase the urine urobilinogen level (see *Drug Influence* above).

pH changes in the urine; strongly acidic urine could cause a decreased urobilinogen level, and strongly alkaline urine could cause an elevated level. Urine sitting for one-half hour or longer may become alkaline.

The urobilinogen level is highest in the afternoon and evening. The 2 hour urine specimen is frequently collected in the afternoon.

NURSING IMPLICATIONS WITH RATIONALE

Inform the patient he may eat and drink before the urine test.

Explain to the patient the procedure for collecting a 2 hour urine specimen or a 24 hour urine specimen. The bladder should be emptied before starting the 2 hour or 24 hour urine test. Inform the patient that all urine must be saved during the specified time.

Keep the collected urine from light in a urine container with a preservative, which should be refrigerated.

Label the container and laboratory slip with the exact times urine collection begins and ends (after the last voiding).

Decreased level (↓ 0.3 mg/dl [adult, random])

Relate clinical problems and drugs to decreased urine urobilinogen. Most antibiotics will reduce the bacterial flora in the intestines, thus decreasing the formation of urobilinogen.

Elevated level (↑ 3.5 mg/dl [adult, random])

Relate clinical problems and drugs to an elevated level of urine urobilinogen.

Check for an elevated urobilinogen level in freshly voided urine with a reagent color dipstick. Record the results of the single test. Note if the patient is receiving drugs that could elevate the urobilinogen level.

Explain to the patient the purpose of the urine urobilinogen test. Explanation could be brief, such as, "to determine the amount of bile substance being excreted." A more detailed explanation may be needed.

Post signs on the patient's bedside and chart and in the Kardex stating the hours of urine collection. The family should be informed not to throw the collected urine away.

Restart the 24 hour urine test if any urine was discarded during the collection time.

List any drugs the patient is taking that could elevate the urobilinogen level on the laboratory slip. If the test is positive, the drugs should be reported and recorded.

V

VANILMANDELIC ACID (VMA) (Urine)

NORMAL RANGE
Adult: 1.5–7.5 mg/24 hours, 7.6–37.9 μmol/24 hours (SI units).
Child: similar to adult.

DESCRIPTION
Vanilmandelic acid (VMA) is the major byproduct of catecholamines (epinephrine and norepinephrine). When a person has severe hypertension, tumors of the adrenal medulla (pheochromocytoma in the adult and neuroblastoma and ganglioneuroblastoma in the child) should be suspected. A high level of VMA excreted in the urine usually indicates an adrenal medulla tumor. Other methods should be used to verify positive VMA results, such as catecholamine and metanephrine assay.

The VMA test is a simple screening method. However, many foods (banana, tea, coffee, chocolate, carbonated drinks, etc.) and drugs (aspirin, sulfonamides, some cough medicines, and others) produce false positive results.[8,9,11,27,30]

CLINICAL PROBLEMS
Decreased level *(< 1.5 mg/24 hours):* uremia. *Drug influence:* clofibrate; antihypertensives—guanethidine (Ismelin), methyldopa (Aldomet), reserpine (Serpasil); monomine (MAO) inhibitors.

Elevated level *(> 7.5 mg/24 hours):* pheochromocytoma; neuroblastoma; ganglioblastoma; myasthenia gravis; muscular dystrophy (progressive); physical and mental stress; foods—fruits (banana), fruit juices, chocolate, tea, coffee, carbonated drinks (except ginger ale), vanilla and vanilla products, candy, mints, jelly, cheese, gelatins, and cough drops. *Drug influence:* salicylates (aspirin), para-aminosalicylic acid (PAS), sulfonamides, penicillin, chlorpromazine (Thorazine), isoproterenol (Isuprel), levodopa, lithium carbonate, nitroglycerin, glyceryl guaiacolate, mephenesin (Tolserol), methenamine (Mandelamine), methocarbamol (Robaxin).

PROCEDURE
No drugs should be taken for 3 days before the test, if possible, especially those listed under *Drug Influence* above.

Insert 10 ml of concentrated hydrochloric acid (HCl) in a large bottle. Some laboratories do not require that a preservative be added to the bottle.

Label the large bottle and laboratory slip with the dates and times the urine collection started and ended. Keep the bottle refrigerated during the 24 hour collection time.

Those foods listed under *Clinical Problems* above should be omitted from the diet for 3 days before the test. Other foods and drinks are not restricted.

FACTORS AFFECTING LABORATORY RESULTS
Drugs (see *Drug Influence* above).
Food (see *Clinical Problems* above).
Strenuous exercise will elevate VMA levels.
Stress will elevate VMA levels.

NURSING IMPLICATIONS WITH RATIONALE

Elevated level (> 7.5 mg/24 hours)

Explain the purpose of the urine test. Explanation may be brief, such as, "to determine the amount of a catecholamine substance" *or* "to determine the cause of the hypertension."

Explain to the patient and family that all urine excreted over the 24 hour period must be saved and kept refrigerated. Tell the patient not to put toilet paper or feces in the urine. Post the urine collection times on the patient's bed or door and in the Kardex.

Instruct the patient not to eat the foods listed under *Clinical Problems* above for 3 days before the test. Write the restricted foods on a piece of paper for the patient's reference. Tell the patient *not* to eat those foods if they are on the meal tray.

Explain to the patient that he should eat well balanced meals. Starvation or severe lack of food could increase the VMA levels.

Encourage the patient to avoid emotional stress and physical activity. Stress and activity increase VMA levels. Encourage the patient to rest during the test.

Monitor vital signs, especially blood pressure. Maintain a blood pressure cahrt.

VDRL (VENEREAL DISEASE RESEARCH LABORATORY) (Serum)
VDRL Screening Test

NORMAL RANGE
Adult: nonreactive.
Child: nonreactive.

DESCRIPTION

Syphilis, a veneral disease caused by the spirochete *Treponema pallidum,* is usually transmitted through sexual contact. There are stages of syphilis (primary, secondary, and tertiary) which, left untreated, could lead to death.

Primary stage: Duration after contact: 3 to 6 weeks. A chancre develops approximately 3 weeks after contact. Spirochetes in the exudate of the chancre lesion (sore) may be visualized with dark-field microscopy. Chancres are generally found in genital areas and in the mouth or on the lips.

Secondary stage: Duration after contact: 2 weeks to 6 months. Secondary lesions are highly contagious and at times may be visualized on dark-field microscopy. The lesions are usually red papular or "snail track" ulcers and may be seen anywhere on the body, especially in the palms of the hands and the soles of the feet. A relapse may occur in 2 to 4 years; this is called latent syphilis. The patient may have a low fever.

Tertiary stage: Duration after contact: 4 to 20 years. This is referred to as late syphilis. Untreated syphilis (tertiary stage) normally does not have clinical signs; however, it does affect the person's cardiovascular system and central nervous system (CNS). The person may develop cardiac valvular disease, aneurysms, general paresis, blindness, slurred speech, delusions, and "insanity."

Two groups of blood tests are used to identify the spirochete *Treponema pallidum:* the nontreponemal antibody test (VDRL and RPR) and the treponemal antibody test (FTA-ABS, TPI).

The VDRL test is useful for detecting primary syphilis 1 to 3 weeks after the presence of a primary lesion and for detecting secondary syphilis.

T. pallidum stimulates the development of nonspecific reaginic antibodies in the serum. If these antibodies are present and react with a lipid antigen (cardiolipin), the VDRL test is positive or reactive. A titer above 1:32 can indicate the secondary stage. With tertiary stage syphilis, the VDRL test is not sensitive and may fail to react or may produce variable titers.

The results of the VDRL test may be negative in the early infectious phase of syphilis or could produce biologic false positives (BFP) due to other acute or chronic diseases. If the VDRL test is negative, weekly VDRL tests may be indicated. RPR (rapid plasma reagin) may be used first as a screening test for syphilis.[4,8,11,26,30,36]

CLINICAL PROBLEMS

Nonreactive *(negative)*: *False negatives:* early primary stage of syphilis, tertiary stage of syphilis.

Reactive *(positive)*: syphilis—*Treponema pallidum* organism. *False positives* (return to nonreactive with 6 months): tuberculosis, pneumonia, infectious mononucleosis, chicken pox, smallpox vaccination (recent), subacute bacterial endocarditis, leprosy. *False positives (chronic;* persist longer than 6 months): malaria, Hashimoto's thyroiditis, rheumatoid arthritis, progressive systemic sclerosis, systemic lupus erythematosus, hepatitis.

PROCEDURE

Collect 5 ml of venous blood in a red-top tube. Prevent hemolysis of the blood sample.

The patient should be NPO for 8 to 12 hours before the test. Some laboratories do not require NPO, so check with the laboratory. Alcohol should not be consumed for 24 hours before the VDRL test.

FACTORS AFFECTING LABORATORY RESULTS

Hemolysis of the blood sample.

Biologic false positives (BFP) due to certain acute or chronic diseases.

Alcoholic intake decreases the test reaction.

NURSING IMPLICATIONS WITH RATIONALE

Explain to the patient that the blood sample is usually part of a routine work-up on medical patients or prior to surgery. A positive test result may not be due to syphilis.

Instruct the patient not to drink alcohol for 24 hours prior to the test. If the patient has consumed alcohol, the test should be postponed for 24 hours.

Inform the patient that he or she should be NPO (have nothing by mouth) after dinner or after midnight, with the exception of water. Check with the laboratory, since most do not require the patient to be NPO.

Obtain a history of any acute or chronic disease. Related biologic false positives (BFP) with certain diseases (see *Clinical Problems* above).

List present acute and/or chronic diseases in the patient's chart and on the laboratory slip. Notify the physician of the patient's current diseases. The physician may be aware of these; however, a reminder may be needed so that other tests may be used or so that a repeat reagin test may be ordered.

Interpretation of tests for syphilis requires skill and experience.

Nonreactive (negative)

Relate a nonreactive VDRL test result to false negative causes if the history and symptoms are suggestive of syphilis. Test should be repeated weekly for several weeks. Nonreactive (negative) results can occur in the early primary stage of syphilis.

Reactive (positive)

Relate a reactive VDRL test result to a positive indication of syphilis or a possible false positive due to acute or chronic diseases (see *Clinical Problems* above). If the history is suggestive of syphilis but an acute or chronic disease is present, the FTA-ABS or TPI test may be performed.

Check with the patient about receiving treatment for syphilis. If primary syphilis persists for weeks before treatment, the VDRL test could remain positive for up to 6 months after treatment. The test results following treatment for secondary syphilis could remain positive for 12 to 18 months. The history of treatment (where, when, how long, and what drugs) is extremely important to know. The health department should be notified when there is a positive test result.

Be supportive of the patient. Be willing to listen and not make a judgment concerning the patient's lifestyle.

Elicit from the patient his contacts (friends) so that they can be properly tested and treated. Explain the importance of preventing the transmission of the disease.

Refer the patient to a venereal disease clinic if one is available (with the physician's permission). Many clinics have case workers and a good follow-up care program.

Emphasize the importance of follow-up care. Frequently, patients are checked every 3 months for 2 years as a preventive measure for detecting a relapse (syphilis).

Observe for signs and symptoms of tertiary (late) syphilis (see *Description* above). These signs and symptoms should be documented and reported. The VDRL test is usually negative with tertiary syphilis.

W

WHITE BLOOD CELLS (WBC) OR LEUKOCYTES; TOTAL (Blood)

NORMAL RANGE
Total WBC count: *Adult:* 5000–10,000 mm³. *Newborn:* 9000–30,000 mm³. *2 years old:* 6000–17,000 mm³.

DESCRIPTION
See *Differential White Blood Cell Count.*

White blood cells (leukocytes) are divided into two groups, the polymorphonuclear leukocytes (neutrophils, eosinophils, and basophils) and the mononuclear leukocytes (monocytes and lymphocytes). Leukocytes are an important part of the body's defense system, and they respond immediately to foreign invaders, going to the site of involvement.

An increase in white blood cells to more than 10,000 mm³ is called leukocytosis, and a decrease in WBC to less than 5000 mm³ is called leukopenia.[8,21,36]

CLINICAL PROBLEMS
Decreased level *(↓ 5000 mm³; leukopenia):* hematopoietic diseases—aplastic anemia, pernicious anemia, hypersplenism, Gaucher's disease; viral infections; malaria; Rickettsia; agranulocytosis; alcoholism; uncontrolled diabetes. *Drug influence:* antibiotics—chloramphenicol, penicillins, cephalothin; analgesics—acetaminophen (Tylenol); sulfonamides; antithyroid drugs—propylthiouracil; barbiturates; cancer chemotherapy agents; diazepam (Valium); diuretics—furosemide (Lasix), ethacrynic acid (Edecrin); chlordiazepoxide (Librium); oral hypoglycemic agents; indomethacin (Indocin); methyldopa (Aldomet); quinine; rifampin.

Elevated level *(↑ 10,000 mm³; leukocytosis):* acute infections—tuberculosis, pneumonia, meningitis, tonsillitis, appendicitis, colitis, peritonitis, pancreatitis, choleaptitis, pyelonephritis, gastritis, diverticulitis, septicemia, rheumatic fever; tissue necrosis—myocardial infarction, cirrhosis of the liver, burns, cancer of the organs, emphysema, peptic ulcer; leukemias—lymphocytic, myelocytic, monocytic; collagen diseases—rheumatoid arthritis, gout; crush injury; renal failure; anemias—sickle cell, hemolytic; parasitic diseases; stress—fever, convulsions, surgery, emotional upset (long-lasting). *Drug influence:* salicylates; isoniazid (INH); antibiotics—ampicillin, erythromycin, kanamycin, methicillin, tetracyclines, streptomycin, vancomycin; gold compounds; procainamide (Pronestyl); triamterene (Dyrenium); atropine (children); allopurinol; potassium iodide; hydantoin derivatives; primaquine; sulfonamides (long-acting).

PROCEDURE
Venous blood: Collect 7 ml of venous blood in a lavender-top tube.
Capillary blood: Collect blood from a finger puncture with a micropipette. Dilute immediately with the proper reagent.
There is no food or drink restriction.

FACTORS AFFECTING LABORATORY RESULTS
Drugs which can increase and decrease the WBC count (see *Drug Influence* above)

The time the blood sample was taken. The WBC count is lower in the morning than in the afternoon.

The age of the individual. Children can have a high WBC count, especially during the first 5 years of life.

NURSING IMPLICATIONS WITH RATIONALE

Explain to the patient the purpose of the test. Explanation could be brief, such as, "to determine the number of white blood cells in circulation."

Explain to the patient the procedure for the test.

Inform the patient that food and drinks are not restricted.

Decreased level (↓ 5000 mm³)

Relate a decreased WBC count to clinical problems and drugs. Leukopenia is a decrease in leukocytes. Certain drugs can cause agranulocytosis, severe leukopenia, and neutropenia. With agranulocytosis, the major body defense system is lost, and the patient is susceptible to severe or long-lasting infections. Alcoholism and uncontrolled diabetes reduce the mobilization of leukocytes, causing the patient to be more prone to infections.

Teach the patient to check the side-effects of patent medicines (i.e., cold medications) which could cause agranulocytosis. Individuals should check with their physician about certain patent drugs—those with many side-effects.

Instruct the patients with leukopenia to avoid persons with colds. Their body resistances are reduced, and they are candidates for severe colds or infections.

List any drugs the patient is taking that can decrease the WBC count on the patient's chart and Kardex.

Elevated level (↑ 10,000 mm³)

Relate elevated WBC levels to clinical problems and drugs. With infections and tissue damage, there is an increased number of leukocytes (leukocytosis) responding to the harmful invaders or the injured site. This is the way in which the body protects itself (defense mechanism).

Check the vital signs and note if the temperature and pulse rate are increased. Also check for other signs and symptoms of inflammation and infection.

Notify the physician of changes in the patient's condition—e.g., fever, increased pulse and respiration rate, and leukocytosis.

REFERENCES: LABORATORY TESTS

1. Billet, E.T., & Welch, M.J. The use of clinical laboratory findings in diagnosing and managing critically ill children. *Critical Care Quarterly*, 1979, *2 (3)*, 19–35.
2. *Bio-Science directory of services*. Van Nuys, Calif.: Bio-Science Laboratories, 1980.
3. Brundage, D. *Nursing management of renal problems* (2nd ed.). St. Louis: Mosby, 1980.
4. Byrne, C.J. et al. *Laboratory tests*. Reading, Mass.: Addison–Wesley, 1981.
5. *Diseases*. Horsham, Penn.: Intermed Communications, 1981.
6. Elbaum, N. Detecting and correcting magnesium imbalance. *Nursing '77*, 1977, *7*, 34–35.
7. Felver, L. Understanding the electrolyte maze. *American Journal of Nursing*, 1980, *80 (9)*, 1591–95.
8. Fischbach, F. *A manual of laboratory diagnostic tests*. Philadelphia: Lippincott, 1980.
9. French, R.M. *Guide to diagnostic procedures* (5th ed.). New York: McGraw-Hill, 1980.
10. Friedman, R.B., et al. Effects of diseases on clinical laboratory tests. *Clinical Chemistry*, 1980, *26 (4)*, 1–243.
11. Garb, S. *Laboratory tests in common use* (6th ed.). New York: Springer, 1976.
12. Grant, M.M., & Winifred, M.K. Assessing a patient's hydration status. *American Journal of Nursing*, 1975, *75 (8)*, 1306–11.
13. Groer, M.E., et al. *Basic pathophsyiology: A conceptual approach*. St. Louis: Mosby, 1979.
14. Henry, J.B. *Todd–Sanford–Davidsohn: Clinical diagnosis and management by laboratory methods* (16th ed.). Philadelphia: Saunders, 1979.
15. Jones, D.A., et al. *Medical–surgical nursing*. New York: McGraw-Hill, 1978.
16. Kee, J.L. Clinical implications of laboratory studies in critical care. *Critical Care Quarterly*, 1979, *2 (3)*, 1–17.
17. Kee, J.L. *Fluids and electrolytes with clinical applications* (2nd ed.). New York: John Wiley and Sons, 1978.
18. Krause, M.V., & Mahan, L.K. *Food, nutrition and diet therapy* (6th ed.). Philadelphia: Saunders, 1979.
19. Lancour, J. Two hormones: Regulators and fluid balance. *In Nursing skillbook: Monitoring fluid and electrolytes precisely*. Horsham, Penn.: Intermed Communications, 1978.
20. Linne, J.J., & Lingsrud, K.M. *Basic techniques for medical laboratory* (2nd ed). New York: McGraw–Hill, 1979.
21. Luckmann, J., & Sorensen, K.C. *Medical–surgical nursing* (2nd ed.). Philadelphia: Saunders, 1980.
22. Menzel, L.K. Clinical problems of electrolyte balance. *Nursing Clinics of North America*, 1980, *15 (3)*, 559–75.
23. Nester, E.W., et al. *Microbiology*. New York: Holt, Rinehart, and Winston, 1973.
24. O'Dorisio, T.M. Hypercalcemic crisis. *Heart and Lung*, 1978, *7 (3)*, 425–32.
25. Patterson, H.R., et al. *Falconer's current drug handbook, 1980–1982*. Philadelphia: Saunders, 1980.
26. Phipps, W., et al. *Shafer's medical–surgical nursing*. (7th ed.) St. Louis: Mosby, 1980.
27. Ravel, R. *Clinical laboratory medicine* (3rd ed.). Chicago: Year Book Medical Publishers, 1978.
28. Robinson, C.H. *Normal and therapeutic nutrition* (14th ed.). New York: Macmillan, 1972.
29. Stark, J. BUN/creatinine: Your keys to kidney function. *Nursing '80*, 1980, *10 (5)*, 33–38.
30. Strand, M.M., & Elmer, L.A. *Clinical laboratory tests* (2nd ed.). St. Louis: Mosby, 1980.
31. Tilkian, S.M., et al. *Clinical implications of laboratory tests* (2nd ed.). St. Louis: Mosby, 1979.
32. Tiongson, J.G., & Woods, A.L. Cardiac isoenzymes: Clinical implications and limitations. *Critical Care Quarterly*, 1979, *2 (3)*, 47–51.
33. Tripp, A. Hyper and hypocalcemia. *American Journal of Nursing*, 1976, *76 (7)*, 1142–45.
34. Wallach, J. *Interpretation of diagnostic tests* (3rd ed.). Boston: Little, Brown, 1978.
35. Whaley, L.F., & Wong, D.L. *Nursing care of infants and children*. St. Louis: Mosby, 1979.
36. Widmann, F. *Clinical interpretation of laboratory tests* (8th ed.). Philadelphia: Davis, 1980.

PART II
Diagnostic Tests

A

AMNIOTIC FLUID ANALYSIS
Amniocentesis, Amnioscopy

NORMAL FINDING
Clear amniotic fluid.

DESCRIPTION
Amniotic fluid analysis is useful for detecting chromosomal abnormality, such as Down's syndrome or mongolism (trisomy 21); fetal sex for sex-linked disorders, such as hemophilia; and fetal maturity. The amniotic fluid is obtained by amniocentesis. This procedure includes an insertion of a needle into the suprapubic area after the fetus has been located and manually elevated and the aspiration of 5 to 15 ml of amniotic fluid. Ultrasound may be used to locate the placenta and fetal positions so that the needle contact can be avoided. Amniocentesis is performed during the 14th to 16th weeks of pregnancy. It usually is not done before the 14th week due to the insufficient amount of amniotic fluid or after the 16th week if a therapeutic abortion would be suggested.

Analysis of the amniotic fluid may also include color, bilirubin (present in the fluid until the 28th week, but absent at full term), meconium (present during stress—e.g., in breech presentation), creatinine, Lecithin/Sphingomyelin (L/S) ratio (a decreased ratio can indicate respiratory distress syndrome), glucose, lipids, and alpha-fetoprotein.

Amnioscopy involves insertion of a fiberoptic lighted instrument (amnioscope) into the cervical canal for direct visualization of the amniotic fluid. The color of the amniotic fluid can indicate fetal hypoxia. This test is normally performed close to full term, since it requires cervical dilation. Since there is a risk of rupturing the amniotic membrane and of intrauterine infection, the test is rarely performed.[3,5,24]

CLINICAL PROBLEMS
Indications: to detect chromosomal disorders (e.g., Down's syndrome), neural tube defects (e.g., spina bifida), hemolytic disease due to Rh incompatibility; to determine fetal sex (important for sex-linked disorders—e.g., hemophilia), fetal maturity, pulmonary maturity of the fetus (L/S ratio).

PROCEDURE
A consent form should be signed by the pregnant woman.

Food and fluids are not restricted.

Have the patient void before the procedure to prevent puncturing the bladder and aspirating urine.

The suprapubic area is cleansed with an antiseptic—e.g., betadine. A local anesthetic (such as 1 percent lidocaine) is injected at the site for the amniocentesis.

The placenta and fetus should be located by ultrasound or manually (fetus only). A 22 gauge spinal needle with stylet is inserted through the skin to the amniotic cavity. From 5 to 15 ml of amniotic fluid are aspirated. The needle is removed and a small dressing is applied to the needle insertion site.

The procedure takes approximately 30 minutes.

FACTORS AFFECTING DIAGNOSTIC RESULTS
A traumatic amniocentesis tap may produce blood in the amniotic fluid.

NURSING IMPLICATIONS WITH RATIONALE

Recognize when amniocentesis for amniotic fluid analysis is indicated—i.e., with a familial history of sex-linked, genetic, or chromosomal disorders; with a history of previous miscarriages; and in advanced maternal age (more than 35 years old). It is not a screening test.

Explain to the patient that the test is to detect possible birth defects or give a similar response. Inform her that normal results from the test do not always guarantee a normal infant, nor do they always predict sex gender correctly. The physician should tell the woman of potential risks, such as premature labor, spontaneous abortion, infection, and fetal or placental bleeding from the needle. These complications rarely occur, but the woman should be told of the risk factors.

Explain the procedure to the patient. Be sure that the patient urinates before the test and the consent form is signed.

Be supportive of the woman and her spouse. Be a good listener. Allow them time to ask questions and express any concerns. Refer questions you can't answer to the appropriate health professionals.

Encourage the woman and her spouse to seek genetic counseling, especially if chromosomal abnormality has been determined. Usually the final decision about terminating a pregnancy rests on the pregnant woman and her spouse.

ANGIOGRAPHY (Angiogram)

Arteriography: Cardiac. (See Cardiac Catheterization, Cerebral Angiography, Pulmonary Angiography, and Renal Angiography.)

NORMAL FINDING
    Normal structure and potency of the blood vessels.

DESCRIPTION
    The terms angiography (examination of the blood vessels) and arteriography (examination of the arteries) are used interchangeably. A catheter is inserted into either the femoral, brachial, or carotid artery and a contrast dye is injected to allow visualization of the blood vessels. This procedure is done with the aid of fluoroscopy. Normally the patient feels a warm, flushed sensation as the dye is injected.

    Angiographies are useful for evaluating patency of blood vessels and for identifying abnormal vascularization resulting from neoplasms (tumors). This test may be indicated when computerized tomography (CT) or radionuclide scanning suggests vascular abnormalities.

    Cerebral angiography: Any of the three arteries (femoral, brachial, or carotid) can be used for the angiography; however, the selection of the artery depends on a previous artery problem. The dye will outline the carotid artery, vertebral artery, large blood vessels of the circle of Willis, and small cerebral arterial branches.

    Pulmonary angiography: The catheter is inserted into the brachial artery (in the arm) or the femoral artery and threaded to the pulmonary artery. The dye is injected for visualizing pulmonary vessels. During the test, the patient should be monitored for cardiac arrhythmias.

    Renal angiography: The catheter is inserted into the femoral artery and passed upward through the iliac artery and the aorta to the renal artery. This test permits visualization of the renal vessels and the parenchyma. An aortogram is sometimes made with renal angiography to detect any vessel abnormality and to show the relationship of the renal arteries to the aorta.[3,5,15,19,23]

CLINICAL PROBLEMS

Type of Angiography	Indications
Cerebral	To detect cerebravascular aneurysm, cerebral thrombosis, hematomas, tumors from increased vascularization, cerebral plaques or spasm, cerebral fistula
	To determine cerebral blood flow, cause of increased intracranial pressure (↑ ICP)
Pulmonary	To detect pulmonary embolism; tumors; aneurysms; congenital defects; vascular changes associated with emphysema, blebs, and bullae; heart abnormality
	To evaluate pulmonary circulation
Renal	To detect renal artery stenosis; renal thrombus or embolus; space-occupying lesions—i.e., tumors, cysts; aneurysms
	To determine the causative factor of hypertension, cause of renal failure
	To evaluate renal circulation

PROCEDURE

Most angiographies require the same patient preparations, so these will be presented first. Differences in preparation for angiography will also be listed.

A consent form should be signed by the patient or a designated family member.

The patient should be NPO for 8 to 12 hours before the angiogram. Anticoagulants (such as heparin) are usually discontinued.

Vital signs should be recorded.

Dentures and metallic objects should be removed before the test.

The injection site should be shaved.

Premedications (i.e., a sedative or narcotic analgesic) are given an hour before the test. If the patient has a history of severe allergic reactions to various substances or drugs, the physician may order steroids and/or antihistamines before and after the procedure as a prophylactic measure.

IV fluids may be started before the procedure so that emergency drugs may be administered, if needed.

The patient lies in a supine position on an x-ray table. A local anesthetic is administered to the injection or incisional site.

The test takes approximately 1 to 2 hours.

Renal: A laxative or cleansing enema is usually ordered the evening before the test.

Pulmonary: ECG (EKG) electrodes are attached to the patient's chest for cardiac monitoring (tracings of heart activity) during the angiography. Pulmonary pressures are recorded and blood samples are obtained before the contrast dye is injected.

FACTORS AFFECTING DIAGNOSTIC RESULTS

Feces and gas can distort or decrease the visualizaton of the kidneys.

Barium sulfate from a recent barium study can interfere with the test results.

Movement during the filming can distort the x-ray picture.

NURSING IMPLICATIONS WITH RATIONALE

Explain to the patient that the purpose of the test is to check the blood circulation in the brain or the lungs or the kidneys.

Explain the procecure to the patient (see *Description* and *Procedure* above). Inform the patient that the radiologist, surgeon or physician will inject a contrast dye into an artery at the groin, elbow, or neck. The area will be numbed and a catheter will be inserted and threaded with the guidance of fluoroscopy to the appropriate site.

Inform the patient that he or she will most likely feel a warm, flushed sensation when the dye is injected which should last for a minute or two. Explain to the patient that the test should not cause pain, but can cause some periodic discomfort during the procedure.

Obtain a patient history of hypersensitivity to iodine, seafood, or contrast dye from other x-ray procedures—e.g., IVP (intravenous pyelography). The physician should also know if the patient is highly sensitive to other substances. Skin testing could be done before the test or prophylactic medications (i.e., steroids, antihistamines) may be given prior to and/or following the test.

Record baseline vital signs.

Give a laxative or cleansing enema, if ordered. Explain to the patient that it will cleanse the lower intestinal tract, allowing better visualization.

Have the patient void, wear a gown, and remove dentures.

Administer premedications (sedative and narcotic analgesic) as ordered. Check that the consent form has been signed before giving premedications. The patient should be in bed with the bedsides up after the premedications are given.

Encourage the patient to ask questions. This test can be frightening to patients and they will need time to express any concerns.

Post-test

Apply pressure on the injection site for 5 to 10 minutes or longer until bleeding has stopped. Check the injection site for bleeding when taking vital signs.

Monitor vital signs (blood pressure, pulse, respiration [BP, P, R]) every 15 minutes for the first hour, every 30 minutes for the next 2 hours, and then every hour for the next 4 hours or until stable. The temperature should be taken every 4 hours for 24 to 48 hours or as ordered.

Enforce bed rest for 12 to 24 hours or as ordered. Activities should be restricted for a day.

Assess the injection site for swelling and for hematoma.

Check peripheral pulses in the extremities—i.e., dorsalis pedis, femoral, and radial. Absence or weakness in pulse volume should be reported immediately.

Note the temperature and color of the extremity. Report changes (e.g., color—pale) to the physician immediately. Arterial occlusion to the extremity could occur.

Apply cold compresses or an ice pack to the injection site for edema or pain with the physician's permission or according to routine orders.

Monitor ECG (electrocardiogram) tracings, urine output, and IV fluids. IV fluids and cardiac monitoring may be discontinued after the angiography.

Inform the patient that coughing usually is not abnormal following a pulmonary angiography.

Assess for dysphagia and for respiratory distress if the carotid artery was used for cerebral angiography.

Assess for weakness or numbness in an extremity, confusion, or slurred speech following a cerebral angiography. These could be symptoms of transient ischemic attack (TIA), known as "small strokes."

Observe for a delayed allergic reaction to the contrast dye—i.e., tachycardia, dyspnea, skin rash, urticaria (hives), decreasing systolic blood pressure, and decreased urine output.

Be supportive of the patient and his or her family. Answer questions and explain your nursing implications.

B

BARIUM ENEMA
Lower Gastrointestinal Test, X-Ray Examination of the Colon

NORMAL FINDING
Adult: normal filling, normal structure of the large colon.

DESCRIPTION
The barium enema test is an x-ray examination of the large intestine (colon) to detect the presence of polyps, an intestinal mass, diverticuli, an intestinal stricture/obstruction, or ulcerations. Barium sulfate (single contrast) or barium sulfate and air (double contrast or air contrast) is given slowly through a rectal tube into the large colon. The filling process is monitored by fluoroscopy and then x-rays are taken. The colon must be free of fecal material so that the barium will outline the large intestine to detect any disorders. The double-contrast technique (barium and air) is useful for identifying polyps.

The barium enema test is indicated for patients complaining of lower abdominal pain and cramps; blood, mucus, or pus in the stool; changes in bowel habits; and changes in stool formation. The test can be performed in a hospital, in a clinic, or at a private laboratory.[5,8,15,16]

CLINICAL PROBLEMS
Abnormal results: carcinoma (tumor or lesion); inflammatory disease—ulcerative colitis, granulomatous colitis, diverticulitis; diverticulae; fistulae; polpys; intussusception.

PROCEDURE
In most institutions, the procedures for the barium enema are similar; however, they usually differ to some degree. Some institutions request that the patient maintain a low-residue diet (tender meats, eggs, bread, clear soup, pureed bland vegetables and fruits, potatoes, and boiled milk) for 2 to 3 days before the test. Abdominal x-rays, ultrasound studies, radionuclide scans, and proctosigmoidoscopy should be done before the barium enema.

Pre-preparation

1. Oral medications should not be given for 24 hours before the test, unless indicated by the physician. Narcotics and barbiturates could interfere with fetal elimination before and after the test.
2. The patient should be on a clear liquid diet for 18 to 24 hours before the test. This would include broth, ginger ale, Coca Cola, black coffee or tea with sugar only, gelatin, and syrup from canned fruit. Some institutions permit a white chicken sandwich (*no* butter, lettuce, or mayonnaise) or hard boiled eggs and gelatin for lunch and dinner; then NPO after dinner.
3. Encourage the patient to increase water and clear liquid intake 24 hours before the test in order to maintain adequate hydration.
4. Castor oil (2 ounces) or magnesium citrate (10 to 12 ounces) should be taken the day before the test in the late afternoon or early evening (4 P.M. to 8 P.M.).
5. A cleansing enema (such as a soap suds enema) should be given the evening before the test.

6. Saline enemas (maximum three enemas) should be given early in the morning (6 A.M.) until the returned solution is clear. Some private laboratories have clients use Dulcolax suppositories in the morning instead of the enemas.

7. Black coffee or tea is permitted 1 hour before the test. Some institutions permit dry toast.

Post-preparation

1. The patient should expel the barium in the bathroom or bedpan immediately after the test.

2. Breakfast or lunch should be given.

3. A laxative (such as, milk of magnesium or magnesium citrate) or an oil retention enema should be given to get the barium out of the colon. Sometimes a laxative may need to be repeated the following day after the test.

FACTORS AFFECTING LABORATORY RESULTS

Inadequate bowel preparation with fecal material remaining in the colon.

The use of barium sulfate in upper gastrointestinal and small bowel studies 2 to 3 days before the barium enema test could affect the results.

NURSING IMPLICATIONS WITH RATIONALE

Explain to the patient that the purpose of the barium enema is to determine the cause of his or her clinical symptoms, or give a similar response.

Review the written procedure for that institution. Explain the procedure to the patient. Procedures do differ from one institution to another. Usually the preparations for a barium enema have similarities (clear liquids, increased fluid intake, laxatives, and cleansing enemas). Fecal material in the large intestine (bowel or colon) should be completely eliminated.

List the procedure step by step for the patient. Most private laboratories have written preparation slips for many of their diagnostic tests, and these slips are given or sent to the client. Many of the hospitals do not have preparation slips, so they depend on the nurse to give the information to the patient.

Emphasize the importance of following dietary restrictions and bowel preparation. With inadequate pre-preparation, the patient will have to repeat the test and the prescribed instructions.

Notify the physician if the patient has severe abdominal cramps and pain prior to the test. The physician may want to check for intestinal perforation. A medication may be indicated to decrease the discomfort. The barium enema test should not be performed if the patient has severe ulcerative colitis, suspected perforation, or tachycardia.

Explain to the patient that he or she will be placed on a tilting x-ray table for positioning purposes to increase the barium flow into the colon. Explain that a technician will be with him or her and will explain each step of the procedure.

Inform the patient that the test takes approximately ½ to 1 hour to complete. Tell the patient to take deep breaths through the mouth, which helps to decrease tension and promote relaxation.

Administer a laxative or cleansing enema after the test. Instruct the patient to check the color of the stools for 2 to 3 days. Stools may be light in color due to the barium sulfate. Absence of stool should be reported. Retention of barium sulfate after the test could cause obstruction and/or fecal impaction.

BLOOD VOLUME DETERMINATION/STUDIES (Blood Volume Measurement)

NORMAL RANGE
Adult: *Total blood volume:* 55–80 ml/kg. Men: 7.5 percent body weight. Women: 6.5 percent body weight. *Red cell volume:* Men: 25–35 ml/kg. Women: 20–30 ml/kg. *Plasma volume:* Men: 32–46 ml/kg. Women: 30–45 ml/kg.

DESCRIPTION
The blood volume determination is commonly used to determine the total blood, red cell, and plasma volumes. Two radioactive substances can be used for measurement: ^{51}Cr-tagged red cells for red blood cell volume and ^{131}I- or ^{125}I-tagged human serum albumin for plasma volume. The patient's blood is mixed with the radioactive substance.

This test is useful for monitoring blood loss during surgery, evaluating gastrointestinal or uterine bleeding, determining the cause of hypotension, determining the blood component lost (i.e., red blood cells, plasma) for replacement therapy, and diagnosing polycythemia vera.[6,8,20]

CLINICAL PROBLEMS
Decreased volume: dehydration (total and plasma volume), hypovolemic shock, hemorrhaging.

Elevated volume: dehydration (RBC volume), polycythemia vera, overhydration (total volume).

PROCEDURE
Obtain the height and weight of the patient.

Obtain a blood sample.

Personnel from the Nuclear Medicine Laboratory will obtain a blood sample and mix a radioisotope (radionuclide—i.e., ^{131}I, ^{125}I, ^{51}Cr) with the blood. After 15 to 30 minutes, the blood containing the radioactive substance will be reinjected into the patient.

Collect another blood sample in 15 minutes.

FACTORS AFFECTING DIAGNOSTIC RESULTS
Intravenous (IV) fluids can affect the test results.

Prolonged time for blood sample collection. If ^{131}I-tagged albumin is used, it will leave the plasma (intravascular fluid compartment) after 15 minutes and enter the extravascular fluid compartment.

NURSING IMPLICATIONS WITH RATIONALE

Recognize the causes associated with decreased and elevated blood volumes (see *Clinical Problems* above).

Explain to the patient the purpose of the test. Explanation may be brief, such as, "to determine the blood volume," *or* "to evaluate blood loss," *or* "to determine the amount for blood and fluid replacement."

Explain the procedure to the patient.

Start intravenous (IV) therapy, if ordered, after the blood volume determination test has been completed.

Explain to the patient that the radioactive substance he or she will receive is of low amount and should be harmless.

Answer the patient's questions or refer them to the appropriate health professionals.

Observe for signs and symptoms of dehydration—i.e., dry mucous membrane, poor skin turgor, and shock-like symptoms.

Observe for signs and symptoms of shock—i.e., tachycardia; tachypnea; pale, cold, clammy skin; and later a drop in blood pressure.

BRONCHOGRAPHY, BRONCHOGRAM

NORMAL FINDING
    Normal tracheobronchial structure.

DESCRIPTION
    Bronchography is an x-ray test to visualize the trachea, bronchi, and the entire bronchial tree after a radiopaque iodine contrast liquid is injected through a catheter into the tracheobronchial space. The bronchi are coated with the contrast dye and a series of x-rays are then taken. Bronchography may be done in conjunction with bronchoscopy.
    Bronchography is contraindicated during pregnancy. This test should also not be done if the patient is hypersensitive to anesthetics, iodine, or x-ray dyes.[3,5,9,19]

CLINICAL PROBLEMS
    Indications: to detect bronchial obstruction—i.e., foreign bodies, tumors; cysts or cavities; bronchietasis.
    Perform with bronchoscopy.

PROCEDURE
    A consent form should be signed by the patient or an appropriate family member.
    NPO for 6 to 8 hours before the test.
    Oral hygiene the night before the test and in the morning. This will decrease the number of bacteria which could be introduced into the lungs.
    Postural drainage is performed for 3 days before the test. This procedure aids in the removal of bronchial mucous and secretions. Potassium iodide or another expectorant may be ordered for 1 to 3 days before the test. This drug will loosen secretions and could detect an allergy to iodine.
    A sedative and atropine are given 1 hour before the test. The sedative/tranquilizer is to promote relaxation and atropine is to reduce secretions during the test.
    A topical anesthetic is sprayed into the pharynx and trachea. A catheter is passed through the nose into the trachea, and a local anesthetic and ionized contrast liquid are injected through the catheter.
    The patient is usually asked to change body positions so that the contrast dye can reach most areas of the bronchial tree.
    Following the bronchography procedure, the patient may receive nebulization and should perform postural drainage to remove contrast dye. Food and fluids are restricted until the gag (cough) reflex is present.

FACTORS AFFECTING DIAGNOSTIC RESULTS
    Secretions in the tracheobronchial tree which can prevent the contrast dye from coating the bronchial walls.

NURSING IMPLICATIONS WITH RATIONALE

Explain to the patient that the purpose of the bronchogram is to visualize the bronchi and to identify abnormal changes, *or* say that the purpose is to take x-rays as part of the bronchoscopy test.

Explain the procedure of the test. Generally, patients are extremely apprehensive about this test and are fearful that they may be unable to breathe. Reassure the patient that the airway will not be blocked. Inform the patient that he or she may have a sore throat after the test as the result of the catheter (irritation).

Obtain a history of hypersensitivity to anesthetics, iodine, and x-ray dyes. Usually the patient will receive an expectorant (e.g., potassium iodide) several days before the test. Potassium iodide would serve two purposes: as an expectorant and to determine if the patient is allergic to iodine, if this is unknown.

Teach the patient how to perform postural drainage (over the side of the bed, or place the bed in the Trendelenberg position for 15 to 20 minutes three times a day). It is important that chest secretions are removed prior to the test to assure good visualization of the bronchial tree.

Encourage the patient to relax and teach relaxation techniques.

Check the consent form to see that it is signed. Administer pre-test medications an hour before the test and and after the consent form has been signed.

Inform the patient that he or she is not to eat for 6 to 8 hours before the test.

Instruct the patient to do good oral hygiene the night before and the morning of the test. Check the oral hygiene procedure. Dentures should be removed before the test.

Record vital signs.

Answer the patient's questions and refer questions you can't answer to other appropriate health professionals. Permit the patient time to express his or her concerns.

Post-test

Assess for signs and symptoms of larygneal edema—i.e., dyspnea, hoarseness, apprehension. This could be due to a traumatic insertion of the catheter.

Assess for allergic reaction to the anesthetic and ionized contrast dye—i.e., apprehension, flushing, rash, urticaria (hives), dyspnea, tachycardia, and/or hypotension.

Check the gag reflex to see that it has returned before offering food and fluids. Have the patient swallow and cough, or tickle the posterior pharynx with a cotton swab; if gag reflex is present, offer ice chips or sips of water before food.

Monitor vital signs. The temperature may be slightly elevated for 1 or 2 days after the test.

Check breath signs. If rhonchi and fever are present, notify the physician and record on the patient's chart.

Have the patient perform postural drainage post-test. This procedure helps with the removal of the contrast dye. Physiologic damage will not occur if some of the dye remains in the lung for a period of time.

Offer throat lozenges or an ordered medication for sore throat.

Be supportive of the patient and family. Be available to answer their questions.

BRONCHOSCOPY

NORMAL FINDING
Normal structure and lining of the trachea and bronchi.

DESCRIPTION
Bronchoscopy is the direct inspection of the larynx, trachea, and bronchi through a standard metal bronchoscope or a flexible fiberoptic bronchoscope called a bronchofibroscope. The flexible fiberoptic bronchoscope has a mirror and light at its distal end, and because of its smallness in width and its flexibility, it allows for visualization of the segmental and subsegmental bronchi.

Through the bronchoscopes, a catheter brush or biopsy forceps can be passed to obtain secretions and tissues for cytologic examination. The two main purposes of bronchoscopy are visualization and specimen collection in the tracheobronchial tree.[3,5,8,19]

CLINICAL PROBLEMS

Indications: to detect tracheobronchial lesion (i.e., a tumor), bleeding site; to remove foreign bodies, secretions (liquid and tissue) for cytologic and bacteriologic examinations, mucus plugs; to improve tracheobronchial drainage.

PROCEDURE

A consent form for bronchoscopy should be signed by the patient or an appropriate family member.

The patient should be NPO for 6 hours before the bronchoscopy, and preferably for 8 to 12 hours before the test.

The patient should remove dentures, contact lenses, jewelry.

Obtain a history of hypersensitivity to analgesics, anesthetics, and antibiotics.

Check vital signs and record. Administer premedications. Record vital signs, premedications, and when the patient voided on the preoperative check list and the patient's chart.

The patient will be lying on a table in the supine or semi-Fowler's position with his head hyperextended, or he will be seated in a chair. Local anesthetic may be sprayed in the patient's throat and the bronchoscope will be inserted through the patient's nose or mouth by the physician. Frequently, it is inserted through the mouth.

Specimen containers should be labelled and specimens should be taken immediately to the laboratory. The procedure takes about 1 hour.

FACTORS AFFECTING DIAGNOSTIC RESULTS

Improper labelling of the specimen.

Failure to take specimens immediately to the laboratory.

NURSING IMPLICATIONS WITH RATIONALE

Explain to the patient that the purpose of the test is to check the bronchial tubes and/or to obtain a specimen.

Explain the procedure to the patient. Explanation is important to help allay the patient's anxiety.

Instruct the patient to relax before and during the test. The premedications will aid in increasing relaxation and decreasing anxiety. Tell the patient the physician will inform him or her of how the procedure is progressing. Bronchoscopy usually is performed under local anesthesia, but could be performed under general anesthesia. The patient should be told whether he or she will receive a local or a general anesthetic.

Advise the patient that the procedure takes about 1 hour.

Check that the consent form is signed and that the patient has voided before giving premedications. Atropine is usually one of the drugs given which causes dryness of the mouth. Inform the patient that the drugs will make him or her feel sleepy and the mouth feel dry. The patient should remain in bed, and the bedsides should be up after premedications are given.

Check that dentures, contact lenses, and jewelry have been removed.

Instruct the patient to practice breathing in and out through the nose with the mouth opened. This is important if the bronchoscope is inserted through the mouth.

Obtain vital signs (VS) and prepare a VS flow chart. Record admission and pre-test vital signs which will service as baseline VS.

Encourage the patient to ask questions and give the patient time to express concerns. Inform the patient that there may be some discomfort but that the spray will help to decrease it. Inform the patient that he will receive adequate air exchange. Oxygen can be given through the side arm of the bronchoscope.

Inform the patient that he may have hoarseness and/or a sore throat after the test.

Post-bronchoscopy

Recognize the complications that can follow bronchoscopy—i.e., laryngeal edema, bronchospasm, pneumothorax, cardiac arrhythmias, and bleeding from the biopsy site.

Check vital signs (BP, P, R) every 15 minutes for 1 hour, every 30 minutes for the next 2 hours, and hourly for 4 hours or until stable. Check the temperature every 4 hours for 24 hours. If the pulse rate greatly increases and the blood pressure begins to fall, these could be signs of shock.

Elevate the head of the bed (semi-Fowler's position). If the patient is unconscious, turn him on his side with the head of the bed slightly elevated.

Assess for signs and symptoms of respiratory difficulty—i.e., dyspnea, wheezing, apprehension, and decreased breath sounds. Notify the physician at once.

Check for hemoptysis (coughing up excessive bloodly secretions) and notify the physician. Inform the patient that he may cough up some blood-tinged mucus and that this is not abnormal. It usually occurs following a biopsy or after a traumatic insertion of the bronchoscope.

Assess the gag (cough) reflex before giving food and liquids. Ask the patient to swallow or cough. It normally takes 2 to 8 hours before the gag reflex returns. Offer ice chips and sips of water before offering food.

Offer the patient lozenges or prescribed medication for mild throat irritaion after the gag reflex is present.

Instruct the patient not to smoke for 6 to 8 hours. Smoking may cause the patient to cough and start bleeding, especially after a biopsy.

Be supportive of the patient. Have physical contact with the patient's hand or arm for reassurance, as necessary.

C

CARDIAC CATHETERIZATION
Cardiac Angiography (Angiocardiography), Coronary Arteriography

NORMAL FINDING
Patency of coronary arteries; normal heart size, structure, valves; normal heart and pulmonary pressures.

DESCRIPTION
The first cardiac catheterization was performed in 1844 on a horse. It was not until 1929 that the first right cardiac catheterization was performed on a human—the young Dr. Werner Forssmann catheterized himself. During the 1930s and 1940s, there were "quite a few" right cardiac catheterizations done, but the first left cardiac catheterization was not performed until the early 1950s. In the late 1960s and during the 1970s the procedure and equipment for cardiac catheterization were greatly improved.

Cardiac catheterization is a procedure in which a long catheter is inserted in a vein or artery of the arm or leg. This catheter is threaded to the heart chambers and/or coronary arteries with the guidance of fluoroscopy. Contrast dye is injected for visualizing the heart structures. During injection of the dye, cineangiography is used for filming heart activity. The terms *angiocardiography* and *coronary arteriography* are used interchangeably with the term *cardiac catheterization;* however, with coronary arteriography, dye is injected directly into the coronary arteries, and with angiocardiography, dye is injected into heart, coronary, and/or pulmonary vessels.

With right cardiac catheterization, the catheter is inserted into the femoral vein or an antecubital vein and threaded through the inferior vena cava into the right atrium to the pulmonary artery. Right atrium, right ventricle, and pulmonary artery pressures are measured and blood samples from the right side of the heart can be obtained. While the dye is being injected, the functions of the tricuspid and pulmonary valves can be observed.

For left cardiac catheterization, the catheter is inserted into the brachial or femoral artery and is advanced retrograde through the aorta to the coronary arteries and/or left ventricle. Dye is injected. The patency of the coronary arteries and/or functions of the aortic and mitral valves and the left ventricle can be observed. This procedure is indicated before heart surgery.

The frequency of complications due to cardiac catheterizations have decreased to less than 2 percent. The complications that can occur, though rare, are myocardial infarction, arrhythmias, cardiac tamponade, pulmonary embolism, and cerebral embolism (CVA).[3,5,8,12,19]

CLINICAL PROBLEMS
Abnormal results: *Right-sided cardiac catheterization:* tricuspid stenosis, pulmonary stenosis, pulmonary hypertension, septal defects. *Left-sided cardiac catheterization:* coronary artery disease—coronary occlusion (partial or complete); valvular heart disease—mitral stenosis, mitral regurgitation, aortic regurgitation; left ventricular hypertrophy; aneurysm—ventricle.

PROCEDURE
A consent form must be signed by the patient or a designated member of the family. The physician should discuss with the patient and/or the family the procedure and possible risk factors before the consent form is signed.

Food and fluids are restricted for 6 to 8 hours before the test, according to the hospital's policy. Some institutions permit clear liquids until 4 hours before the test.

Skin tests may be performed if the patient is allergic to iodine products. Antihistamines (e.g., Benadryl) may be ordered the evening before and the morning of the test if an allergic reaction is suspected.

Medications are restricted for 6 to 8 hours before the test unless otherwise ordered by the physician. Oral anticoagulants are discontinued or the dosage is reduced to prevent excessive bleeding. Heparin may be ordered to prevent thrombi.

The injection site of the arm or groin is shaved and cleansed with antiseptics.

The weight and height of the patient should be recorded. These are used to calculate the amount of dye needed—i.e., 1 ml/kg of body weight.

The patient should void before receiving the premedications. Dentures should be removed unless this is not indicated.

Record baseline vital signs (VS). Note the volume intensity of pulses. Vital signs should be monitored during the test.

Premedications should be given ½ to 1 hour before the cardiac catheterization. Usually a sedative or tranquilizer (e.g., Valium [diazepam]) and/or an analgesic are given.

The patient is taken to the cardiac catheterization room and is strapped to a padded table that tilts. The patient should lie still during the insertion of the catheter and the filming of coronary arteries and heart.

A 5 percent dextrose in water infusion is started at a "keep vein open" (KVO) rate for giving emergency drugs, if needed.

ECG (EKG) leads are applied to the chest skin surface to monitor heart activity.

A local skin anesthetic is injected at the catheter insertion site. A cutdown to locate the vessel may be needed. The patient will feel a hot, flushing sensation for several seconds or a minute as the dye is injected.

The patient may be instructed during the procedure to cough and breathe deeply. Coughing can also help to decrease nausea and dizziness.

The procedure takes 1.5 to 3 hours.

FACTORS AFFECTING DIAGNOSTIC RESULTS
Insufficient amount of contrast dye.
Movement by the patient could cause complications and interfere with the filming.

NURSING IMPLICATIONS WITH RATIONALE

Explain to the patient that the purpose of the test is to check the coronary arteries for blockage *or* to check for heart valve defects. This test is almost always done before heart surgery, mostly to determine if heart surgery is necessary.

Explain the procedure to the patient. Ask the patients what they know about the test and what the physician has told them. The cardiologist or cardiac surgeon should explain the risk factors to the patient.

Inform the patient that he will be in a special cardiac catheterization room. Give information about the padded table, the ECG leads to monitor heart activity, the IV fluids which will run slowly, the local skin anesthetic, and instructions that he may receive (such as to cough and breathe deeply). Inform the patient that there should be no pain except some discomfort at the catheter insertion site and from lying on his back. Instruct the patient to ask any questions he may have during the test. Tell the patient to tell the physician if he has chest pain or difficulty in breathing during the procedure. The patient's ECG and VS are monitored; however, the patient should speak out if he is experiencing chest pain or dyspnea.

Tell the patient that he may feel a hot, flushing sensation for a minute or two because of the dye. The reason for this is a brief vasodilation due to the dye.

Inform the patient that food, drinks, and medications are restricted for 6 to 8 hours before the test unless otherwise ordered by the physician.

Encourage the patient to ask questions and allow the patient and family time to express any concerns. Refer questions you cannot answer to the cardiologist or other health professionals.

Advise the patient that the doctors and nurses will be wearing hospital gowns and masks.

Obtain a patient history of allergic reactions to seafood, iodine, or iodine contrast dye used in other x-ray tests (e.g., IVP). A skin test may be performed to determine the severity of the allergy. An antihistamine (e.g., Benadryl) may be given the day before and/or the day of the test as a prophylactic measure.

Record baseline vital signs. Vital signs will be monitored during the procedure. Record the patient's height and weight for calculating the amount of dye to be given.

Have the patient void and remove dentures before the test. Check that the catheter insertion sites has been prepped (shaved and cleansed with an antiseptic).

Administer premedications ½ to 1 hour before the test. Make sure that the patient has voided and that the consent form has been signed before giving the premedications.

Tell the patient that the test takes approximately 1.5 to 3 hours.

Post-test

Monitor vital signs (BP, P, R) every 15 minutes the first hour, every 30 minutes for the next 2 hours, and every hour for 4 hours or until stable, or as ordered. Temperatures should be taken every 4 hours while the patient is awake for several days.

Observe the catheter insertion site for bleeding or hematoma. Change dressings as needed.

Check peripheral pulses below the insertion site; if the femoral artery was used, then check the popliteal and dorsalis pedis pulses, and if the bracheal artery was used, then check the radial pulse. Note the strength of the pulse beat.

Assess the patient's skin color and temperature.

Tell the patient that he is to remain on bed rest for 12 hours. The patient can turn from side to side, but the bed should not be elevated for 6 hours if the femoral artery was used for the cardiac catheterization. The leg should be extended. If the brachial artery was used, the head of the bed can be slightly elevated; however, the arm should be immobilized for 3 hours.

Be supportive of the patient and family. Answer questions or refer them to the appropriate health professionals. Communicate with the patient about the nursing care being given.

Administer narcotic analgesics or analgesics as ordered. Give antibiotics, if ordered.

Encourage fluid intake after the test, unless contraindicated (e.g., CHF).

CHOLANGIOGRAPHY (IV), PERCUTANEOUS CHOLANGIOGRAPHY, T-TUBE CHOLANGIOGRAPHY

NORMAL FINDING
Patent biliary ducts (absence of stones and strictures).

DESCRIPTION
Intravenous IV cholangiography examines the biliary ducts (hepatic ducts within the liver, the common hepatic duct, the cystic duct, and the common hepatic duct, the cystic duct, and the common bile duct) by radiographic and tomographic visualization.

Often the gallbladder is not well visualized. The contrast substance, an iodine prepara-tion such as Cholografin, is injected intravenously and approximately 15 minutes later x-rays are taken. IV cholangiography is a tedious and time-consuming test, and toxic reactions are more common with the IV contrast substance than with the oral agents.

Precutaneous cholangiography is indicated when biliary obstruction is suspected. The contrast substance is directly instilled into the biliary tree. The process is visualized by fluoroscopy and spot films are taken.

T-tube cholangiography, also known as postoperative cholangiography, may be done 7 to 8 hours after a cholecystectomy to explore the common bile duct for patency of the duct and to see if any gallstones are left. During the operation, a T-shaped tube is placed in the common bile duct to promote drainage. The contrast substance is in-jected into the T-tube. A stone or two could be missed during a cholecystectomy, caus-ing occlusion of the duct.[3,5,8,9,23]

CLINICAL PROBLEMS

Test	Indications
IV cholangiography	To detect stricture, stones in the biliary system, tumor in the biliary system, cause of jaundice
Percutaneous cholangiography	To detect obstruction of the biliary system, cause of severe jaundice
T-tube cholangiography	To detect obstruction of the common bile duct from stones, stricture

PROCEDURE

IV cholangiography: A consent form for IV cholangiography should be signed by the patient or an appropriate family member.

The patient should be NPO for 8 hours before the test. Some radiologists encourage fat-free liquids before the test to prevent renal toxicity due to the injected dye.

A laxative (i.e., citrate of magnesium or castor oil) may be given the night before the test and a cleansing enema may be given in the morning. Keeping the GI tract clear can prevent shadows on the x-ray films. Check with the radiology department for the exact preparation needed.

A contrast agent, Cholografin, is injected intravenously while the patient is lying on a tilting x-ray table. X-rays are taken every 15 to 30 minutes until the common bile duct is visualized.

Tomographic studies may be performed after the biliary ducts have been visualized.

Percutaneous cholangiography: A consent form for percutaneous cholangiography should be signed by the patient or an appropriate family member.

The patient should be NPO for 8 hours before the test.

A laxative the night before and cleansing enema the morning of the test may be ordered.

Preoperative medications usually include sedatives/tranquilizers. An antibiotic may be ordered for 24 to 72 hours before the test for prophylactic purposes.

The patient is placed on a tilting x-ray table that rotates. The upper right quadrant of the abdomen is cleansed and draped. A local (skin) anesthetic is given.

The patient should exhale and hold his breath while a needle is inserted with the guidance of fluoroscopy into the biliary tree. Bile is withdrawn and the contrast sub-stance is then injected. Spot films are taken.

A sterile dressing will be applied to the puncture site.

T-tube cholangiography: A consent form for T-tube cholangiography should be signed by the patient or an appropriate family member.

The patient should be NPO for 8 hours before the test.

A cleansing enema may be ordered in the morning before the test.

The patient lies on an x-ray table and a contrast agent, such as Hypaque, is injected into the T-tube and an x-ray is taken. The final x-ray is taken 15 minutes later.

The T-tube may be removed following the procedure or it may be left in place.

FACTORS AFFECTING DIAGNOSTIC RESULTS

Obesity, gas, or fecal material in the intestines can affect the clarity of the x-ray.

NURSING IMPLICATIONS WITH RATIONALE

Explain to the patient that the purpose of the test is to determine if the biliary ducts (above and below the gallbladder) are patent.

Explain to the patient the procedure for the IV cholangiography, percutaneous cholangiography, and T-tube cholangiography. Check with your institution to see if procedures differ and make modifications in your explanation to the patient. List the procedure step by step for the patient, as requested. This can decrease high levels of anxiety.

Obtain a patient history of allergies to seafood, iodine, or x-ray dye. Report a history of allergies to these substances to the physician and record in the patient's chart.

Permit the patient to ventilate his concerns. Answer questions, if possible. Refer questions you cannot answer to the physician or radiologist.

Check that the consent form has been signed by the patient before giving a sedative and before the test.

Administer the pre-test orders—i.e., laxatives, sedatives, etc.

Inform the patient having IV cholangiography that the test may take several hours (up to 4 hours).

Observe for signs and symptoms of allergic reaction to contrast agents—i.e., nausea; vomiting; flushing; rash; urticaria (hives); hypotension; slurred, thick speech; and dyspnea.

Check the infusion site for signs of phlebitis—i.e., pain, redness, swelling. Apply warm compresses to the infusion site if symptoms are present, as ordered.

Check vital signs as ordered for percutaneous cholangiography—e.g., every 15 minutes for the first hour, every 30 minutes for the second hour, and then every hour for 4 hours. Notify the physician if the temperature is 100°F (or 37.9°C) or over.

Instruct the patient to remain in bed for 6 hours following percutaneous cholangiography.

CHOLECYSTOGRAPHY (ORAL), GALLBLADDER RADIOGRAPHY, GALLBLADDER (GB) SERIES

NORMAL FINDING

A gallbladder of normal size and structure without stones.

DESCRIPTION

Oral cholecystography is an x-ray test frequently used to visualize gallstones in the gallbladder. There are two types of gallstones: radiopaque, usually composed of calcium carbonate, and radiolucent, composed of cholesterol or bile pigment. The radiolucent stones are the most common ones and can be visualized using contrast material (radiopaque dye) absorbed by the gallbladder. It takes 12 to 14 hours for the process of dye absorption. The dye is (1) absorbed by the small intestine, then absorbed by the liver, (2) excreted in the bile, and (3) concentrated in the gallbladder. Nonfunctioning liver cells can hamper the excretion of the radiopaque dye.

Failure to visualize the gallbladder could be due to: hypermotility of the bowel (diarrhea), liver disease, obstruction of the cystic duct, and inadequate patient preparation—i.e., a high-fat diet the night before will cause the gallbladder to empty, thus losing the dye. If the gallbladder cannot be visualized using an oral contrast substance, the IV cholangiography may be ordered.

Immediately after the oral cholecystography test, the patient may be given a fat stimulus meal. Fluoroscopic examination and x-rays are taken to observe the ability of the gallbladder to empty the dye. If GI x-rays are ordered, the gallbladder x-ray should be obtained first, since barium could interfere with the test results.[3,5,8,9,16,23]

CLINICAL PROBLEMS

Cholelithiasis (gallstones), neoplasms (tumors) of the gallbladder, cholecystitis (inflammation of the gallbladder, with or without stones), obstruction of the cystic duct.

PROCEDURE

The patient should have a fat-free diet 24 hours before the x-ray. Some x-ray departments suggest a high-fat meal at noon to empty the gallbladder and then a low-fat meal in the evening. After the dinner meal the night before the test, the patient should be NPO except for sips of water.

Two hours after the dinner meal, radiopaque tablets are given according to the directions on the folder. There are various commercial contrast agents—i.e., Telepaque (iopanoic acid), Oragrafin (calcium or sodium ipodate), Cholebrine, Priodax, Teridax, and Monophen. The patient should take the tablets or capsules (6 tablets of Telepaque) 5 minutes apart with a full glass of water (240 ml total).

No laxatives until after the x-ray tests. Some x-ray departments request a saline enema the morning of the test to clear the gastrointestinal tract so that fecal material does not interfere with the gallbladder test.

A high-fat meal (cream, butter, eggs) or synthetic fat-containing substances (Bilevac) may be given in the x-ray department after the fasting x-rays are taken. Post-fatty meal films will be taken at intervals to determine how fast the gallbladder expels the dye.

The fasting x-ray tests (Stage I) take from 45 minutes to 1 hour, and the post-fatty meal tests (Stage II) take another hour or two.

FACTORS AFFECTING DIAGNOSTIC RESULTS

Inadequate patient preparation—i.e., a high-fat meal the night before, not taking all the tablets. Check with the radiology department for the correct preparation.

GI series, barium enema, thyroid scan, ^{131}I uptake before the cholecystography test.

Diarrhea or vomiting can inhibit absorption of the contrast substance.

Liver disease.

NURSING IMPLICATIONS WITH RATIONALE

Explain to the patient that the purpose of the test is to check for gallstones or to determine the cause of the pain in the upper-right quadrant.

Explain the test procedure to the patient. Check your x-ray department's procedure before describing the preparation for the test to the patient. A written procedure list would be a helpful reminder.

Obtain a history of allergies the patient may have to seafood, iodine, or x-ray dye.

Observe for signs and symptoms of jaundice—i.e., yellow sclera of the eyes, yellow skin, and a serum bilirubin level greater than 3 mg/dl.

Inform the patient that the evening meal before the test should be fat-free. If there are foods high in fat on the tray (i.e., whole milk, cream, butter, sauces, fatty meats, etc.), he should not eat them. In some institutions coffee or tea with sugar is given in the morning.

Administer the radiopaque tablets every 5 minutes with a full glass of water 2 hours after the dinner meal. The patient may take the tablets on his own, but he may need to be reminded.

Inform the patient that it is not uncommon for the test to be repeated and that he should not be alarmed. If the test is repeated, the patient should remain on a low-fat diet and the radiopaque tablets should be taken again as directed.

Observe for signs and symptoms of allergic reaction to the radiopaque tablets—i.e., elevated temperature, rash, urticaria (hives), hypotension, thick speech, or dyspnea.

Report vomiting and diarrhea prior to the test to the physician. The tablets may not be absorbed because of hypermotility. Usually the test is cancelled.

Report to the physician and/or the x-ray department if the patient is scheduled for a barium enema, GI series, thyroid scan, or ^{131}I uptake before the gallbladder (GB) series. These tests should be done after the GB series to prevent test interference.

Inform the patient that the test does not hurt. Tell him the test is usually in two parts—the first part takes approximately 45 minutes to 1 hour and, if the second part is ordered, he will receive a high-fat meal or a fat-containing agent and then more x-ray pictures will be taken.

COLONOSCOPY

NORMAL FINDING
Normal mucosa of the large intestine; absence of pathology.

DESCRIPTION
Colonoscopy is an inspection of the large intestine (colon) using a long flexible fiber-scope (colonoscope). This instrument is inserted anally and advanced with extreme care through the rectum, the sigmoid colon, and the large intestine to the cecum. Occasionally fluoroscopy may be used to guide the colonoscope through the intestine and to locate the tip of the colonoscope when it does not advance.

This test is performed when the barium enema and proctosigmoidoscopy results are negative and a lesion is still suspected, or it can be used to confirm results of these tests. A biopsy forceps or cytologic brush can be passed through the scope for obtaining specimens and removing foreign bodies. Polyps can be removed with the use of an electrocautery snare.

Colonoscopy should not be done on pregnant women near term, following an acute myocardial infarction, after recent abdominal surgery, in acute diverticulitis, in severe (active) ulcerative colitis, or in a confused/uncooperative patient. Occasionally, colon perforation occurs due to the fiberscope; however, this is rare. Bleeding may be a side-effect of the biopsy or polypectomy.[5,8,18]

CLINICAL PROBLEMS
Indications: to detect the origin of lower intestinal bleeding, diverticular disease, or benign or malignant lesions—i.e., polyps or tumors; to diagnose and follow-up ulcerative colitis; and screening and follow-up of patients with "high risk colons."

PROCEDURE

A consent form should be signed by the patient or a designated member of the family.

Specific laboratory tests (hemoglobin, hematocrit, PT, PTT, and platelet count) should be done within the 2 days before the test.

The medication list should be checked and iron therapy held until after the procedure.

Patient should receive a clear liquid diet for 2 to 3 days before the test and should be NPO for 8 hours prior to the test.

Dulcolax tablets may be ordered every night for 3 days prior to the procedure.

A laxative (i.e., castor oil 1 to 2 oz. or magnesium citrate 10 oz.) is usually given the night before the test. In the morning, warm water or saline enemas are given until the returning fluid is clear. Soapsud enemas should not be given, since they can irritate the intestinal mucosa.

A sedative/tranquilizer may be ordered prior to the test to promote relaxation. A narcotic analgesic may also be given.

An endoscopist and a radiologist usually perform the colonoscopy. The procedure takes from 30 minutes to 1.5 hours.

The patient lies in Sim's position on his left side. A well-lubricated colonoscope is inserted. A small amount of air is insufflated for better visualization. Fluoroscopy could be used and x-rays are taken.

Glucagon or IV anticholinergics may be given to decrease bowel spasms.

If specimens are obtained, place the tissue specimens in 10 percent formalin and place cytology smears in 95 percent ethyl alcohol or Carnoy's solution or use a commercial fixation spray. The latter can distort cells.

The procedure can be done in the hospital (the x-ray department or the endoscopy room), clinics, or the physician's office.

FACTORS AFFECTING DIAGNOSTIC RESULTS

A soapsud enema can cause intestinal irritation.

Barium sulfate from other diagnostic studies can decrease visualization; therefore, the study should not be attempted within 10 days to 2 weeks of a barium study.

Failure to use appropriate preservatives on specimens.

NURSING IMPLICATIONS WITH RATIONALE

Explain to the patient that the purpose of the test is to identify the cause of his bowel problem *or* to examine the lining of the large intestine.

Explain the procedure to the patient. Permit the patient time to express concerns and feelings about his clinical problem or the test.

Administer the laxatives and enema as ordered (see *Procedure* above).

Check that the laboratory test (Hgb, HCT, PT, PTT, platelets) results are posted in the patient's chart.

Have the patient sign a consent form for having the colonoscopy before administering premedication(s)—i.e., a sedative/tranquilizer and/or narcotic analgesic.

Record baseline vital signs.

Encourage the patient to relax during the test. Instruct the patient to breathe deeply and slowly through the mouth during the insertion of the colonoscope.

Inform the patient that he most likely will be lying on his left side and may be asked to change body positions.

Post-test

Monitor vital signs (VS) every ½ hour for 2 hours, hourly for 4 hours, or until stable, or as ordered.

Inform the patient that he may have flatus because of air insertion.

Check for excessive anal bleeding and report findings. Removal of polyps may cause increased bleeding. Severe abdominal cramps and hemorrhaging should be reported immediately, for they could indicate perforation. Hemoglobin and hematocrit tests may be ordered for 1 to 2 days post-test.

Check for abdominal distention and report findings.

Instruct the patient to remain on bed rest for 6 to 8 hours after the test or as ordered by the physician.

Strain all stools for polyps if any were removed but not recovered. As requested, place specimens in formalin solution and send them to the pathology laboratory.

COLPOSCOPY

NORMAL FINDING
Normal appearance of the vagina and cervical structures.

DESCRIPTION
Colposcopy is the examination of the vagina and cervix using a binocular instrument (colposcope) which has a magnifying lens and a light. This test is for identifying pre-cancerous lesions of the cervix and can be performed in the gynecologist's office or in the hospital. After a positive Papanicolaou (Pap) smear or a suspicious cervical lesion, colposcopy is indicated for examining the vagina and cervix more thoroughly. A typical epithelium, leukoplakia vulvae, and irregular blood vessels can be identified with this procedure, and photographs and a biopsy specimen can be obtained.

Since this test has become more popular, there has been a decreased need for coniza-tion (surgical removal of a cone of tissue from the cervical os). Colposcopy is also useful for monitoring women whose mothers received diethylstilbestrol during pregnancy; these women are prone to develop precancerous and cancerous lesions of the vagina and cervix. Colposcopy is used to monitor female patients who have had cervical lesions removed.[5,8,15,23]

CLINICAL PROBLEMS
Indications: to identify vaginal and cervical lesions, abnormal cervical tissue after a positive Pap smear, irregular blood vessels, leukoplakia vulvae; to monitor previous treatment for dysplasia and cervical lesions, vaginal and cervical tissue changes for women whose mothers took diethylstilbestrol during pregnancy.

PROCEDURE
Food and drinks are not restricted.

The patient's clothes should be removed, and the patient should wear a gown and be properly draped.

The patient assumes a lithotomy position (legs in stirrups). A speculum is inserted into the vagina and a long, dry cotton swab applicator is used to clear away any cervical secretions. Another long cotton swab applicator with saline may be used to swab the cervix for visualizing vascular patterns.

Acetic acid (3 percent) is applied to the vagina and cervix. This produces color changes in the cervical epithelium and helps in detecting abnormal changes.

A biopsy specimen of suspicious tissues and photographs may be taken. Pressure should be applied to control bleeding at the biopsy site, or cautery may be used.

A vaginal tampon may be worn after the procedure.

The test takes approximately 15 to 20 minutes.

FACTORS AFFECTING DIAGNOSTIC RESULTS
Mucus, cervical secretions, creams, and medications can decrease visualization.

NURSING IMPLICATIONS WITH RATIONALE

Explain to the patient that the purpose of the test is to improve visualization of the vagina and cervix *or* to monitor or identify possible tissue changes in the cervix.

Explain the procedure to the patient—e.g., the fact that food and drinks are not restricted, the lithotomy position, the speculum insertion, the fact that the instrument (colposcope) is not inserted into the vagina and is used to magnify cervical tissue, and that a biopsy specimen and photographs may thus be taken.

Inform the patient that she should not experience pain but that there may be some discomfort with the insertion of the speculum or when the biopsy specimen is taken.

Tell the patient that the test takes 15 to 20 minutes.

Encourage the patient to ask questions and express any concerns or fears. Reducing anxiety is important for the patient and for the test. Remain with the patient during the procedure.

Place the biopsy tissue into a bottle containing 10 percent formalin, and place the cells, if obtained, on a slide and spray them with a fixation solution.

Post-test

Inform the patient that she may have some bleeding for a few hours because of the biopsy. Tell the patient that she can use tampons and that if bleeding becomes heavy and it is not her menstrual period, she should call the gynecologist.

Instruct the patient not to have intercourse for a week until the biopsy site is healed or as ordered by the physician.

Inform the patient that the doctor will notify her of the results and tell her if she hasn't heard from the office in a week, to call.

COMPUTERIZED TOMOGRAPHY (CT) SCAN
COMPUTERIZED AXIAL TOMOGRAPHY (CAT);
Cat Scan, Computerized Transaxial Tomography (CTT), EMI Scan

NORMAL FINDING
Normal tissue; no pathologic findings.

DESCRIPTION
The computerized tomography (CT) scan was developed in England in 1972 by the Electric Music Industries, Ltd. and was originally called the EMI scan. Other names for the CT scan are: computerized axial tomography, or CAT scan; computerized transaxial (transverse) tomography, or CTT scan; and computer-assisted transaxial tomography, or CATT scan. The preferred term is computerized tomography, or CT scan.

The CT scanner produces a narrow x-ray beam which examines body sections from many different angles. It produces a series of cross-sectional images in sequence that build up a three-dimensional picture of the organ—e.g., the brain. The traditional x-ray takes a flat or frontal picture which gives a two-dimensional view. The computerized tomography scanner is about 100 times more sensitive than the x-ray machine. Although it is a costly diagnostic test, CT scanning is popular since it can diagnose an early stage of disease and other tests are not needed.

CT technique was first used to detect diseases of the brain. Today computerized tomography is an accurate and valuable technique for identifying brain lesions. It is replacing pneumoencephalography. Recently, orders for radionuclide brain scans and cerebral angiography have greatly decreased. CT scanning frequently is used following head trauma with neurologic symptoms to determine its severity.

The CT scan can be performed with or without iodine contrast dye. The iodine in the contrast dye causes a greater tissue absorption and is referred to as contrast enhancement. Small tumors may not be seen if contrast enhancement is not used. Tissues are identified according to their density. A dense substance such as bone appears white; a low-density substance, such as cerebral fluid, appears dark; and tissues show varying shades of gray.

Computed tomography of the body is commonly used, but CT's ability to identify abnormalities in the body is not always as good as its ability to identify abnormalities in the brain. Back-up diagnostic tests are usually needed. With body tomography, structures of the thorax with the great vessels (lungs, heart, aorta, vena cava), of the abdomen (liver, pancreas, gallbladder, kidney), and of the pelvis (uterus, ovaries, testes, bladder) can be examined. CT of the body has not replaced the use of ultrasonography (ultrasound) for examining abdominal organs.[5,8,13,15,23,25]

CLINICAL PROBLEMS

Type of Computed Tomography	Abnormal Results
Head	Cerebral lesions
	Hematomas
	Tumors (meningioma, glioblastoma)
	Cysts
	Hydrocephalus
	Cerebral atrophy
	Cerebral infarction (obstruction)
	Cerebral edema
Body	Tumors of the lung, liver, pancreas, kidney, and adrenals
	Cysts or abscesses of the lung, liver, pancreas, and kidneys
	Pancreatitis (enlargement of the pancreas)
	Liver cirrhosis with ascites
	Renal calculi
	Polycystic kidney disease
	Aortic aneurysm
	Enlarged lymph nodes
	Pleural effusion

PROCEDURE

The procedure for patient preparation will be divided into head CT and body CT.

Head computerized tomography: A consent form should be signed by the patient or a designated family member.

The patient should be NPO for 3 to 4 hours before the test. If contrast enhancement is not performed, the patient does not need to restrict food or fluids. However, the need for contrast dye is not always known, so it is better for the patient to be NPO, if possible. Contrast dye can cause nausea and vomiting.

The patient should remove hairpins, clips, and jewelry (earrings) before the test.

Steroids or antihistamines may be ordered several days before the test if the patient has known allergies to iodine, shellfish, or contrast dye used in other x-ray tests. Emergency drugs and equipment should be readily available to treat severe allergic reactions—e.g., anaphylactic shock.

The patient lies on a special table with his or her head positioned in a cradle. A wide rubberized strap is wrapped snugly around the head to keep it immobilized during the test. The patient's head is moved into a circular (doughnut-like opening) scanner. Various sounds are heard, such as clicking noises and gears shifting.

If contrast enhancement is needed, an iodine contast agent (i.e., meglumine diatrizoate or sodium diatrizoate) is injected intravenously over a period of 2 minutes. The patient will feel warm and flushed and experience a metallic or salty taste. Nausea is not uncommon. These symptoms usually last for only a minute.

A mild sedative or analgesic may be ordered for restless patients or those who have aches and pains of the neck or back.

The test takes approximately 45 minutes to 1.5 hours.

Body computerized tomography: A consent form should be signed by the patient or a designated family member.

The patient should be NPO for 3 to 4 hours before the body CT scan.

For patients with a lot of flatus or fecal material, an enema may be ordered.

The patient should wear a hospital gown and remove jewelry and metal objects.

Steroids or antihistamines are given several days before the test if the patient has allergies to iodine products. If a patient with hypersensitivity to iodine has not received one of the drugs to avoid allergic reaction, the antihistamine Benadryl could be given orally several hours before or intravenously during the CT scan.

The patient lies in a supine position on a special table with his or her body in the circular opening (doughnut-like) of the scanner. A strap will be placed around the waist to keep the patient securely on the table. The circular scanner revolves around the body area that is to be examined. Usually the patient is requested several times to hold his or her breath to decrease movement of the abdominal organs. The patient is alone in the room and the radiologist or specialized technician is in the control room. The technician can observe the patient and can communicate through an intercom system. Clicking noises will be heard from the scanner.

A needle aspiration or biopsy can be performed in conjunction with computerized tomography.

Usually contrast enhancement is indicated for body CT. To visualize the gastrointestinal tract and separate it from other abdominal organs, the patient may be asked to drink 2 cups of a barium-like substance. IV contrast dye could be injected before or during the scanning. Contrast dye is usually not given for chest or spinal CTs.

Patients who are pregnant or think they are pregnant should not have this test done. Ultrasound examinations are safe during pregnancy.

The test takes approximately 1.5 hours.

FACTORS AFFECTING DIAGNOSTIC RESULTS

Barium sulfate can obscure visualization of the abdominal organs. Barium studies should be performed 4 days before the CT or after the CT.

Excessive flatus can cause patient discomfort and may cause an inaccurate reading.

Movement can cause artifacts.

NURSING IMPLICATIONS WITH RATIONALE

Explain the purpose of the test. Explanation could be brief, such as, "to examine for abnormalities in the head (brain) or body (chest or abdomen)."

Explain the procedure to the patient. Describe the CT room and the scanner to the patient. Some radiology departments have pictures of the circular scanner. Tell the patient that he or she will hear clicking noises. Inform the patient that the amount of radiation received should be no more than he or she would receive from a series of x-rays. Inform the patient that the test is not painful. Tell the patient that head CT takes approximately 45 minutes to 1.5 hours; 45 minutes for head scanning and an additional 45 minutes if contrast enhancement is indicated during the procedure. For body CT, the test takes 1.5 hours.

Obtain a patient history of allergies to seafood, iodine, and contrast dye from other x-ray tests. For hypersensitivity to iodine products, steroids may be ordered for 3 days before CT scanning. For emergency CT scans (e.g., for head injury), an antihistamine, Benadryl, may be given orally or intravenously with a history of iodine or seafood hypersensitiveness. Contrast enhancement is not always done with computerized tomography, especially for head, chest, and spinal CT scanning.

Inform the patient that food and drinks are restricted for 3 to 4 hours before the test. For abdominal CT, a low-residue diet may be ordered for 2 days before the test to decrease flatus. If contrast enhancement definitely is not indicated, the patient does not need to be NPO. Frequently the scanning is done without contrast dye; however, contrast enhancement may be indicated during the procedure for better visualization of a small lesion. Contrast dye injection can cause nausea and vomiting.

Advise the patient that if IV contrast dye is injected, he or she will feel a warm, flushed sensation of the face or body and may have some nausea. This should last for only a minute or two. Observe the patient for signs and symptoms of an allergic reaction to the dye—i.e., dyspnea, palpitations, tachycardia, blood pressure drop, itching, and urticaria (hives). Emergency drugs should always be available to counteract severe allergic reactions, such as anaphylactic shock.

Inform the patient that he may be asked to hold his breath several times during an abdominal CT scan.

Observe for a delayed allergic reaction to the contrast dye—i.e., skin rash, urticaria (hives), headache, and vomiting. An oral antihistamine may be ordered for mild reactions.

Be supportive of the patient and family. The use of CT (CAT) scan can be frightening. The major risk involved is an allergic reaction to the dye.

Instruct the patient to resume his usual level of activity and diet, unless otherwise indicated.

CYSTOSCOPY, CYSTOGRAPHY (CYSTOGRAM)

NORMAL FINDING
Normal structure of the urethra, bladder, prostatic urethra, and ureter orifices.

DESCRIPTION
Cystoscopy is the direct visualization of the bladder wall and urethra with the use of a cystoscope (a tubular lighted telescopic lens). Usually this diagnosis test is performed by a urologist. Small renal calculi can be removed from the ureter, bladder, or urethra with this procedure and a tissue biopsy can be obtained. In addition, a retrograde pyelography may be performed during the cystoscopy.

Cystoscopy is performed in a cystoscopy room of a hospital or in a urologist's office under general or local anesthesia. Premedications are adminstered an hour prior to the test.

Cystography is the instillation of a contrast dye into the bladder via a catheter. This procedure can detect a rupture in the bladder, a neurogenic bladder, fistulas, and tumors. The test is useful when x-rays are needed and a cystoscopy or retrograde pyelography are contraindicated.[2,3,5,8,19]

CLINICAL PROBLEMS
    Indications: to determine the cause of hematuria or the cause of urinary tract in-
    fection; to detect renal calculi (stones), tumors, or prostatic hyperplasia; to remove
    renal stones.

PROCEDURE
    A consent form should be signed by the patient or an appropriate family member.
    The patient can have a full liquid breakfast the morning of the cystoscopy. The
    urologist may want the patient to have several glasses of water before the test. If the
    patient is to have general anesthesia, he or she would be NPO for 5 to 8 hours before
    cystoscopy.
    Record baseline vital signs.
    A sedative/tranquilizer (Valium, barbiturate) and a narcotic analgesic (Demerol,
    morphine) are usually given an hour before the cystoscopy. The procedure is done
    under local or general anesthesia.
    The patient is placed in a lithotomy position (feet or legs in stirrups). A local anesthetic
    is injected into the urethra. Water may be instilled to enhance better visualization.
    The cystoscopy takes approximately 1 hour.

FACTORS AFFECTING DIAGNOSTIC RESULTS
    None reported.

NURSING IMPLICATIONS WITH RATIONALE

Explain to the patient the purpose of the test. Explanation can be brief, such as, "to
    determine the cause of your problem (bleeding, etc.)" *or* "to examine the interior
    part of the bladder."
Explain the procedure to the patient. Tell the patient the procedure should cause little
    or no pain or discomfort. Answer questions and refer questions you cannot answer
    to the urologist.
Check with the urologist about the form of anesthesia the patient will receive—local or
    general. Inform the patient that a local anesthetic will be injected into the urethra
    several minutes before the cystoscope is inserted.
Check that the consent form has been signed before administering the premedications.
    Normally the drugs are given 1 hour before the test.
Offer fluids as ordered before the test.
Encourage the patient to ask questions and express any concerns to the nurse and to
    the urologist.

Post-test
Recognize the complications that can occur as the result of a cystoscopy—i.e.,
    hemorrhaging, perforation of the bladder, urinary retention, and infection.
Monitor vital signs (VS). Compare VS with baseline VS. Blood pressure, pulse, and
    respirations may be ordered every 15 minutes for the first hour, every 30 minutes
    for the second hour, and every hour for 4 hours or longer. The patient's temperature
    should be taken every 4 hours while awake for several days.
Inform the patient that a slight burning sensation when voiding for a day or two is
    considered normal. Usually the urologist leaves an order for an analgesic.
Monitor the urinary output for 48 hours following a cystoscopy. If urine output is less
    than 200 ml in 8 hours, encourage fluid intake. Anuria could indicate urinary reten-
    tion due to blood clots or urethral stricture. Report findings to the urologist. An
    indwelling catheter may be ordered.

Report and record gross hematuria. Inform the patient that blood-tinged urine is not uncommon after a cystoscopic examination.

Observe for signs and symptoms of an infection—i.e., fever, chills, an increased pulse rate, and pain. Antibiotics may be given before and after the test as a prophylactic measure.

Apply heat to the lower abdomen to relieve pain and muscle spasm as ordered. A warm sitz bath may be ordered.

E

ELECTROCARDIOGRAPHY (ELECTROCARDIOGRAM—ECG or EKG), VECTORCARDIOGRAPHY

NORMAL FINDING
Normal electrocardiogram deflections (P, PR, QRS, ST, and T).

DESCRIPTION
An electrocardiogram (ECG or EKG) records the electrical impulses of the heart by the means of electrodes and a galvanometer (ECG machine). These electrodes are placed on the legs, arms, and chest. Combinations of two electrodes are called bipolar leads—i.e., lead I is the combination of both arm electrodes, lead II is the combination of the right arm and left leg electrodes, and lead III is the combination of the left arm and left leg electrodes. The unipolar leads are AVF, AVL, and AVR; the A means augmented, V is the voltage, and F is left foot, L is left arm, and R is right arm. There are at least 6 unipolar chest or precordial leads. A standard electrocardiogram consists of 12 leads: 6 limb leads (I, II, III, AVF, AVL, AVF) and 6 chest (precordial) leads (V_1, V_2, V_3, V_4, V_5, V_6).

With each cardiac cycle or heartbeat, the SA node (sinoatrial or sinus node) sends an electrical impulse through the atrium, causing atrial contraction or atrial depolarization. The SA node is called the pacemaker, since it controls the heart beat. The impulse is then transmitted to the AV (atrioventricular) node and the bundle of His and travels down the ventricles, causing ventricular contraction or ventricular depolarization. When the atria and the ventricles relax, repolarization and recovery occurs.

The electrical activity that the ECG records is in form of waves and complexes: P-wave (atrial depolarization); QRS complex (ventricular depolarization); and S-T segment, T-wave, and U-wave (ventricular repolarization). An abnormal ECG indicates a disturbance in the electrical activity of the myocardium. A person could have heart disease and have a normal ECG as long as the cardiac problem did not affect the transmission of electrical impulses.

P-wave (atrial contraction): The normal time is 0.12 seconds or three small blocks. An enlarged P-wave deflection could indicate atrial enlargement, which could be the result of mitral stenosis.

An absent or altered P-wave could suggest that the electrical impulse did not come from the SA node.

PR interval (from the P-wave to the onset of the Q-wave): The normal time interval is 0.2 seconds or five small blocks.

An increased interval could imply a conduction delay in the AV node. It could be the result of rheumatic fever or arteriosclerotic heart disease.

A short interval could indicate Wolff–Parkinson–White syndrome.

QRS complex (ventricular contraction): The normal time is less than 0.12 seconds or three small blocks.

An enlarged Q-wave may imply an old myocardial infarction.

An enlarged R-wave deflection could indicate ventricular hypertrophy (enlargement).

An increased time duration may indicate a bundle branch block.

S-T segment (beginning ventricular repolarization): A depressed S-T segment indicates myocardial ischemia (decreased supply of oxygen to the myocardium).

An elevated S-T segment can indicate acute myocardial infarction or pericarditis.

A prolonged S-T segment may imply hypocalcemia or hypokalemia.

A short S-T segment may be due to hypercalcemia.

T-wave (ventricular repolarization): A flat or inverted T-wave can indicate myocardial ischemia, myocardial infarction, or hypokalemia.

A tall, peaked T-wave (>10 mm or 10 small blocks in precordial leads, or >5 mm or 5 small blocks in limb leads) can indicate hyperkalemia.

Vectorcardiography (vectorcardiogram, VCG): This records electrical impulses from the cardiac cycle, making it similar to the ECG.

However, it shows a three-dimensional view (frontal, horizontal, and sagittal planes) of the heart, whereas the ECG shows a two-dimensional view (frontal and horizontal planes). The vectorcardiogram is considered more sensitive than the electrocardiogram for diagnosing a myocardial infarction. It is useful for assessing ventricular hypertrophy in adults and children.[3,5,8,9,11,15]

CLINICAL PROBLEMS

Indications: to detect cardiac arrhythmias, cardiac hypertrophies, myocardial ischemia, electrolyte imbalances (potassium, calcium, and magnesium), myocardial infarction, pericarditis; to determine the effects of drugs (i.e., digitalis, quinidine, etc.); to monitor ECG changes during the stress/exercise test and the recovery phase after a myocardial infarction.

PROCEDURE

Food, drinks, and medications are not restricted, unless otherwise indicated.

Clothing should be removed to the waist and the female patient should wear a gown. Nylon stockings should be removed and trouser bottoms should be raised.

The patient should lie in a supine position.

The skin surface should be prepared. Excess hair should be shaved from the chest, if necessary.

Electrodes with electropaste or pads are strapped to the four extremities. The color-coded lead wires are inserted into the correct electrodes—i.e., white (right arm), etc. Chest electrodes are applied. The lead selector is turned to record the 12 standard leads unless the ECG machine automatically records the lead strips.

The ECG takes approximately 15 minutes.

FACTORS AFFECTING DIAGNOSTIC RESULTS

Body movement and electromagnetic interference during the ECG recording could distort the tracing.

NURSING IMPLICATIONS WITH RATIONALE

Explain to the patient that the purpose of the ECG is to record the electrical impulses of the heart. A more detailed explanation may be necessary.

Explain the procedure to the patient in regards to food, removal of clothing, body position for the test, and electrode placements. Tell the patient that the ECG takes about 15 minutes.

Record the list of medications the patient is taking. The physician may want to compare ECG readings to check for improvement and changes; therefore, knowing the drugs the patient is taking at the time of the ECG would be helpful.

Instruct the patient to relax and breathe normally during the ECG procedure. Tell the patient to avoid tightening the muscles, grasping bedrails or other objects, and talking during the ECG tracing.

Tell the patient that the ECG should not cause pain or any great discomfort.

Inform the patient that he should tell you if he is having chest pain during the ECG tracing. Mark the ECG paper at the time the patient is having chest pain.

Allow the patient time to ask questions. Refer questions you cannot answer to the physician or cardiologist.

Remove the electropaste or jelly, if used, from the electrode sites. Assist the patient with dressing, if necessary.

Cleanse the electrode discs with alcohol.

ELECTROENCEPHALOGRAPHY (ELECTROENCEPHALOGRAM—EEG)

NORMAL FINDING
Adult and child: Normal tracing—regular short waves.

DESCRIPTION
The EEG test measures the electrical impulses produced by brain cells. Electrodes are applied to the scalp surface at predetermined measured positions which record brain wave activity on moving paper. Electroencephalogram (EEG) tracings can detect patterns characteristic of some diseases—i.e., seizure disorders, neoplasms, cerebral vascular accidents, head trauma, and infections of the nervous system. At times, recorded brain waves may be normal when there is pathology.

Another use for the EEG is to determine cerebral death. If the EEG recording gives a flat or straight line for many hours, this usually indicates severe hypoxia and brain death. The cardiovascular functions are usually being maintained through the use of life-support systems—e.g., a respirator, oxygen, and IV's. The neurologist interprets the EEG readings and gives suggestions.[3,5,7,8,11,12,13]

CLINICAL PROBLEMS
Abnormal tracing: epilepsy, seizures—grand mal, petit mal, psychomotor; brain neoplasms (tumors); brain abscesses; head injury (trauma); intracranial hemorrhage; encephalitis; unconsciousness, coma.

PROCEDURE
The procedure may be performed while the patient is: (1) awake (2) drowsy, (3) asleep, (4) undergoing stimuli (hyperventilation or rhythmic flashes of bright light), or (5) a combination of any of these.

Pre-EEG: Shampoo the hair the night before. Instruct the patient not to use oil or hair spray on the hair.

The decision concerning withdrawal of medications before the EEG is made by the physician. Sleeping pills and other sedatives should not be given the night before the test, since they can affect the EEG recording.

Food and drinks are not restricted except for coffee, tea, cola, and alcohol.

The EEG tracing is usually obtained with the patient lying down; however, the patient could be seated in a reclining chair.

For a sleep recording, keep the patient awake 2 to 3 hours later the night before the test and wake the patient up at 6 A.M. A sedative such as chloral hydrate may be ordered.

The EEG test takes approximately 1.5 to 2 hours. Flat electrodes will be applied to the scalp.

Post-EEG: Remove the collodion or paste from the patient's head. Acetone may be used to remove the paste.

The patient should resume normal activity unless he has been sedated.

FACTORS AFFECTING DIAGNOSTIC RESULTS
Drugs—i.e., sedatives, barbiturates, anticonvulsants, and tranquilizers.

Alcohol could decrease cerebral impulses.

Oily hair or the use of hair spray can affect test reults.

NURSING IMPLICATIONS WITH RATIONALE

Explain to the patient that the purpose of the test is to record brain activity *or* to determine a seizure disorder.

Explain the procedure to the patient, step by step. List the important steps on paper for the patient.

Inform the patient that he will *not* get an electric shock from the machine (electroencephalograph) and that the machine does not determine the patient's intelligence and cannot read the patient's mind. Many patients are apprehensive and fearful of this test.

Encourage the patient to eat a meal before the test. Hypoglycemia should be prevented, since it can affect normal brain activity. Coffee, tea, cola, and any other stimulants should be avoided. Alcohol is a depressant and can affect the test result.

Inform the patient that the test does not produce pain.

Report to the physician if the patient is taking medications which could change the EEG result.

Check with the physician and/or EEG department in regards to the type or types of recordings ordered—i.e., awake, sleep, stimuli. Advise the patient to be calm and to relax during the test. If rest and stimuli (flashing lights) recordings are ordered, inform the patient that there will be a brief time when there are flashing lights. Prepare the patient but do not increase the patient's apprehension, if possible.

Be supportive of the patient. Answer questions and permit the patient to express concerns.

Report to the physician and inform the EEG lab if the patient is extremely anxious, restless, or upset.

Inform the patient that the test takes 1.5 to 2 hours. The room is quiet where the EEG recording is made and is conducive to rest and sleep.

Instruct the patient that following the test, normal activity can be resumed.

Observe for seizures and describe the seizure activity—the movements and how long they last. Have a tongue blade by the bedside at all times. Chart all seizure activity and the time of its occurrence, because it is very important for the technologist and electroencephalographer to know this.

ELECTROMYOGRAPHY (ELECTROMYOGRAM—EMG)

NORMAL FINDING

At rest: minimal electrical activity.

Voluntary muscle contraction: markedly increased electrical activity.

DESCRIPTION

Electromyography, known as EMG, measures electrical activity of skeletal muscles at rest and during voluntary muscle contraction. A needle electrode is inserted into the skeletal muscle to pick up electrical activity, which can be heard over a loudspeaker, viewed on an oscilloscope, and recorded on graphic paper all at the same time. Normally there is no electrical activity when the muscle is at rest; however, in motor disorders abnormal patterns can occur. With voluntary muscle contraction, there is a loud popping sound and increased electrical activity (wave) is recorded.

Since the nerves innervate muscles, nerve conduction studies are usually done at the same time; thus the EMG may consist of two parts. The test is most helpful in diagnosing neuromuscular, peripheral nerve, and muscular disorders. The EMG can be used to differentiate between myopathy and neuropathy.[3,5,8,19]

CLINICAL PROBLEMS

Abnormal results: muscle disorders—muscular dystrophy; neuromuscular disorders—peripheral neuropathy (i.e., diabetes mellitus, alcoholism), myasthenia gravis, myotonia; central neuronal degeneration—amyotrophic lateral sclerosis (ALS), anterior poliomyelitis.

PROCEDURE

A consent form should be signed by the patient or the appropriate family member.

Food and drinks are not restricted, with the exceptions of coffee, tea, colas, or other caffeine drinks, and smoking is restricted for at least 3 hours before the EMG.

Medications such as muscle relaxants, anticholinergics, and cholinergics should be withheld before the test with the approval of the physician. If the patient needs the specific medication, the time for the test should be rearranged.

The patient lies on a table or stretcher or sits in a chair in a room free of noise. The EMG takes 1 hour but could take longer if a group of muscles are to be tested.

Needle electrodes are inserted in selected or affected muscles. If the patient experiences pain, the needle should be removed and reinserted.

If enzyme tests are ordered (i.e., serum SGOT, CPK, LDH) the samples should be drawn before the EMG or 5 to 10 days after the test.

FACTORS AFFECTING DIAGNOSTIC RESULTS

Pain could cause false results.

Age of the patient: electrical activity may be decreased in some elderly persons.

Drugs: muscle relaxants, anticholinergics, and cholinergics could affect the results.

NURSING IMPLICATIONS WITH RATIONALE

Explain to the patient that the purpose of the test is to check muscle activity or to determine the electrical activity of the muscle, or give a similar response.

Explain the procedure to the patient. Inform the patient that the test will not cause electrocution; however, there may be a slight temporary discomfort when the needle electrodes are inserted. If pain persists for several minutes, the patient should tell the technician.

Ask the physician about withholding patient medications that could affect EMG results. If the patient takes drugs that could interfere with test results prior to the test, the drugs should be listed on the request slip and recorded in the chart.

Instruct the patient to follow the technician's instructions—i.e., to relax the specified muscle(s) and to contract the muscle(s) when requested. An analgesic may be ordered before and after the test.

Inform the patient that the EMG test usually takes 1 hour, but it could take longer.

Check the physician's order for a serum enzyme request. Blood needed for serum enzyme determinations (i.e., AST [SGOT], CKP, LDH) should be drawn before the EMG test.

F

FLUOROSCOPY, FLUOROSCOPIC EXAMINATION

NORMAL FINDING
Normal size, structure, and physiologic function of the organ(s) being examined (chest, heart, intestines).

DESCRIPTION
The fluoroscopic examination allows the radiologist and physician to view in motion the physiologic function of organs on a fluorescent screen. Usually the patient is between the x-ray tube and the fluorescent screen. The x-ray beam penetrates the patient and then strikes the screen. Unfortunately, the patient can receive substantially more radiation than he would receive from standard radiography. The benefits of fluoroscopic examination should outweigh the effects of excessive radiation. Today fluoroscopy is used with many diagnostic tests for visualization and for guidance.

During cardiac catheterization, the fluoroscopic procedure is essential for visualizing the coronary arteries. The moving images can be recorded on videotape and can be a valuable aid to diagnosis.

During fluoroscopic examination, the room is dark for contrast and visualization purposes. If the radiologist and assistant remain in the room, lead aprons should be worn.[5,8,9,15,23]

CLINICAL PROBLEMS

Test Area	Indications
Thorax	To visualize lung expansion, diaphragm movement or paralysis, bronchiolar obstruction
Abdomen	To detect bowel obstruction (stricture or tumor), filling defects, active bleeding and ulceration (peptic ulcer), Meckel's diverticulum, intra-abdominal hernias
Heart	To detect coronary occlusion (partial or total)

PROCEDURE
Thorax:
Food and drinks are usually not restricted.
Jewelry should be removed. A patient gown should be worn.
The patient should breathe deeply and cough as instructed.
Abdomen:
NPO after midnight.
A patient gown should be worn.
The patient swallows a chalky substance, barium sulfate.
Food and fluids are permitted after the examination.
A laxative is usually ordered after the test or that evening.
Heart:
NPO after midnight.
Follow the procedure for Cardiac Catheterization.

FACTORS AFFECTING DIAGNOSTIC RESULTS
Jewelry and metal objects.
Nausea and vomiting.
Medications: narcotics, barbiturates.

NURSING IMPLICATIONS WITH RATIONALE

Explain to the patient the purpose of the test. Explanation may be brief, such as, "to determine if there is a clinical problem" or give a similar response.

Explain the procedure to the patient.

Inform the patient that the fluoroscopic examination should *not* cause discomfort.

Discuss the patient's anxiety and fears. Refer questions you cannot answer to other appropriate health professionals.

Explain to the patient that the chest fluoroscopy should take approximately 10 minutes and the abdominal fluoroscopy 30 minutes to 1 hour.

Determine if the patient is pregnant or if pregnancy is suspected. Report findings immediately to the physician. Fluoroscopy should not be done during pregnancy.

Inform the patient that the radiologist or x-ray personnel will give step-by-step instructions during the procedure. Tell the patient to ask questions if he has any.

Determine if the patient has had extensive x-rays in the last few years or during his lifetime. Excessive radiation can be cumulative. Notify the physician of previous prolonged exposure to radiation.

G

GASTRIC ACID SECRETION, GASTRIC ACID STIMULATION (GASTRIC ANALYSIS—TUBE), TUBELESS GASTRIC ANALYSIS (DIAGNEX BLUE)

NORMAL RANGE
Fasting: 1.0–5.0 mEq/L/hour.
Stimulation: 10–25 mEq/L/hour.
Tubeless: detectable dye in the urine.

DESCRIPTION

The gastric analysis test examines the acidity of the gastric secretions in the basal state (without stimulation) and the maximal secretory ability (with stimulation; i.e., with histamine phosphate, histalog [betazole HCl], pentagastrin, alcohol, caffeine, or insulin—the latter three are seldom used today for testing.) An increased amount of free hydrochloric acid could indicate a peptic ulcer (stomach or duodenal), and an absence of free hydrochloric acid (achlorhydria) could indicate gastric atrophy (possibly due to gastric malignancy) or pernicious anemia. In addition, gastric contents can be collected for cytologic examination.

Gastric analysis by tube (basal and stimulation) and tubeless gastric analysis (urine examination after a resin dye and stimulant are administered) are the methods used for evaluating gastric secretions. The *Hollander test*, an insulin test utilizing the gastric analysis method, evaluates the effects of IV insulin on vagus nerve stimulation. Normally, IV insulin causes hypoglycemia, which increases vagus stimulation and acid secretion. This test is usually done before and after a vagotomy to determine the effect of vagus nerve resection in decreasing vagal stimulation and acid secretion. The Hollander test can be dangerous and is rarely performed.

Tube gastric analysis (basal): Gastric secretions are aspirated through a nasogastric tube after a period of fasting. Specimens are obtained to evaluate the acidity of the gastric content first (basal) and the gastric stimulation test follows.

Tube gastric analysis (stimulation): The stimulation test is usually a continuation of the basal gastric analysis. After samples of gastric secretions are obtained, a gastric stimulant (i.e., histalog or pentagastrin) is administered and gastric contents are aspirated every 15 to 20 minutes until several samples are obtained.

Tubeless gastric analysis: This test is for screening purposes to detect the presence or absence of hydrochloric acid; however, it will *not* give the amount of free acid in the stomach. A gastric stimulant (caffeine, histalog) is given and an hour later a resin dye (Azuresin, Diagnex Blue) is taken orally by the patient. The free hydrochloric acid (HCl) releases the dye from the resin base; the dye is absorbed by the gastrointestinal tract and is excreted in the urine. Absence of the dye in the urine 2 hours later is indicative of gastric achlorhydria. This test method saves the patient the discomfort of being intubated with a nasogastric tube; however, it does lack accuracy.

There is controversy over the usefulness of gastric acid secretory tests; however, they are still used to document gastric acid hypersecretions—e.g., Zollinger–Ellison syndrome and hypergastrinemia.[3,5,9,10,19]

CLINICAL PROBLEMS
Decreased level: pernicious anemia, gastric malignancy (atrophy), atrophic gastritis.
Elevated level: peptic ulcer (duodenal), Zollinger–Ellison syndrome.

PROCEDURE

Tube gastric analysis (basal and stimulation): Usually the basal and stimulation gastric analysis tests are performed by a gastroenterologist or physician.

The patient should be NPO for 8 to 12 hours prior to the test. Smoking should be restricted for 8 hours.

Certain groups of drugs (i.e., anticholinergics, cholinergics, adrenergic blockers, antacids, steroids) and alcohol and coffee should be restricted for at least 24 hours before the test. It should be noted on the request slip if the drugs cannot be withheld.

Baseline vital signs should be recorded.

Loose dentures should be removed.

A lubricated nasogastric tube is inserted through the nose or mouth.

A residual gastric specimen and four additional specimens taken 15 minutes apart should be aspirated and labelled with the patient's name, the time, and a specimen number. The nasogastric tube may be attached to low intermittent suction.

Stimulation test: This is usually a continuation of the basal gastric analysis test.

A gastric stimulant is administered—i.e., histalog (betazole HCl) or histamine phosphate intramuscularly; pentagastrin subcutaneously; or caffeine solution 500 mg or 7 percent ethyl alcohol 50 ml through the tube.

Several gastric specimens are obtained over a period of 1 to 2 hours (histamine four 15 minute specimens in 1 hour and histalog eight fifteen minute specimens in 2 hours). Specimens should be labelled with the patient's name, the date, the time, and specimen numbers.

Vital signs should be monitored. Emergency drugs such as epinephrine (adrenalin) should be available.

The test usually takes 2.5 hours for both parts (basal and stimulation).

Tubeless gastric analysis: The patient should be NPO for 8 to 12 hours before the test. The morning urine specimen is discarded.

Certain drugs are withheld for 48 hours before the test—i.e., antacids, electrolyte preparations (potassium, calcium, sodium, magnesium), quinidine, quinine, iron, vitamin B complex.

Give the patient caffeine sodium benzoate 500 mg in a glass of water.

Collect a urine specimen 1 hour later. This is the control urine specimen.

Give the patient the resin dye agent (Azuresin or Diagnex Blue) in a glass of water.

Collect a urine specimen 2 hours later. The urine may be colored blue or blue-green for several days. Absence of blue color in the urine usually indicates absence of hydrochloric acid in the stomach.

FACTORS AFFECTING DIAGNOSTIC RESULTS

Incorrect labelling of specimens.

Drugs: antacids, anticholinergics, and cimetidine could decrease HCl levels; adrenergic blockers, cholinergics, steroids, and alcohol could elevate HCl levels; antacids, electrolyte and iron preparations, vitamin B complex, and quinidine could falsely elevate the Diagnex Blue level.

Stress, smoking, and sensory stimulation could increase HCl secretion.

NURSING IMPLICATIONS WITH RATIONALE

Recognize the purpose of the tube or tubeless gastric analysis test (see *Description* and *Clinical Problems* above).

Explain the purpose of the test. Explanation could be brief, such as, "to determine if the stomach is secreting an excess or a decreased amount of hydrochloric acid."

Explain the procedure of the tube or tubeless gastric analysis test to the patient. Check with the physician before you give your explanation to find out whether he or she will perform both parts—both basal and stimulation gastric analysis (see *Procedure* above). List the steps of the test on paper for the patient, as needed.

Tell the patient how the nasogastric tube is inserted (i.e., the tube is lubricated and passes through the nose or mouth), that he will be asked to swallow or will be given sips of water as the tube is passed into the stomach, and that the end of the tube is attached in most cases to low intermittent suction.

Notify the physician if the patient is receiving the following categories of drugs: antacids, antispasmodics, anticholinergics, adrenergic blockers, cholinergics, and steroids. Drugs from the above groups and a few others should be withheld for 24 to 48 hours before the gastric analysis. Drugs that cannot be withheld should be listed on the request slip.

Monitor vital signs. Observe for possible side-effects from use of stimulants—i.e., dizziness, flushing, tachycardia, headache, and a lower systolic blood pressure.

Label the specimens (gastric or urine) with the patient's name, the date, the time, and the specimen number.

Be supportive of the patient. Encourage the patient to express his or her concerns or fears. Answer questions or refer them to the physician or to other appropriate health professionals.

GASTROINTESTINAL (GI) SERIES, UPPER GI SERIES, BARIUM SWALLOW, SMALL BOWEL SERIES, HYPOTONIC DUODENOGRAPHY

NORMAL FINDING

Normal structure of the esophagus, stomach, and small intestine, and normal peristalsis.

DESCRIPTION

Many names are given to the upper GI series, which includes a fluoroscopic and x-ray examinations of the esophagus, stomach, and small intestine. The patient is given orally a barium meal (barium sulfate) or a water-soluble contrast agent, Gastrografin (meglucamine diatrizoate). By means of fluoroscopy, the barium is observed as it passes through the digestive tract and spot films are taken. Inflammation, ulcerations, and tumors of the stomach and duodenum can be detected through this procedure.

Upper GI series are performed in hospitals or in privates laboratories. A preparation sheet is given or sent to the patient prior to the test.

If increased peristalsis, a spastic duodenal bulb, a space-occupying lesion is observed or suspected in the duodenal area during the GI series, a *hypotonic duodenography* procedure can be performed by giving glucagon, atropine, or probanthine to slow down the action of the small intestine. Preparations for the hypotonic duodenography are similar to those for the upper GI series. Because of the anticholinergic effect of the drug, the patient should be observed closely for urinary retention.[5,8,9,16,19,23]

CLINICAL PROBLEMS

Hiatal hernia; esophageal varices; esophageal or small-bowel strictures; gastric or duodenal ulcer; gastritis or gastroenteritis; gastric polyps; neoplasms (benign or malignant tumor) of the esophagus, stomach, or duodenum; diverticula of the stomach and duodenum; pyloric stenosis; malabsorption syndrome; volvulus of the stomach; foreign bodies.

PROCEDURE

The patient should be NPO (food and fluid), should take no medications, and should not smoke for 8 to 12 hours before the test. A low-residue diet may be ordered for the 2 to 3 days before the test. If medications cannot be withheld the evening before or the morning of the test, then the drugs should be listed on the request slip and the radiologist should be notified.

The patient swallows a chalk-flavored (chocolate, strawberry) barium meal or Gastrografin in the calculated amount.

Spot films are taken during the fluoroscopic examination. The procedure takes approximately 1 to 2 hours but could take 4 to 6 hours if the test is to include the bowel series. A 24 hour x-ray film, post GI series, may be requested.

A laxative is usually ordered after the completion of the test to get the barium out of the GI tract.

FACTORS AFFECTING DIAGNOSTIC RESULTS

Barium in the gastrointestinal tract from a recent barium study.

Retention of food and liquids, which would decrease visualization.

Excessive air in the stomach and small intestine.

NURSING IMPLICATIONS WITH RATIONALE

Explain to the patient that the purpose of the test is to visualize the gastrointestinal tract *or* to observe the abnormalities in the gastrointestinal tract.

Explain the procedure to the patient concerning diet; food, drink, and medication restrictions; no smoking; the length of time required to complete the procedure; and the post-test laxative, if ordered (see *Procedure* above).

Inform the patient that all of the chalk-flavored liquid must be swallowed. Tell the patient the tests should not cause pain or any significant discomfort.

Encourage the patient to ask questions or express any concerns. Refer questions you cannot answer to other appropriate health professionals. Tell the patient that if, during the test, he has any questions, he should feel free to ask them.

Record vital signs. Note in the chart any epigastric pain or discomfort.

Post-test

Check with the radiology department to make sure that the upper GI series and/or small bowel studies are completed before giving the late breakfast or late lunch. Usually the x-ray department will send a slip with the patient stating that the test is finished or a 24 hour x-ray film will be needed.

Administer the ordered laxative (e.g., milk of magnesia) after the test. Inform the patient that the stools should be light in color for the next several days. Instruct the patient to notify the physician if he or she does not have a bowel movement in 2 to 3 days. Barium can cause fecal impaction.

GASTROSCOPY, ESOPHAGOSCOPY, DUODENOSCOPY, ENDOSCOPY

Esophagogastroscopy, Esophagogastroduodenoscopy

NORMAL FINDING

Normal mucous membranes of the esophagus, stomach, and duodenum; absence of pathology.

DESCRIPTION

Gastroscopy usually includes an esophagoscopy, and the two tests are called esophagogastroscopy. If duodenoscopy is included with the endoscopic examination, then the term is esophagogastroduodenoscopy. For this test, a flexible fiberoptic endoscope is used for direct visualization of the internal structures of the esophagus, stomach, and duodenum. A camera can be attached to the fiberoptic endoscope, and biopsy forceps or a cytology brush can also be inserted through a channel of the endoscope. Suction can be applied for the removal of secretions and foreign bodies.

This test is performed under local anesthesia in a gastroscopic room of the hospital or in the clinic, usually by a gastroenterologist. This procedure can be done on an emergency basis by removal of foreign objects (a bone, a pin, etc.) and for diagnostic purposes. The major complications that can occur from esophagogastroduodenoscopy are perforation and hemorrhage.

With the improvement of the instrument, this test is more sensitive and specific for identifying pathologic changes and lesions than the upper GI series.[5,8,9]

CLINICAL PROBLEMS

Esophageal: Esophagitis, hiatal hernia, esophageal stenoses, achalasia, esophageal neoplasms (benign or malignant tumors), esophageal varices, Mallory–Weiss tear.

Gastic: gastritis, gastric neoplasm (benign or malignant), gastric ulcer (acute or chronic), gastric varices.

Duodenal (small intestine): duodenitis, diverticula, duodenal ulcer, neoplasm (benign or malignant).

PROCEDURE

A consent form should be signed by the patient or a designated family member.

The patient should be NPO for 8 to 12 hours. When this procedure is used during an emergency, NPO cannot be enforced, so the patient's stomach is lavaged (suctioned) to prevent aspiration.

A sedative/tranquilizer, a narcotic analgesic, and atropine are given an hour before the test, or they can be titrated IV immediately prior to the procedure and during the procedure as needed.

A local anesthetic (i.e., Pontocaine, cocaine) may be sprayed into the patient's posterior pharynx. Because of the side-effects of swallowed local anesthetics, this practice is being abandoned increasingly.

Dentures, jewelry, and clothing should be removed from the neck to the waist.

Specimen containers (10 percent formaldehyde and 95 percent ethyl alcohol) should be labelled with the patient's name, the date, and the type of tissue.

Emergency drugs and equipment should be available for hypersensitivity to medications (premedications and anesthetic) and for severe laryngospasms.

Record baseline vital signs. The patient should void before the procedure.

The test takes approximately 1 hour or less.

FACTORS AFFECTING DIAGNOSTIC RESULTS

Barium from a recent gastrointestinal (GI) series can decrease visualization of the mucosa. This test should not be performed within 2 days after a GI series. An x-ray film of the abdomen can be taken to see if barium is in the stomach or duodenum.

NURSING IMPLICATIONS WITH RATIONALE

Recognize that a gastroscopy test for visualizing the esophageal, gastric, and duodenal mucosa is actually an esophagogastroduodenoscopy. These names are frequently used interchangeably.

Explain to the patient the purpose of the test. Explanation can be brief, such as, "to visualize the gastrointestinal mucosa" or "to determine the cause of the symptoms."

Explain the procedure to the patient. Inform the patient that the instrument is flexible; the procedure will be done under local anesthesia (the throat will be sprayed); premedications will be given before the test; dentures and jewelry should be removed; and food and drinks will be restricted for 8 to 12 hours before the test.

Check that the patient's dentures, eyeglasses, and jewelry are removed. Give the patient a hospital gown.

Have the patient void. Take vital signs.

Check that a consent form has been signed before giving the patient premedications. Once the sedative and the narcotic analgesic are given, the patient should remain in bed with the bedsides up. Tell him or her that these medications will cause drowsiness.

Explain to the patient that he or she may feel some pressure with the insertion of the endoscope and may feel some fullness in the stomach when air is injected for better visualization of the stomach and intestine areas.

Be a good listener. Allow the patient time to ask questions and to express concerns or fears. Refer questions you cannot answer to the gastroenterologist or physician.

Place the biopsy (tissue) specimen in a bottle container with 10 percent formaldehyde solution. The cells from the cytology brush should be placed in a bottle containing 95 percent ethyl alcohol or Carnoy's solution or on a slide and sprayed with a commercial fixation solution. Commercial fixatives tend to distort the cells.

Post-test

Keep the patient NPO for 2 to 4 hours after the test, as ordered. Check the gag reflex before offering food and fluids by asking the patient to swallow and by touching the posterior pharynx with a cotton swab or tongue blade, if the throat was sprayed with an anesthetic.

Monitor vital signs (BP, P, R) every 15 minutes for the first hour, every 30 minutes for the next 2 hours, and every hour for 4 hours or until stable. The temperature should be taken every 4 hours for 2 days or as ordered.

Give the patient throat lozenges or analgesics for throat discomfort. Inform the patient that he or she may have flatus or "burp-up gas," which is normal. This is caused by the instillation of air during the procedure for visualization purposes.

Observe the patient for possible complications—e.g., perforation in the GI tract from the endoscope. Symptoms could include pain (epigastric, abdominal, back pain), dyspnea, fever, tachycardia, and subcutaneous emphysema in the neck.

Be supportive of the patient and family.

H

HYSTEROSALPINGOGRAPHY (HYSTEROSALPINGOGRAM)

NORMAL FINDING
Normal structure of the uterus and patent fallopian tubes.

DESCRIPTION
Hysterosalpingography is a radiologic examination (fluoroscopy and x-ray) of the uterus and fallopian tubes. A contrast substance (either oil-base Ethiodol or Lipiodol or water-soluble Salpix) is injected into the cervical canal. It then flows through the uterus and into the fallopian tubes and spills into the abdominal area for visualizing the uterus, the fallopian tubes, and the body of the uterus. Usually both a radiologist and a physician (gynecologist) perform the procedure; the gynecologist inserts the speculum into the vagina and remains so that he or she can fluoroscopically view the flow of the contrast substance. X-ray films are taken.

The hysterosalpingogram should be done on the seventh to the ninth day after the menstrual cycle. The patient should not be pregnant, have active bleeding, or have an acute infection; if any of these conditions exist the test should be cancelled.

There may be some abdominal cramping, and sometimes there are chills and transient dizziness; chills as the contrast substance spills into the abdominal area. Normally the spillage is not harmful and is expected.

The amount of radiation exposure is high due to the fluoroscopic examination. Today, ultrasonography is replacing hysterosalpingography, except that the latter test is more effective in determining tubal patency.[5,8,9,23]

CLINICAL PROBLEMS
Indications: to identify uterine abnormalities—uterine masses (i.e., fibroids, tumor), uterine fistulas, cause of bleeding (e.g., traumatic injury); to identify fallopian tubal abnormalities—tubal occlusion (partial or complete)—i.e., adhesions, stricture); to identify extrauterine pregnancy.

PROCEDURE
A consent form for hysterosalpingography should be signed by the patient.

Food and drinks are not restricted.

A cleansing enema and douche may be ordered prior to the test.

A mild sedative—e.g., diazepam (Valium)—may be ordered prior to the test.

The patient lies on an examining table in the lithotomy position. The gynecologist, physician, or radiologist inserts the speculum into the vaginal canal and the contrast substance is injected into the cervix under fluoroscopic control. X-rays are taken throughout the 15 to 30 minute procedure.

FACTORS AFFECTING DIAGNOSTIC RESULTS
Tubal spasm may cause tubal stricture, which could give the appearance of a partial or complete tubal obstruction in a normal fallopian tube.

NURSING IMPLICATIONS WITH RATIONALE

Explain to the patient that the purpose of the test is to visualize the uterus and tubes for any abnormalities *or* to determine the patency of the fallopian tubes.

Explain the procedure to the patient. The procedure may slightly differ in your institution, so check before explaining to the patient.

Check to see that the consent form is signed. Ask the patient when she had her last menstrual period. Record the information. If pregnancy is suspected, the procedure should not be done.

Administer pre-test orders—enema, douche, or sedative. If the patient comes from home, check that she has prepared herself as ordered.

Inform the patient that the test takes about 15 to 30 minutes. If the patient's physician will be present, let her know. It may be either alarming or comforting to see him or her "pop in."

Inform the patient that she may experience some abdominal cramping and some dizziness. Explain that this is normal, but that if there is continuous and severe cramping, she should tell the examiners.

Encourage the patient to ask questions and express concerns. Be a good listener. Refer questions and concerns you cannot handle adequately to other appropriate health professionals.

Inform the patient that there may be some bloody discharge for several days following the test. If it is continuous, then after 3 to 4 days she should notify her physician.

Check for signs and symptoms of infection following the test, such as fever, increased pulse rate, and pain. Notify the physician. If the patient is at home, inform the patient to call the physician and report these symptoms.

I

INTRAVENOUS PYELOGRAPHY (IVP)
Intravenous Pyelogram, Excretory Urography

NORMAL FINDING
Normal size, structure, and functions of the kidneys, ureters, and bladder.

DESCRIPTION
IV pyelography (pyelogram) is more properly called *excretory urography*, since this test is used for visualizing the entire urinary tract and not just the kidney pelvis. A radiopaque substance (sodium diatrizoate) or Renografin-60 (meglumine diatrizoate) is injected intravenously and a series of x-rays are taken at specific times. The test usually takes 30 to 45 minutes.

Excretory urography is useful for locating stones and tumors and for diagnosing kidney diseases—i.e., polycystic kidney, renovascular hypertension. A few patients may be hypersensitive to the radiopaque iodine dye, especially if they have a history of allergy to many substances. An intradermal skin test may be done prior to the IVP to determine the patient's sensitivity to the dye. Emergency drugs (epinephrine, vasopressors, etc.), a tracheostomy set, a suction machine, and oxygen should be available for treating anaphylactoid reaction if it should occur.[2,3,5,8,9,19]

CLINICAL PROBLEMS
Abnormal findings: renal calculi; neoplasm (tumor) of the kidney, bladder; kidney diseases—polycystic kidney, hydronephrosis, renovascular hypertension.

PROCEDURE
A consent form for IVP should be signed by the patient or an appropriate member of the family.

The patient should be NPO for 8 to 12 hours before the test. Usually the patient is NPO after dinner. In the morning, the patient may be slightly dehydrated; however, this will help the kidney to concentrate the dye.

A laxative is ordered the night before and a cleansing enema(s) is ordered the morning of the test. These preparations may vary, so check with the radiology department for exact preps.

An antihistamine or a steroid may be given prior to the test to patients who are hypersensitive to iodine, seafood, and contrast dye used in other diagnostic tests, as well as for those who have histories of asthma and severe allergies.

Baseline vital signs should be recorded.

The patient lies in the supine position on an x-ray table. X-rays are taken 3, 5, 10, 15, and 20 minutes after the dye is injected. Tomography may be used for identifying a mass.

Emergency drugs and equipment should be available at all times.

The test takes approximately 30 to 45 minutes. A delay in visualizing the kidneys could indicate kidney dysfunction.

The patient voids at the end of the test and another x-ray is taken to visualize the residual dye in the bladder.

FACTORS AFFECTING DIAGNOSTIC RESULTS
Feces, gas, and barium in the intestinal tract can decrease visualization of the kidney, ureters, and bladder.

NURSING IMPLICATIONS WITH RATIONALE

Explain to the patient that the purpose of the test is to detect any kidney disorder *or* to observe the size, shape, and structure of the kidney, ureters, and bladder, or give a similar response.

Explain the procedure to the patient. As a reminder, the procedural steps could be listed for the patient.

Obtain a patient history of known allergies. Notify the physician if the patient is allergic to seafood, iodine preparations, and contrast dye. As a precaution, the physician may order an antihistamine or a steroid drug if the patient has an allergic reaction to drugs. A skin test may be performed to determine how hypersensitive the patient is to the radiopaque contrast dye.

Instruct the patient that he or she is not to eat or drink after dinner. Mild dehydration usually occurs. This could be harmful to patients with poor renal output, especially the aged and the debilitated. Sips of water or a glass of water may be indicated to avoid complications.

Inform the patient that he or she may feel a transient flushing or burning sensation and a salty or metallic taste during or following the intravenous injection of the contrast dye.

Check the BUN (blood urea nitrogen). If BUN levels are greater than 40 mg/dl, notify the physician. Normally the test would not be done.

Encourage the patient to ask questions and express any concerns before and during the procedure to the nurse, radiologist, and technician.

Post-test

Monitor vital signs and urinary output.

Observe, report, and record possible delayed reactions to the contrast dye—i.e. dyspnea, rashes, flushing, urticaria (hives), tachycardia, and others.

Check the site where the dye was injected. Usually it is in the antecubital fossa vein. For pain, warmth, redness at the injection site, apply warm compresses, with the physician's permission.

Administer oral antihistamines or steroids as ordered for treating dye reactions.

L

LYMPHANGIOGRAPHY (LYMPHANGIOGRAM), LYMPHOGRAPHY

NORMAL FINDING
Normal lymphatic vessels and lymph nodes.

DESCRIPTION
Lymphangiography is an x-ray examination of the lymphatic system—lymphatic vessels and lymph nodes. A radiopaque iodine contrast oil substance (e.g., Ethiodol) is injected into the lymphatic vessels of each foot; the dye can also be injected into the hands to visualize axillary and supraclavicular nodes. Normally, fluoroscopy is used with x-ray filming to check on lymphatic filling of the contrast dye and to determine when the infusion of the contrast dye should be stopped. The infusion rate is controlled by a lymphangiographic pump, and approximately 1.5 hours are required for dye to reach the level of the third and fourth lumbar vertebrae. The entire test takes 2.5 to 3 hours.

This test is useful to identifying malignant lymphoma (Hodgkin's disease) and metastasis to the lymph nodes. Lymphangiograms are also used for staging malignant lymphoma, from Stage I (a single lymph node area of involvement) to Stage IV (diffuse extranodol involvement). Other tests, such as ultrasonography, computerized tomography, and/or biopsy may be used to confirm the diagnosis and to stage lymphoma involvement.

Lymphangiography is usually contraindicated if the patient is hypersensitive to iodine or has severe chronic lung disease, cardiac disease, or advanced liver or kidney disease. Persons with possible allergies to iodine and/or contrast dye used in other diagnostic tests (e.g., IVP) should receive antihistamines or steroids before the test, and emergency drugs should be available during the test. Lipid pneumonia may occur if the contrast dye flows into the thoracic duct and sets up microemboli in the lungs. The small emboli that can occur will gradually disappear after several weeks or months.[5,8,23]

CLINICAL PROBLEMS
Indications: to identify malignant lymphoma (Hodgkin's disease), metastasis to the lymph nodes, the cause of lymphedema, primary (decreased number of lymphatic vessels) or secondary (tumor or surgical removal); to assist with the staging of malignant lymphoma.

PROCEDURE
A consent form should be signed by the patient.

Food and drinks are not restricted.

Antihistamines and a sedative may be ordered prior to the test.

Contrast dye (blue) is injected intradermally between several toes of each foot, staining the lymphatic vessels of the feet in 15 to 20 minutes.

A local skin anesthetic is injected and small incisions are made on the dorsum of each foot.

A 30 gauge lymphangiographic needle with polyethylene tubing is inserted carefully into the identified lymphatic vessel. The contrast dye is slowly infused with the aid of the infusion pump over a period of 1.5 hours until it reaches the third and fourth lumbar vertebrae. The patient should remain still during the procedure. X-rays are taken of the lymphatics in the leg, pelvic, abdominal, and chest areas.

Twenty-four hours later, a second set of films is taken to visualize the lymph nodes. X-ray filming usually takes 30 minutes. The contrast dye remains in the lymph nodes for 6 months to a year; thus repeated x-rays can be taken to determine the disease process and the response to treatment.

FACTORS AFFECTING DIAGNOSTIC RESULTS
None known.

NURSING IMPLICATIONS WITH RATIONALE

Explain to the patient that the purpose of the test is to visualize the lymph vessels and lymph nodes (lymphatic system).

Explain the procedure to the patient. Be available to answer questions and be supportive of the patient and family.

Check that the consent form was signed by the patient before giving the sedative for the test.

Inform the patient that he or she should remain still during the test, as instructed. Inform the patient that there may be some discomfort with the injection of the local skin anesthetic into each foot. The sedative is given to promote relaxation and to decrease movement during the test.

Obtain a patient history of allergies to seafood, iodine preparations, or contrast dye used in another x-ray test.

Inform the patient that the blue contrast dye discolors the urine and stool for several days and could cause the skin to have a bluish tinge for 24 to 48 hours.

Tell the patient that the test takes 2.5 to 3 hours and that he or she will be told to return the next day for additional x-rays. Tell the patient that the procedure will *not* be repeated the next day; only x-rays will be taken.

Record baseline vital signs (VS) and have the patient void before the test.

Post-test

Keep the patient on bed rest for 24 hours or as ordered.

Monitor vital signs. Check blood pressure, pulse, and respirations every 15 minutes for the first hour, every 30 minutes for the second hour, and then hourly for 4 hours or until stable. Continue monitoring vital signs (BP, T, P, R) every 4 hours for 48 hours. Observe for dyspnea, pain, and hypotension, which could be due to microemboli from the spillage of the contrast dye.

Assess the incisional site for signs of an infection—i.e., redness, oozing, and swelling. Report and record findings. The dressing is usually not changed for the first 48 hours.

Check for leg edema. Elevate lower extremities as indicated

M

MAMMOGRAPHY (MAMMOGRAM)

NORMAL FINDING
Normal ducts and glandular tissue; no abnormal masses.

DESCRIPTION
Mammography is an x-ray examination of the breast to detect cysts or tumors. Benign cysts are seen on the mammogram as well-outlined, clear lesions and tend to be bilateral, whereas malignant tumors are irregular and poorly defined and tend to be unilateral. A breast mass (neoplasm) cannot be clinically palpable until it is 1 cm in size, so it may take 5 years or longer to grow and be detectable. A mammogram can detect a breast lesion approximately 2 years before it is palpable.

There is much controversy on how often a woman should receive a mammogram and whether this x-ray test should be only for symptomatic women having a palpable mass, nipple discharge, skin thickening of the breast, or a markedly asymmetric breast rather than for those who are asymptomatic. Several authorities feel that some asymptomatic women may be prone to cancer of the breast because of a familial history of breast cancer—i.e., in the mother, grandmother, or sister. Usually these women and those who have been treated for other types of cancer are requested to have mammograms yearly, beginning at the age of 35 to 40, or as recommended by their physicians.

The American Cancer Society and the American College of Radiologists have suggested guidelines for mammography. Both organizations suggest having a baseline mammogram for women between the ages of 35 and 40 and repeat mammograms annually after the age of 50.

Mammography exposes the breast to a large amount of radiation. A low-energy x-ray beam is used today, which may decrease the amount of radiation received by the breast. The mammogram can detect approximately 90 percent of breast malignancies; however, the test carries a 10 percent false-positive rate. A positive test should be confirmed by biopsy, ultrasonography (ultrasound technique), or diaphanography (transillumination technique).[5,8,9,23]

CLINICAL PROBLEMS
Indications: to detect a palpable breast mass (cyst or tumor); to identify women who are at high risk—those with a familial history of breast cancer or a history of cancer of the uterus, ovaries, or gastrointestinal tract; to examine the breast periodically, as indicated by the physician.

PROCEDURE
Food and drinks are not restricted.

The patient removes clothes and jewelry from the neck to the waist and wears a paper or cloth gown which opens in the front.

The patient is seated and each breast (one at a time) rests on a x-ray cassette table. As the breast is compressed, the patient will be asked to hold her breath while the x-ray is taken. Two x-rays are taken of each breast.

The procedure usually takes 15 to 30 minutes.

FACTORS AFFECTING DIAGNOSTIC RESULTS
Previous breast surgery can affect the reading of the x-ray film.

Jewelry, metals, ointment, and powder could cause false positive results.

NURSING IMPLICATIONS WITH RATIONALE

Explain to the patient that the purpose of the test is routine breast filming *or* to identify the palpable lesion in the breast.

Explain the procedure to the patient. Explain that the test will not hurt but may cause a little discomfort when the breast is compressed during the x-ray.

Inform the patient that the test takes 15 to 30 minutes; however, the patient will be asked to wait until the x-rays are developed and readable. Inform the the patient not to be alarmed if an additional x-ray is needed.

Ascertain whether the patient is pregnant or suspected of being pregnant. A mammogram is contraindicated during pregnancy.

Instruct the patient not to use ointment, powder, or deodorant on the breast or under the arms on the day of the mammogram.

Ask the patient to identify the lump in the breast if one is present.

Be supportive of the patient. Allow the patient time to express her fears and concerns. Notify the physician of her concerns, especially if they cause her great anxiety. Have the physician speak to the patient.

Answer the patient's questions when possible or refer the question(s) to her physician or to the radiologist.

Encourage the patient to self-examine the breast after each menstrual period. Demonstrate breast examination, if necessary.

MYELOGRAPHY (Myelogram)

NORMAL FINDING
Normal spinal subarachnoid space; no obstructions.

DESCRIPTION

Myelography is an fluoroscopic and radiologic examination of the spinal subarachnoid space (spinal canal) using air or a radiopaque contrast agent (oil- and water-soluble). This procedure is performed in an x-ray department by a radiologist, a neurologist, and/or a neurosurgeon. After the contrast dye is injected into the lumbar area, the fluoroscopic table is tilted until the suspected problem area can be visualized and spot films are taken.

If the contrast agent is an oil (i.e., Pantopaque or isophendylate), then the contrast agent must be removed at the end of the test. Since oil is heavier than spinal fluid, it does not mix and tends to sink to the lower part of the spinal canal. Water-soluble contrast agents (e.g., metrizoate sodium) do not have to be removed; however, after the procedure the patient should remain in a high Fowler's position (60° elevation of the head) for 8 hours. With patients who are hypersensitive to iodine and seafood, air is the contrast agent used.

The myelogram is usually performed to detect spinal lesions—i.e., intervertebral disks, tumors, or cysts. This procedure is contraindicated if increased intracranial pressure is suspected.[3,5,8,19,23]

CLINICAL PROBLEMS

Indications: to identify herniated intervertebral disks, metastatic tumors, cysts, astrocytomas and ependymomas (within the spinal cord), neurofibromas and meningiomas (within the subarachnoid space); to detect spinal nerve root injury, arachnoiditis.

PROCEDURE

A consent form should be signed by the patient or a designated family member.

The patient should be NPO for 4 to 8 hours before the test. If the myelogram is scheduled for the afternoon, then the patient may have a light breakfast or clear liquids in the morning, as ordered.

A cleansing enema may be ordered the night before or early in the morning of the test to remove feces and gas for improving visualization.

Premedications include a sedative and/or narcotic analgesic and usually atropine. The drugs are prescribed by the physician.

The patient is placed in the prone position on a fluoroscopic table and is secured to the table with the use of several straps. A spinal puncture is performed and contrast dye is injected. As the dye enters the spinal canal, the table is tilted.

After the test, the radiopaque oil is removed and the patient should remain flat for 6 to 8 hours. If a water-soluble radiopaque agent was used, then the patient's head should be elevated at 60° for 8 hours.

The myelogram takes approximatley 1 hour.

FACTORS AFFECTING DIAGNOSTIC RESULTS

Gas or fecal material in the gastrointestinal tract.

NURSING IMPLICATIONS WITH RATIONALE

Explain to the patient that the purpose of the test is to determine if there is a lesion, such as a disc.

Explain the procedure to the patient. Inform the patient that he or she will most likely lie on his abdomen and will be strapped to a table. The physician will tilt the table as the dye circulates in the spinal canal.

Inform the patient that he may have a transient burning sensation and/or a flushed, warm feeling as the dye is injected and afterwards. Tell the patient that if he has any discomfort (i.e., pain down the legs), he should let the physician know. The test takes about 1 hour.

Obtain a patient history of allergies to iodine, seafood, and radiopaque dye used in other x-ray tests. Inform the physician, for air or oxygen may then be used as the contrast agent instead of the dye. A skin test may be performed.

Follow the prescribed pre-test regime—i.e., NPO, a cleansing enema, and premedications (sedative or narcotic analgesic). Check that the consent form has been signed before giving a sedative or narcotic.

Allow the patient the time to ask questions and express concerns or fears. Refer questions you cannot answer to the physician or to other health professionals.

Recognize conditions in which myelography would be contraindicated—i.e., multiple sclerosis (could cause an exacerbation) and increased intracranial pressure (↑ ICP). The radiologist and/or neurosurgeon should be notified if they are unaware of the patient's condition.

Record baseline vital signs.

Post-test

Monitor vital signs every 30 minutes for the first 2 hours and every hour for the next 4 hours until stable or as ordered. Temperature should be taken every 4 hours while awake for 24 to 48 hours.

Instruct the patient to lie in the prone and/or supine position for 6 to 8 hours, as ordered. If the patient received a water-soluble contrast agent, or if all the contrast oil was not removed, the head of the bed should be elevated at a 60° angle for 8 hours or longer.

Monitor urinary output. The patient should void in 8 hours.

Encourage the patient to increase fluid intake. The fluids will help restore the cerebrospinal fluid loss. Increased fluid intake may decrease a postlumbar puncture headache, which could be due to a loss of spinal fluid.

Observe for signs and symptoms of chemical or bacterial meningitis—i.e., severe headache, fever, stiff neck, irritability, photophobia, and convulsions.

Instruct the patient about preventure measures for avoiding back injury—i.e., principles of good body mechanics, such as flexing the knees and keeping the back straight when lifting.

P

PAPANICOLAOU SMEAR (PAP SMEAR—CYTOLOGY TEST FOR CERVICAL CANCER)

NORMAL FINDING
No abnormal or atypical cells.

DESCRIPTION
The Pap (Papanicolaou) smear became nationally known and used in the early 1950s for detecting cervical cancer and precancerous and cancerous tissues. Dr. George Papanicolaou developed the cytology test in 1928 after spending 18 years in research. Today he is referred to as the father of modern cytology. As the result of his work, there are many cytology studies done on body tissues and secretions.

Since malignant tissue changes usually take many years, yearly examination of exfoliative cervical cells (cells that have sloughed off) allows detection of early precancerous conditions. It is suggested that women from age 18 to 40 have yearly Pap smears and that women from age 40 on have either twice-a-year or yearly smears. How often the Pap smear test should be performed is determined by the patient's physician.

The Pap smear (cytology) results are reported on a five-point scale:
Grade (Class) I: Absence of atypical or abnormal cells.
Grade (Class) II: Atypical cells, but no evidence of malignancy.
Grade (Class) III: Suggestive of but not conclusive for malignancy.
Grade (Class) IV: Strongly suggestive of malignancy.
Grade (Class) V: Conclusive for malignancy.

For suggestive or positive Pap smears, colposcopy and/or a cervical biopsy are frequently ordered to confirm the test results. Atypical cells can occur due to cervicitis and excessive or prolonged use of hormones.

Cytologic samples from the vagina and cervix may be used to determine the effects of taking sex hormones.[5,8,9,10]

CLINICAL PROBLEMS
Indications: to detect precancerous and cancerous cells and cervicitis; to identify viral, fungal, and parasitic conditions; to assess the effects of sex hormonal replacement and the response to the chemotherapy and radiation therapy.

PROCEDURE
Food and drinks are not restricted.

The patient should not douche, insert vaginal medications, or have sexual intercourse for at least 24 hours (preferably 48 hours) before the test. The test should be done between menstrual periods.

The patient should remove all clothes from the waist down, except for her shoes. The patient is generally asked to remove all clothes, since the breasts are examined after the Pap smear is taken. A paper or cloth gown is worn.

Instruct the patient to lie on the examining table in the lithotomy position (heels in the stirrups).

A speculum is inserted into the vagina. The speculum may be lubricated with warm running water.

A curved wooden spatula (Pap stick) is used to scrape the cervix. The obtained specimen is transferred onto a slide and is immersed immediately in a fixative solution (e.g.,

95 percent ethyl alcohol) or sprayed with a commercial fixation spray.
The Pap smear procedure takes approximately 10 minutes.

FACTORS AFFECTING DIAGNOSTIC RESULTS
Allowing cells to dry on the slide before using the fixation solution or spray.
Douching, use of vaginal suppositories, or sexual intercourse within the 24 hours before the test.
Menstruation can interfere with the test results.
Drugs (i.e., digitalis preparations and tetracycline) could change cellular structure.
Lubricating jelly on the speculum can interfere with test results.

NURSING IMPLICATIONS WITH RATIONALE

Explain to the patient that the purpose of the test is to detect abnormal cervical cells.
  Explain to the patient that the test should be done yearly or twice a year, as determined by her physician. High-risk patients (with a familial history of cervical cancer or a previous Grade II test) and women over 40 years old usually have the Pap smear taken twice a year.
Explain the procedure to the patient. Emphasize to the patient that she should not douche, insert vaginal suppositories, or have sexual intercourse for at least 24 hours (some say 48 hours) before the Pap smear. Douching could wash away the cervical cells.
Obtain a patient history regarding menstruation and any menstrual problems—i.e., the last menstrual period, bleeding flow, vaginal discharge, itching, and whether she is taking hormones or oral contraceptives.
Answer the patient's questions and refer questions you cannot answer to the physician. Try to alleviate the patient's anxiety, if at all possible. Be a good listener.
Inform the patient that a bimanual examination of the vagina, lower abdomen, and rectum may or will follow the Pap smear.
Tell the patient that test results should be back in 2 to 3 days. Physicians differ in reporting test results; some send cards to the patient stating that the Pap smear is normal, while other physicians will send cards only if the test is abnormal and the patient needs to make another appointment.
Label the slide with the patient's name and the date. The lab slip should include the patient's age and the specimen site(s).

PNEUMOENCEPHALOGRAPHY (Pneumoencephalogram, Fractional Pneumoencephalogram)

NORMAL FINDING
Normal size, structure and patency of the cerebral ventricles and cisterns.

DESCRIPTION
Pneumoencephalography is a radiologic examination of the cerebral ventricles and cisterns by repeatedly replacing a small amount of spinal fluid with air in the lumbar (spinal) area. This test is also referred to as air encephalography. If only a small amount of spinal fluid is removed and the fluid is replaced with air (*not* repeatedly), then the test is called fractional pneumoencephalography. A *ventriculography* test is the injection of air through burr holes into the ventricles in the skull.

Though pneumoencephalography is being replaced by computerized tomography (CT) scan and cerebral angiography (arteriography), it is still performed occasionally when a pituitary tumor or a cerebral ventricular or cisternal tumor is suspected. The test should not be performed if increased intracranial pressure is present.

Usually patients have severe headaches, nausea, and vomiting during and after the test. Strict bed rest, increased fluid intake, and analgesics are necessary for 24 to 48 hours after the procedure.[3,5,23]

CLINICAL PROBLEMS
Indications: to detect lesions (e.g., tumors) of the pituitary gland, cerebral ventricles, or cisterns.

PROCEDURE
A consent form should be signed by the patient or a designated family member.

The patient should be NPO for 8 hours before the test.

Premedications include a sedative and atropine. Normally, analgesics are not prescribed, since they can mask signs and symptoms of brain stem herniation which could occur during the procedure.

Dentures and jewelry should be removed before the procedure.

The patient is strapped to a motorized chair or a radiograph table. X-rays are taken as small amounts of spinal fluid are removed and air is injected repeatedly into the spinal canal. The chair is rotated so that the air enters the ventricles.

Vital signs are taken during the procedure. An IV with dextrose in water may be started to keep the vein open (KVO) as a lifeline for administering emergency drugs, if necessary.

The procedure takes 1 to 2 hours to complete.

FACTORS AFFECTING DIAGNOSTIC RESULTS
Narcotic analgesics given prior to the test could mask signs and symptoms of herniation; in such a case, the test would be immediately discontinued.

NURSING IMPLICATIONS WITH RATIONALE

Explain to the patient that the purpose of the test is to identify any abnormalities or lesions in the brain, or give a similar response.

Explain the procedure to the patient. Inform the patient that a lumbar puncture will be performed and small amounts of air will be injected into the spinal canal. Explain that he or she may experience some headache and nausea during and after the procedure.

Tell the patient that he will be strapped to a motorized chair or table and that the chair will be rotated or that his head will be moved frequently if he is on the table.

Allow the patient time to ask questions or express concerns or fears. Refer questions you cannot answer to the physician or other appropriate health professionals.

Instruct the patient that food and drinks are restricted after midnight or for 8 hours before the test.

Record baseline vital signs.

Administer premedications. If analgesics are ordered, check with the physician, since analgesics may mask signs and symptoms of brain stem herniation.

Post-test

Keep the patient flat in bed or, if necessary, elevate the head no more than 30° for 24 hours or as ordered. Instruct the patient to turn from side to side slowly every 2 hours. Quick movements could cause dizziness or nausea or intensify the headache.

Monitor vital signs every 15 minutes for the first hour, every 30 minutes for the next 2 hours, and every hour for 4 hours or until stable, or as ordered. Report any changes to the physican and record results in the patient's chart.

Encourage the patient to increase his or her fluid intake. Hydration is important for restoring spinal fluid.

Administer analgesics for headache as needed.

Be supportive of the patient and the family. Explain to the family that the patient needs to be quiet and that their visits should be short. Tell the family not to engage the patient in a long conversation.

PROCTOSIGMOIDOSCOPY, PROCTOSCOPY, SIGMOIDOSCOPY

NORMAL FINDING
Normal mucosa and structure of the rectum and sigmoid colon.

DESCRIPTION

The new term for proctoscopy, an examination of the anus and rectum, and sigmoidoscopy, an examination of the anus, rectum, and sigmoid colon, is *proctosigmoidoscopy*. There are three types of instruments used: (1) a 7 cm rigid proctoscope or anoscope, (2) a 25 to 30 cm rigid sigmoidoscope, and (3) a 60 cm flexible sigmoidoscope used to visualize the descending colon. A proctosigmoidoscopy is another type of endoscopic examination which can be performed in the hospital, in a clinic, or in the physician's office.

With this procedure, the rectum and distal sigmoid colon can be visualized, and specimens can be obtained by a biopsy forcep or a snare, cytology brush, or culture swab. This test is usually indicated when there are changes in bowel habits, chronic constipation, or bright blood or mucus in the stool, or it can be done as part of an annual physical examination in patients over 40 years old.[3,5,8,19]

CLINICAL PROBLEMS

Abnormal findings: hemorrhoids; rectal and sigmoid colon polyps; fistulas, fissures; rectal abscess; neoplasms (benign or malignant); ulcerative or granulomatous proctitis; infection and/or inflammation of the rectosigmoid area.

PROCEDURE

A consent form should be signed by the patient or a designated family member.

A light dinner the night before the test and a light breakfast are permitted. Policies in some institutions do not allow breakfast the morning of the test. Usually heavy meals, vegetables, and fruits are prohibited within 24 hours of the test.

A saline or warm tap water enema(s) or a small hypertonic salt enema (Fleet enema) is given the morning of the test. If enemas are contraindicated, then a rectal suppository, such as Dulcolax (bisacodyl), could be given. Fecal material must be evacuated before the examination. Oral cathartics are seldom used, for they may increase fecal flow from the small intestine during the test.

The patient should assume either a knee–chest position or Sim's (side-lying) position for the proctosigmoidoscopy. The patient will be strapped to the table and properly draped to avoid embarrassment.

As the lubricated endoscope (proctoscope, sigmoidoscope, or proctosigmoidoscope) is inserted into the rectum, the patient should be instructed to breathe deeply and slowly. Sometimes air is injected into the bowel to improve visualization. The air can cause gas pains, and use of air is avoided, if possible. Cotton swabs and suction should be available.

Specimens can be obtained during the procedure. Tissue specimen(s) should be placed in a bottle containing 10 percent formalin, and cells from a cytology brush should be placed in a bottle containing 95 percent ethyl alcohol or Carnoy's solution or on a slide and sprayed with a fixation solution. The commercial fixative sprays may cause distortion of cells.

The procedure takes approximately 15 to 30 minutes.

FACTORS AFFECTING DIAGNOSTIC RESULTS

Barium can decrease the visualization, and so barium studies should be performed a week before the test or afterwards.

Fecal material in the lower colon can decrease visualization.

Placement of tissue and cell specimens in solutions without preservative solutions can cause false results. Fixative sprays could distort the cells.

NURSING IMPLICATIONS WITH RATIONALE

Explain to the patient that the purpose of the test is to determine the cause of his or her symptoms (i.e., bright blood or mucus in stools, constipation, bowel changes) *or* tell him that it is part of the routine physical examination for preventive health care.

Explain the procedure to the patient in regards to body position, pre-test preparation (enema and diet), and the time required for the procedure.

Inform the patient that the procedure may cause some discomfort but should not cause severe pain. Encourage the patient to breathe deeply and slowly and to relax during the test. Explain that he or she may have some gas pains if a small amount of air is injected during the procedure for the purpose of better visualization.

Check the chart to determine if the patient has had a barium study within 3 days before the scheduled proctosigmoidoscopy. If so, the physician should be notified.

Obtain a patient history in regard to being pregnant or having ulcerative colitis. Frequently, enemas and suppositories are contraindicated during pregnancy and with ulcerative colitis. In addition, rigid proctosigmoidoscopy may be contraindicated during pregnancy, especially near term.

Record baseline vital signs before the test. Vital signs may be monitored during the examination.

Allow the patient time to ask questions and express concerns. Refer questions you cannot answer to a physician or to the appropriate health professional.

Post-test

Monitor vital signs as indicated or at least every 30 minutes for the first 2 hours.

Encourage the patient to rest for several hours after the test if possible. This procedure may be done in a clinic, in a physician's office, or in the hospital. If the test is done on an out-patient basis, the patient should rest for 1 hour before leaving.

Observe the signs and symptoms of bowel perforation—i.e., pain, abdominal distention, and rectal bleeding due to the endoscopic procedure. This problem rarely occurs. Also observe for shocklike symptoms—i.e., paleness, diaphoresis, tachycardia, and later a drop in blood pressure. Report all symptoms immediately to the physician.

Be supportive of the patient and his or her family.

PULMONARY FUNCTION TESTS

NORMAL FINDING

Normal values vary with the person's age, sex, and height; greater than 80 percent of the predicted value.

DESCRIPTION

Pulmonary function tests may be divided into two groups of tests; the ventilatory function tests for differentiating between obstructive and restrictive lung diseases and the arterial blood gases (ABG) tests for evaluating the distribution and diffusion of gases across the alveolar capillary membrane. Arterial blood gases are discussed in Part I of this text. The ABGs are not always a part of the pulmonary function tests and frequently are ordered to monitor the respiratory status in relation to gas exchange. Ventilatory function tests that are performed with a spirometer and a recording device will be presented in this section.

There are various reasons why pulmonary tests are ordered—i.e., as baseline screening tests to compare with future pulmonary tests, to evaluate pulmonary disability (for insurance), to evaluate pulmonary status before surgery, to determine the severity of lung disease (either obstructive or restrictive), to follow the course of pulmonary disease with treatment, and to detect early respiratory failure. They cannot identify the type of lung tumor or give its location. With the use of spirometry, pulmonary volumes, capacities, and flow rates can be measured.

The spirometer measures and records tidal volume (V_t or TV), vital capacity (VC), forced expiratory volume (FEV), forced inspiratory volume (FIV), and many other ventilatory parameters. Some of the important measurements for detecting disease entities are as follows.

Tidal volume (TV, V_t): Normal breathing with approximately 500 ml of inspired and expired gas.

Vital capacity (VC): The is one of the important test readings. The VC is the maximal amount of air exhaled after a maximal inspiration. A forced vital capacity (FVC) is the greatest amount of air exhaled quickly and forcefully after a deep inspiration. With obstructive lung disease, the FVC and FEV_1 are decreased, and with restrictive lung disease, they could be normal or decreased.

Forced expiratory volume (FEV): This test is part of the forced vital capacity test, giving the total volume of air exhaled in 1 second (FEV_1), 2 seconds (FEV_2), 3 seconds (FEV_3), and 4 seconds (FEV_4).

Expiratory reserve volume (ERV): This is the maximal amount of air that can be exhaled after normal breathing.

Inspiratory capacity (IC): This is the greatest amount of air inhaled after exhaling in normal breathing.

Forced inspiratory volume (FIV): This is the greatest amount of air inhaled after a maximal expiration from a forced vital capacity (FVC).

Residual volume (RV): After a maximal expiration, the amount of air left in the lungs is referred to as the RV. Chronic air trapping from COLD will cause an increased RV. In restrictive lung disease, the residual volume may be decreased.

Functional residual capacity (FRC): This test gives the amount of air left in the lungs after normal expiration. This is calculated by adding expiratory reserve volume and residual volume (ERV + RV = FRC). With obstructive lung disease, the FRC is increased due to hyperinflation of the lungs through air trapping. The FRC can be normal or decreased in restrictive lung disease.

Maximal voluntary ventilation (MVV): This is the maximal rate and depth of respiration after breathing fast and deep for 10 to 15 seconds. It tests the air flow and airway resistance. A decreased MVV can indicate obstructive lung disease and a normal or decreased MVV can be suggestive of restrictive lung disease.

Total lung capacity (TLC): This is the total amount of air in the lungs at the end of a maximal inspiration. The total lung capacity (TLC) can be measured by adding the vital capacity and the residual volume (VC + RV = TLC) or by adding the inspiratory capacity, tidal volume, expiratory reserve volume, and residual volume (IC + Vt + ERV + RV = TLC).

Flow volume loop (F–V loop): The F–V loop is a forced expiratory volume and followed by a forced inspiratory volume (FEV + FIV = F–V loop). This test is useful for detecting small airway obstructive disease—i.e., emphysema or advanced restrictive disease.[4,5,8,15,19]

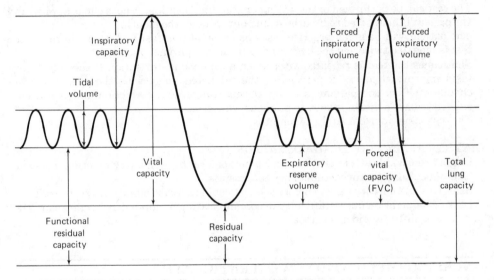

Graphic of lung volume and capacity.

CLINICAL PROBLEMS

Obstructive diseases *(expiration affected):* emphysema, chronic bronchitis, bronchiectasis, allergic response, edema of the bronchial tree, smoke inhalation and noxious gas, airway inflammation due to bacterial or viral infections, bronchospasm, bronchial secretions.

Restrictive diseases *(inspiration affected):* pulmonary fibrosis, pneumonia, lung tumors, kyphoscolosis (restrictive lung expansion), neuromuscular diseases, chest trauma, obesity, scleroderma, pulmonary edema, surgical removal of part of the lung.

PROCEDURE

Food and drink are restricted before the pulmonary function test. Heavy meals before the test should be discouraged.

The patient should not smoke for 4 to 6 hours before the tests.

The request slip should indicate the types of tests that are to be performed—i.e., ventilatory function tests with use of spirometry and/or arterial blood gas tests with or without rest and exercise.

The clothes that the patient is wearing should not restrict his performance. If the patient is hospitalized, he should wear pajamas and/or a robe.

The patient's age, height, and weight should be recorded. These data are used to predict the normal range.

Medications are not restricted unless indicated by the physician. Usually sedatives and narcotics are not given before the test. Intermittent positive pressure breathing (IPPB), with or without a bronchodilator, should not be given within 2 hours (preferably 4 hours) of the test. If the patient is taking nitroglycerin (NTG) for angina pectoris, he or she should bring the tablets along.

The procedure should be postponed if the patient has an active cold or is under the influence of alcohol. If a patient has had recent cardiac catheterization or acute myocardial infarction (MI), the test is usually not performed until 4 days to 1 week after the cardiac catheterization and not until 6 weeks post-MI.

The patient should void before the test. If the patient wears dentures, they should be left in.

The test can be performed in the sitting or standing position. A nose clip is applied and the patient is instructed to breathe in and out through the mouth.

The patient will be given practice sessions on breathing fast and deep. Normally the test is repeated twice and the best tracing from the spirometer is used.

Sometimes the test is repeated after using a bronchodilator spray. If the ventilatory tests improve to over 80 percent of the predicted value with the use of a bronchodilator, then the patient is in the normal range with correction and is not considered to have a disability due to pulmonary disease.

The test takes approximately 45 minutes.

FACTORS AFFECTING DIAGNOSTIC TESTS

Use of bronchodilators in IPPB up to 2 hours before the pulmonary function tests may produce false improved pulmonary test results.

Sedatives and narcotics given before the test could decrease pulmonary test results.

Lack of cooperation due to difficulty in communicating or not understanding can make testing difficult and inaccurate.

NURSING IMPLICATIONS WITH RATIONALE

Explain to the patient that the purpose of the test is to check baseline pulmonary function *or* to identify lung pathology.

Explain the procedure to the patient. Inform the patient that before the test he should eat breakfast, take medications (with the exception of sedatives and narcotics), omit IPPB treatment for 2 to 4 hours, and avoid smoking for 4 to 6 hours. He should be properly clothed, and wear his dentures during the test. Tell the patient that the test should not be performed if he has an active cold or communicable disease.

Note on the request slip the last IPPB treatment the patient has received. List the oral bronchodilators and steroids that the patient is taking. Record the patient's age, height, and weight.

Practice breathing patterns for the pulmonary function test with the patient—i.e., normal breathing, rapid breathing, and forced deep inspiration and forced deep expiration. Patients are apprehensive of their first pulmonary function test.

Be supportive of the patients and answer their questions. Questions you cannot answer should be referred to the physician or to the personnel in the pulmonary function laboratory.

Record pulse and respiration rates on the patient's chart. Assess for signs and symptoms of respiratory distress—i.e., breathlessness, dyspnea (rapid or slow, labored respirations), tachycardia, severe apprehension, and grayish or cyanotic color.

R

RADIOACTIVE IODINE (RAI) UPTAKE TEST

[131]I Uptake Test, Radioiodine Thyroid Uptake Test

NORMAL RANGE

Adult: *2 hours:* 1–13 percent (thyroid gland). *6 hours:* 2–25 percent (thyroid gland). *24 hours:* 15–45 percent (thyroid gland).

DESCRIPTION

The radioactive iodine uptake test is used to determine the metabolic activity of the thyroid gland by measuring the absorption of ^{131}I or ^{123}I in the thyroid. The uptake test is one of the tests used in diagnosing hypothyroidism and hyperthyroidism. Examples of others are the T_3 resin uptake, the T_4 test, and the thyroid scan. It is also useful for differentiating between hyperthyroidism (Graves' disease) and an overactive toxic adenoma. This test tends to be more accurate for diagnosing hyperthyroidism than for diagnosing hypothyroidism.

A calculated dose of ^{131}I or [123]I (in capsule or liquid form) is given orally. The patient's thyroid is scanned at three different times. The tracer dose has small amount of radioactivity and is considered harmless.

In addition to the ^{131}I uptake test, the patient's urine output may be checked for radioactive iodine excretion.[5,8,10,15,20,26]

CLINICAL PROBLEMS

Decreased level: hypothyroidism (myxedema). *Drug influence:* Lugol's solution, vitamins, expectorants (i.e., SSKI), antithyroid agents, cortisone preparation, ACTH, aspirin, antihistamines, phenylbutazone (Butazolidin), anticoagulants (i.e., Coumarin), thiopental (Pentothal). *Foods:* seafood, cabbage, ionized salt.

Elevated level: hyperthyroidism (Graves' disease), thyroiditis, cirrhosis of the liver. *Drug influence:* barbiturates, estrogens, lithium carbonate, phenothiazines.

PROCEDURE

The patient should be NPO for 8 hours prior to the test. The patient can eat an hour after the radioiodine capsule or liquid has been taken.

The amount of radioactivity in the thyroid gland may be measured three times (after 2, 6, and 24 hours).

The patient should return to the nuclear medicine laboratory at specified times to measure the ^{131}I uptake level with the scintillation counter.

FACTORS AFFECTING DIAGNOSTIC RESULTS

Drugs and foods—see *Clinical Problems* above.

Severe diarrhea, intestinal malabsorption, and x-ray contrast media studies may cause a decreased ^{131}I uptake level, even in normal thyroid glands.

Rapid diuresis during the test could cause iodine excretion and a low iodine uptake in the thyroid gland.

Renal failure could cause an increased iodine uptake.

NURSING IMPLICATIONS WITH RATIONALE

Explain to the patient that the purpose of the test is to determine the function of the thyroid gland *or* to determine if the thyroid gland is overactive.

Explain to the patient the procedure for the test.

Ask the patient if he or she has allergies to iodine products.

Instruct the patient not to eat for 8 hours before the test.

Inform the patient that he may eat an hour after the radioiodine capsule or liquid has been taken, according to the nuclear medicine laboratory's procedure.

Inform the patient that a technician from the nuclear medicine lab will give the radioactive substance and that he or she must go to the laboratory 2, 6, and 24 hours after taking the iodine preparation. Explain to the patient that the procedure is to determine the percent of ^{131}I or ^{123}I uptake, that the test should not be painful, and that the amount of radiation received should be harmless. Emphasize the importance of being on time for each determination.

List on the request slip for the ^{131}I uptake test the x-ray studies and drugs the patient has received in the last week, which could affect test results. These drugs should, if possible, be discontinued for 3 or more days before the test (see *Drug Influence* above).

Draw blood for T_3 and/or T_4 tests, if ordered, before the patient takes the radioiodine capsule or liquid.

Tell the patient when it is time to return to the nuclear medicine laboratory. Post signs, if necessary. The testing should be done on time.

Answer the patient's questions. Encourage the patient to communicate concerns.

Inform the patient that the radioactive substance should not harm family members, visitors, or other patients, since the dosage is low and gives off very little radiation. Women who are pregnant definitely should not be given this test or any other radioactive tests.

Observe for signs and symptoms of hyperthyroidism—i.e., nervousness, tachycardia, excessive hyperactivity, exophthalmos, mood swings (euphoria to depression), and weight loss. Report these to the physician and record them in the patient's chart.

RETROGRADE PYELOGRAPHY (RETROGRADE PYELOGRAM)
Retrograde Ureteropyelography

NORMAL FINDING
Normal size and structure of the bladder, ureters, and kidneys.

DESCRIPTION
A retrograde pyelography test may be performed after intravenous pyelography (IVP) or in place of IVP. The contrast dye is injected through a catheter into the ureters and the renal pelvis. The visualization of the urinary tract is exceptionally good, since the dye is injected directly. Usually, this test is done in conjunction with cystoscopy.

Though retrograde pyelograms are not done too frequently today, this test is still performed when there is a suspected nonfunctioning kidney, an unlocated stone, or an allergy to intravenous contrast dye. Only a small amount of the dye that is injected directly into the ureters will be absorbed through the membranes.[2,3,5,8,19]

CLINICAL PROBLEMS
Abnormal findings: renal calculi, neoplasm (tumor), renal stricture, absence of nonfunctioning kidney.

PROCEDURE
A consent form should be signed by the patient or an appropriate member of the family.

The patient should be NPO for 8 hours before the retrograde pyelography. The patient should not be dehydrated before the test.

Laxatives and cleansing enemas may be ordered prior to the test.

Baseline vital signs should be recorded.

Sedatives/tranquilizers and narcotic analgesics are given approximately 1 hour before the test.

The patient is usually placed in the lithotomy position (feet and legs in stirrups).

Radiopaque contrast dye is injected through a ureteral catheter into the renal pelvis and x-rays are taken. As the catheter is removed, additional x-rays may be taken.

This procedure is usually done under local or general anesthesia and the test takes approximately 1 hour.

FACTORS AFFECTING DIAGNOSTIC RESULTS

Barium in the GI tract could interfere with good visualization. Barium studies should be done after a retrograde pyelogram.

NURSING IMPLICATIONS WITH RATIONALE

Explain to the patient that the purpose of the test is to identify kidney stones *or* to determine the cause of his kidney problems, or give a similar response related to the symptoms.

Explain the procedure to the patient. Explain to the patient that he or she will be placed in stirrups. If the patient is having the test done under local anesthesia, tell the patient that he or she will most likely feel pressure with the insertion of the cystoscope and may feel the urge to urinate. Inform him or her that there should be little to no pain or discomfort. Tell the patient that the test takes about 1 hour.

Inform the patient that food and drinks are restricted for 8 hours before the test. Some physicians may not restrict water unless the patient is to have general anesthesia. Check for symptoms of dehydration—i.e., dry mouth and mucous membranes, poor skin turgor, decreased urine output, and fast pulse and respirations. Report symptoms to the physician and record them on the patient's chart.

Record baseline vital signs.

Obtain a patient history of allergies to seafood, iodine, and/or radiopaque dye used in other diagnostic tests.

Administer laxatives, cleansing enemas, and premedications as prescribed. If the patient is not hospitalized, check that the prescribed orders were completed at home or in another institution. Check that the consent form has been signed before giving premedications.

Post-test

Monitor vital signs q15 minutes × 4, q30 minutes × 2, and qh × 4 or until stable. The patient's temperature should be taken q4h while awake for 1 to 3 days.

Observe for allergic reactions to the contrast dye—i.e., skin rash, urticaria (hives), flushing, dyspnea, and tachycardia.

Monitor urinary output. Report and record gross hematuria. Blood-tinged urine usually is normal. Report to the physician if the patient has not voided in 8 hours or the urinary output is less than 200 ml in 8 hours.

Give an analgesic for discomfort or pain. Report severe pain to the physician.

Observe for signs and symptoms of infection (sepsis)—i.e., fever, chills, abdominal pain, tachycardia, and, later, hypotension.

Be supportive of the patient and family. Answer the patient's questions or refer them to the physician or urologist.

S

SCANS (NUCLEAR) (Bone, Brain, Heart, Kidney, Liver and Spleen, Lung, and Thyroid)
Radioisotope Scans, Radionuclide Imaging

NORMAL FINDING
Adult: normal; no observed pathology.

DESCRIPTION
Nuclear medicine is the clinical field concerned with the diagnostic and therapeutic uses of radioactive materials or isotopes (one or more atoms of the same chemical element but with different atomic weights). A radioactive isotope is an unstable isotope which decays or disintegrates, emitting radiation or energy. In many institutions, radioisotopes are referred to as radionuclides. Radioactive materials are concentrated by certain organs of the body, and their distribution in normal tissue differs from the distribution in diseased tissue.

Examples of radionuclides or radiopharmaceuticals used for studying the function, anatomy, and morphology of the organs are: ^{99m}Tc (technetium) labelled phosphate, sulfur colloid, aggregated normal serum albumin (MAA), Glucoheptonate, Iprofenin, ^{125}I, ^{123}I, ^{201}Tl (Thallium), and ^{133}Xe.

Rectilinear scanners or scintillation (gamma) camera detectors are used for imaging, and the results usually are recorded on x-ray film. Equal or uniform gray distribution is normal, but darker areas can be referred to as hot spots (hyperfunction) and lighter areas as cold spots (hypofunction).[1,5,6,8,19,20]

CLINICAL PROBLEMS

Organ	Indications
Bone	To detect early bone disease (i.e., osteomyelitis); carcinoma metastasis to the bone; bone response to therapeutic regimens—i.e., radiation therapy, chemotherapy (antineoplastic agents)
	To determine unexplained bone pain
	To detect fractures and abnormal healing of fractures; degenerative bone disorders
Brain	To detect an intracranial mass—i.e., tumors (malignant or benign), abscess; cancer metastasis to the brain; head trauma (i.e., subdural hematoma); cerebral vascular accident (CVA—stroke) after the third or fourth week; aneurysms
Heart (cardiac)	To identify cardiac hypertrophy (cardiomegaly)
	To quantitate cardiac output (ejection fraction)
	To detect myocardial infarction (MI); ischemic heart disease
Kidney (renal)	To detect parenchymal renal disease—i.e., tumor, cysts, glomerulonephritis; obstruction of the urinary tract
	An iodine-sensitive patient when IVP cannot be performed
	To assess the function of renal transplantation

Organ	Indications
Liver and spleen	To detect tumors, cysts, or abscesses of the liver or spleen; hepatic metastasis
	To assess liver response to therapeutic regimens—i.e., radiation therapy, chemotherapy
	To identify hepatomegaly and splenomegaly
	To identify liver position and shape
Lung	To detect pulmonary emboli; tumors; pulmonary diseases with perfusion changes—i.e., emphysema, bronchitis, pneumonia
	To assess arterial perfusion changes secondary to cardiac disease
Thyroid	To detect thyroid mass (i.e., tumors); diseases of the thyroid gland (i.e., Graves', Hashimoto's thyroiditis)
	To determine the size, structure, and position of the thyroid gland
	To evaluate thyroid function resulting from hyper-thyroidism and hypothyroidism[1,3,4,5]

PROCEDURE

The radionuclide (radioisotope) is administered orally or intravenously. The interval from the time the radioactive substance is given to the time of the imaging can differ according to the radionuclide and organ in question. The scintillation camera detects the radiation that comes from the organ. Normally masses such as tumors absorb more of the radioactive substance than does normal tissue.

For diagnostic purposes, the dose of radionuclide is low (<30 mCi) and should have little effect on the patient's visitors, other patients, and nursing and medical personnel. Usually food and drinks are not restricted.

The procedures for the organ scans are listed according to the radionuclides used, the method of administration, the waiting period after injection, the food and drinks allowed, and other instructions.

1. Bone.
   a. Radionuclides: ^{99m}Tc-labelled phosphate compounds (technetium-99m diphosphonate, pyrophosphate, medronate sodium).
   b. Administration: Intravenously.
   c. Waiting period after injection: Waiting periods can differ according to the radionuclides used—e.g., for ^{99m}Tc the period is 2 to 3 hours (3 hours for an edematous person).
   d. Food and drinks: No restrictions; for ^{99m}Tc, water is encouraged during the waiting period (at least 6 glasses).
   e. Other instructions: The patient should void before the imaging begins. Imaging usually takes $\frac{1}{2}$ to 1 hour to complete. A sedative may be ordered if the patient has difficulty lying quietly during imaging.
2. Brain: For cerebral blood dynamic study or static imaging flow.
   a. Radionuclides: ^{99m}TcO$_4$, ^{99m}Tc DTPA (technetium 99m diethylenetriamine penta-acetic acid), ^{99m}Tc glucoheptonate.
   b. Administration: Intravenously.
   c. Waiting period after injection: ^{99m}TcO$_4$, 1 to 3 hours; ^{99m}Tc DTPA (Sn), 45 minutes to 1 hour. Frequently, a few photo scans are taken before the waiting period.
   d. Food and drinks: No restrictions.
   e. Other instructions: When using ^{99m}TcO$_4$, the patient may be given 10 drops of

Lugol's solution the night before or at least 1 hour before the injection or potassium perchlorate 200 mg to 1 gram 1 to 3 hours before the scheduled scan. These drugs block the uptake of $^{99m}TcO_4$ in the salivary glands, thyroid, and choroid plexus. With ^{99m}Tc DTPA (Sn), blocking agents are not necessary. The patient should remain still during the imaging (for ½ to 1 hour).

3. Heart (Cardiac).
   a. Radionuclides: ^{99m}Tc-pyrophosphate (technetium-99m pyrophosphate) testing for myocardial infarction (MI) 1 to 6 days after suspected MI; ^{201}Tl (thallium-201) testing for ischemic heart disease. ^{201}Tl testing can be done as part of the stress test. ^{99m}Tc-labelled red blood cells are used for ejection fraction studies.
   b. Administration: Intravenously.
   c. Waiting period after injection: ^{99m}Tc, 30 minutes to 1 hour; ^{201}Tl, 10 to 15 minutes. After the patient reaches maximum heart stress on the treadmill, IV radioactive thallium is given.
   d. Food and drinks: For thallium and stress ejection fraction studies, patients should be NPO from midnight until the study.
   e. Other instructions: The patient should lie quietly for 15 to 30 minutes during the imaging for an MI and for 1 hour during the imaging for ischemic heart disease.

4. Kidney: For renal blood flow (renogram) studies and imaging.
   a. Radionuclides: ^{99m}Tc (technetium) compounds (^{99m}Tc pertechnetate), ^{99m}Tc DTPA (diethylenetriamine-penta-acetic acid), ^{99m}Tc glucoheptonate, ^{131}I hippuran—usually ^{131}I hippuran for perfusion studies and ^{99m}Tc DTPA for renal disorders.
   b. Administration: Intravenously.
   c. Waiting period after injection:
      (1) Renal perfusion study: Imaging is done immediately after ^{131}hippuran is given intravenously. Renogram curves are plotted.
      (2) Kidney area: 3 to 30 minutes after ^{99m}Tc DTPA is injected.
   d. Food and drinks: No restrictions. The patient should be well hydrated, drinking at least 2 to 3 glasses of water 30 minutes before the scheduled scan. Dehydration could cause abnormal results in normal patients.
   e. Other instructions: The patient should void before the scan. If the patient has had x-ray procedures of the kidneys (i.e., IVP), the renogram or scan should be delayed 24 hours. Lugol's solution, 10 drops, may be ordered if ^{131}I hippuran is given. The patient should lie quietly for 30 minutes to 1 hour during imaging.

5. Liver and spleen.
   a. Radionuclides: ^{99m}Tc (technetium) compounds (^{99m}Tc pertechnetate, ^{99m}Tc sulfur colloid, ^{99m}Tc-Sn phytate), and ^{113m}In colloid.
   b. Administration: Intravenously.
   c. Waiting period after injections: ^{99m}Tc pertechnetate, 15 minutes before imaging (a spleen scan can be done at the same time); ^{99m}Tc sulfur colloid, 15 minutes.
   d. Food and drinks: No restriction. Some institutions may require the patient to be NPO after midnight.
   e. Other instructions: The patient should lie quietly for 30 minutes to 1 hour during the imaging. He may be asked to return at specified times. The patient may be asked to turn from side to side and onto his abdomen during imaging.

6. Lung.
   a. Radionuclides: ^{99m}Tc (technetium) compounds—i.e., ^{99m}Tc-MAA (macroaggregated albumin), ^{99m}Tc-HAM (human albumin microspheres).
   b. Administration: Intravenously.

      c. Waiting period after injection: ^{99m}Tc compounds, 5 minutes after the injection of the radionuclide.

      d. Food and drinks: No restrictions.

      e. Other instructions: A chest radiograph is usually ordered for comparison with the nuclear medicine study. The patient should lie quietly for 30 minutes during the imaging.

  7. Thyroid.

      a. Radionuclides: ^{131}I sodium iodide, ^{123}I, ^{125}I, ^{99m}Tc (technetium) pertechnetate.

      b. Administration: ^{123}I, ^{125}I, ^{131}I (orally, liquid or capsule), ^{99m}Tc pertechnetate (intravenously).

      c. Waiting period after injection: ^{123}I, ^{125}I, ^{131}I—24 hours. ^{123}I is the radionuclide most commonly used, since it has a shorter half-life. ^{99m}Tc pertechnetate, 30 minutes.

      d. Food and drinks: No restrictions.

      e. Other instructions: Three days before the scan (imaging), discontinue, with the physician's permission, iodine preparations, thyroid hormones, phenothiazines, corticosteroids, aspirin, sodium nitroprusside, cough syrups containing iodides, and multivitamins. Seafoods and iodized salt should be avoided. If the drugs cannot be withheld for 3 days, the drugs should be listed on the nuclear medicine request slip. The patient should lie quietly for 30 minutes during the imaging procedure.[1,3,4,5]

FACTORS AFFECTING DIAGNOSTIC RESULTS

Antihypertensives may affect results.

Two radionuclides administered in 1 day may interfere with each other.

Movement by the patient may distort the image.

A distended bladder could decrease visibility of the pelvic (bone) area.

Diet and drugs containing iodine could interfere with the results of the thyroid scan (see *Procedure* for the thyroid above).

Too short or too long a waiting period after injection of the radionuclide could affect the results.

Dehydration prior to imaging could affect the results.

NURSING IMPLICATIONS WITH RATIONALE

Explain to the patient that the purpose of the study or scan is to detect various disease entities. Radionuclide imaging is used in conjunction with radiologic studies and with other diagnostic tests to identify pathologic disorders. However, a positive brain scan can detect a lesion but it cannot provide histologic information about the lesion. Usually abnormal tissues concentrate the radionuclide.

Explain to the patient the procedure for the ordered study. Procedures will differ according to the type of study (see *Procedure* above). In most cases, food and drinks are not restricted. For the bone scan (^{99m}Tc), water is encouraged during the waiting period. For the renal scan, the patient should be well hydrated before the scheduled scan. Blocking agents (i.e., Lugol's solution and potassium perchlorate) are usually ordered before studies that use radioiodine, except for the thyroid scan.

Have the patient sign the consent form, if required.

Inform the patient that there could be a waiting period after the injection of the radioactive substance. Some of the tissues take longer than others to concentrate the substance.

Instruct the patient to void (urinate) before the study. Voiding will diminish bladder activity and increase visibility.

Obtain a brief health history prior to radionuclide imaging in regards to recent exposure to radioisotopes (radionuclides), allergies which could cause an adverse reaction, being pregnant, and breastfeeding an infant.

Explain to the patient that the dose of radiation he or she will receive from radionuclide imaging is usually less than the amount of radiation he or she would receive from diagnostic x-rays.

Inform the patient that the injected radionuclide should not affect the family, visitors, other patients, or hospital staff members. The radioactive substance usually leaves the body in 6 to 24 hours. The dose of radionuclide is very low.

Explain to the patient that the detection equipment will be moved over a section or sections of the body; however, there should not be any discomfort from the imaging equipment.

Inform the patient that he or she may be asked to change body positions during the test. Other than that, he or she should lie still during the procedure.

Inform the patient that the imaging may take 30 minutes to 1 hour, depending on which organ is being studied. The patient should be informed that he or she may need to return for additional imaging at specified intervals. If returning is necessary, the technician will inform the patient and the nurse.

Instruct the patient to remove jewelry or any metal object in the area of the study.

Adhere to the instructions from the nuclear medicine lab concerning the patient and the radionuclide procedure. The patient should arrive on time. This is especially true if he or she has received the injection. The waiting periods for each study have specified times.

Be supportive of the patient and family. Answer questions, if possible, and refer question you cannot answer to appropriate personnel.

Advise the patient to ask questions and to communicate any concerns. Be available when the patient wishes to discuss his or her concerns and fears.

Inform the patient that the personnel in nuclear medicine will give step-by-step directions concerning the procedure. Tell the patient to "speak up" if he or she does not understand.

Report to the physician if the patient is extremely apprehensive. The physician may wish to see the patient and/or order a sedative.

Notify the dietitian and/or dietary department not to send foods high in iodine content for 3 days to the patient who is to receive a thyroid scan, unless otherwise indicated. This also includes iodized salt. Inform the patient not to eat rich foods rich is iodine—i.e., seafood, table salt.

List restricted drugs containing iodine that the patient is taking on the nuclear medicine slip (see *Procedure* for the thyroid above). This is important if the radionuclide is iodine. Usually drugs containing small amounts of iodine are discontinued 3 days before the test. In certain cases, discontinuing the medication may be impossible.

Inform the patient that heart (cardiac) imaging may be done during the stress test as part of the testing for ischemic heart disease.

SCHILLING'S TEST (VITAMIN B12)

^{57}Co-tagged Vitamin B12 (Cobalt-57-tagged Cyanocobalamine)

NORMAL RANGE
  Adult: >7 percent.

DESCRIPTION

Vitamin B12 is essential for red blood cell maturation and for gastrointestinal and neurologic function. The extrinsic factor of vitamin B12 is obtained from foods and is absorbed in the small intestines when the intrinsic factor is present. The intrinsic factor is produced by the gastric mucosa, and when this factor is missing, pernicious anemia, a megaloblastic anemia, develops.

The Schilling test is used to determine whether there is a defect in vitamin B12 absorption (extrinsic factor) or a deficiency in the intrinsic factor. With normal absorption of vitamin B12, the small intestines absorb more than is needed and the excess is excreted by the kidneys. With impaired absorption, B12 cannot be absorbed and therefore cannot be excreted in the urine.

A vitamin B12 deficiency affects the bone marrow, the gastrointestinal tract, and the neurologic system. The bone marrow becomes hyperplastic, having many bizarre red blood cell forms. The leukocytes (WBC) are large but reduced in number; likewise, the platelets are bizarre in form and reduced in number. A beefy, red tongue; indigestion; abdominal pain; and diarrhea occur as the result of GI mucosal atrophy and decreased hydrochloric acid. A lack of vitamin B12 also causes tingling, numbness of the hands and feet, paralysis, and behavioral changes due to degeneration of the dorsolateral columns of the spinal cord and peripheral nerves.

Radioactive ^{57}Co-tagged vitamin B12 is given orally and followed an hour later by an intramuscular injection of nonradioactive vitamin B12. The IM vitamin B12 will saturate the liver and the protein-binding sites, thus permitting the cobalt-tagged vitamin B12 to be absorbed by the small intestines and excreted in the urine. There are various types of radioactive cobalt (^{57}Co, ^{56}Co, ^{60}Co,), but ^{57}Co is preferred because of its shorter half-life and its low-energy gamma radiation. Usually a Schilling test is performed after a plasma vitamin B12 assay (RIA) test; however, the Schilling test for diagnosing pernicious anemia is considered to be more accurate.[6,8,9,10,15,20,26]

CLINICAL PROBLEMS

Decreased level *(<5 percent)*: pernicious anemia (<3 percent), malabsorption syndrome, liver diseases, hypothyroidism (myxedema), pancreatic insufficiency, sprue.

PROCEDURE

Phase I: The patient should be NPO for 8 to 12 hours before the test.

A sample of urine (25 to 50 ml) should be collected before cobalt-tagged vitamin B12 is given to determine if there are radionuclide contaminants.

Radioactive ^{57}Co-tagged vitamin B12 capsule(s) or liquid is/are administered orally by a technician from nuclear medicine.

Nonradioactive vitamin B12 is given intramuscularly by the nurse 1 hour after the radioactive dose.

The patient can eat after the IM vitamin B12 injection.

Collect urine for 24 to 48 hours, according to the institution's procedure, in a special large container. No preservative is needed in the urine container and the container does not need to be refrigerated.

Label the urine container with the patient's name, the room number, the date, and the time.

Phase II: This is performed when there is a decreased percentage of radioactive vitamin B12 in the excreted urine. It will determine if the problem is due to pernicious anemia or malabsorption syndrome.

Phase II may be performed a week after Phase I.

^{57}Co-tagged vitamin B12 bound to human intrinsic factor (IF) is administered orally by the technician from nuclear medicine.

Repeat the Phase I procedure—i.e., NPO, nonradioactive vitamin B12, urine collection.

FACTORS AFFECTING DIAGNOSTIC RESULTS
A recent radionuclide scan.

If nonradioactive vitamin B12 is not given IM or is not given on time, the [57]Co-tagged vitamin B12 will be absorbed in the liver.

Food and drinks taken within 1 to 8 hours before the test.

Urinary excretion of B12 is decreased in the elderly and in patients with urinary insufficiency, diabetes mellitus, and hypothyroidism.

NURSING IMPLICATIONS WITH RATIONALE

Explain to the patient the purpose of the Schilling test. Explain that the test is to determine the cause of his or her symptoms—i.e., pernicious anemia, malabsorption syndrome, or others.

Explain the procedure to the patient. Tell the patient that he or she will be NPO for 8 to 12 hours before the test and that food should not be eaten until after the IM injection. Explain that a tracer dose of radioactive liquid or capsule(s) will be given by a person from nuclear medicine. An hour later, an IM injection will be given and then urine will be collected for 24 hours or longer.

Instruct the patient to put all urine in the special urine container. Inform the patient not to put feces or toilet paper in the urine.

Post a sign to save all urine on the patient's door or bed, in the utility room, and in the Kardex.

Tell the patient's family or visitors not to throw urine away.

Explain to the patient that the radioactive substance should not be harmful to him or her, family members, visitors, or other patients. Explain that the radiation dose is extremely low.

Give the nonradioactive vitamin B12 injection at the specified time, *on time*.

Notify the dietary department to release the breakfast tray after the nonradioactive vitamin B12 is given.

Report to the physician if the patient has had a decrease in urine output. This could affect the results of the test and the physician may wish to have the urine collected for 48 to 72 hours.

Do not administer laxatives the night before the test. Laxatives could decrease the absorption rate.

Inform the patient that foods high in vitamin B12 are mostly animal products (i.e., milk, eggs, meat, and liver) and that B12 levels are low in vegetables. If the patient has pernicious anemia, he or she should be advised to eat more animal products and the dietitian should be notified. IM vitamin B12 may be ordered.

Label the special urine container with the exact dates and times of collection, (e.g., 2/3/83 at 8:00 A.M. to 2/5/83 at 8:00 A.M.) and notify the nuclear medicine department.

Report signs and symptoms of pernicious anemia to the physician and record them in the patient's chart—i.e., pallor; fatigue; dyspnea; sore mouth; smooth, beefy, red tongue; indigestion; tingling numbness in the hands and feet; and behavioral changes.

SEX CHROMATIN MASS, BUCCAL SMEAR, BARR BODY ANALYSIS

NORMAL RANGE
Barr body in 25 to 50 percent of the female buccal mucosal cells.

DESCRIPTION
The sex chromatin test is a screening method to detect the presence or absence of Barr body (an inactivated X chromosome in a mass lying at the periphery of the cell nucleus) in the buccal mucosal cells. Buccal smears are used to check for Barr body when chromosomal abnormalities are suspected—e.g., Turner's syndrome (absent or <20 percent Barr body in females) and Klinefelter's syndrome (presence of Barr body in males). This test is also indicated if amenorrhea or abnormal sexual development is present.

Abnormal findings should be followed up by chromosome analysis (karyotype). The sex chromatin test should not be used for sex determinations.[5,8,24]

CLINICAL PROBLEMS
Abnormal findings: *Turner's syndrome* (female): absence of Barr body, amenorrhea, sterility, underdeveloped breasts. *Klinefelter's syndrome* (male): presence of Barr body, small penis and testes, sparse facial hair, gynecomastia, sterility.

PROCEDURE
There is no food or drink restriction.

The patient should rinse his or her mouth well.

A wooden or metal spatula is used to scrape the buccal mucosa twice; the first scraping is discarded and the second is spread over a glass slide. The slide should be sprayed with a fixation solution and sent to the laboratory for identifying a Barr body in the cells. The specimen should be labelled with the patient's name, sex, and age, as well as the date and the specimen site.

Check that the specimen is not saliva. The smear is stained and examined under a microscope.

The procedure usually takes 10 to 20 minutes.

FACTORS AFFECTING DIAGNOSTIC RESULTS
If the specimen is saliva and not cells, the test result could be inaccurate.

Failure to use a presevative (spray) on the buccal smear specimen will cause cell deterioration.

NURSING IMPLICATIONS WITH RATIONALE

Explain to the patient and/or parents that the purpose of the test is to determine the cause of abnormal sexual development. Inform them that this is a screening test and that other tests, such as chromosome analysis, may be indicated.

Explain the procedure to the patient and parents. Inform the patient that the cells from inside the mouth (buccal smear) are used, since they are easy to obtain. Tell them that the test has a high percentage of accuracy. The procedure usually takes 10 to 20 minutes; however, the results from the test may take several weeks.

Inform the patient that there should be a minimal amount of discomfort. Light pressure will be applied when scraping the mucosa.

Be supportive of the patient and his or her family. Be a good listener. Answer questions or refer them to the appropriate health professionals.

Record in the chart any abnormal sexual characteristics or problems and note them on the request slip—e.g., amenorrhea, gynecomastia.

SKIN TESTS (Tuberculin, Blastomycosis, Coccidioidomycosis, Histoplasmosis, Trichinosis, and Toxoplasmosis)

NORMAL FINDING
  Negative results.

DESCRIPTION
  Skin testing is useful for determining present or past exposure to an infectious organism—bacterial (tuberculosis), mycotic (blastomycosis, coccidioidomycosis, histoplasmosis), or parasitic (trichinosis and toxoplasmosis). The types of skin tests include scratch, patch, multipuncture, and intradermal. Generally the intradermal injection is the method most commonly used for skin testing. The antigen of the organism is injected under the skin, and if the test is positive in 24 to 72 hours, the injection site becomes red, hard, and edematous.
  Bacterial organism and disease: *Tuberculosis:* The tuberculin (antigen) skin test indicates whether a person has been infected by the tubercle bacilli. A negative test usually rules out the disease.
  The methods for skin testing include:

1. Mantoux test: Either PPD (purified protein derivative tuberculin) or OT (old tuberculin) is injected intradermally. PPD has several strengths, but the intermediate strength is usually used unless the patient is known to be hypersensitive to skin tests. The patient should not receive PPD or OT if he or she has had a previous positive test. The test is read in 48 to 72 hours.
2. The tine test or Mono-Vacc test: These are multipuncture tests which use tines impregnated with PPD or OT. This method is used for mass screening. The tine test is read in 48 to 72 hours, and the Mono-Vacc Test is read in 48 to 96 hours.
3. Vollmer's patch test: This test resembles a bandaid; however, the center piece is impregnated with concentrated OT. The patch is removed in 48 hours and the test is read 48 hours later.

  Mycotic organisms and diseases: *Blastomycosis:* The organism *Blastomyces dermatitidis* causes blastomycosis. The antigen blastomycin is injected intradermally, and if an erythematic area greater than 5 mm in diameter occurs, the test is positive. The skin test should be read in 48 hours. Positive sputum and tissue specimens will confirm the blastomycin skin test.
  Coccidioidomycosis: The coccidioidin skin test is useful for diagnosing coccidioidomycosis, a fungus disease caused by *Coccidioides immitis*. The antigen coccidioidin is injected intradermally and the skin test should be read in 24 to 72 hours. If the patient has been treated for coccidioidomycosis, he or she may remain positive during his or her life span.
  Histoplasmosis: Histoplasmosis is caused by the organism *Histoplasma capsulatum*, which, on a lung x-ray, resembles tuberculosis. The histoplasmin skin test for histoplasmosis is not always reliable. The antigen is injected intradermally and should be read in 24 to 48 hours. A positive test result occurs when an erythematic area is over 5 mm in diameter. To confirm the skin test results, sputum and tissue specimens should be obtained.
  Parasites: *Trichinosis:* *Trichinella spiralis* is the parasitic organism that causes trichinosis. This organism is present in uncooked meat, especially pork. Symptoms

occur approximately 2 weeks after ingesting the organism; the patient complains of nausea, diarrhea, pain, colic, fever, and swelling of the muscles. The antigen is injected intradermally and the test should be read in 15 to 20 minutes. A positive test is a blanched wheal with an erythematic area surrounding it.

Toxoplasmosis: Toxoplasma gondii is the organism causing toxoplasmosis. This organism is found in the eye ground and brain tissue of man. It can cause blindness and brain damage. The antigen, toxoplasmin, is injected intradermally and the test result should be read in 24 to 48 hours. A positive test is an erythematic area over 10 mm in diameter.[3,5,8,15]

CLINICAL PROBLEMS

Antigen Skin Test	Organism	Disease
Tuberculin	Tubercle bacilli	Tuberculosis
Blastomycin	*Blastomyces dermatitidis*	Blastomycosis
Coccidioidin	*Coccidioides immitis*	Coccidioidomycosis
Histoplasmin	*Histoplasma capsulatum*	Histoplasmosis
Trichinellin	*Trichinella spiralis*	Trichinosis
Toxoplasmin	*Toxoplasma gondii*	Toxoplasmosis

PROCEDURE

Food and drinks are not restricted.

Cleanse the inner aspect of the forearm with alcohol and let it dry.

Inject intradermally 0.1 ml of the antigen into the inner aspect used for the forearm.

Record the patient's name, the name of the test, the site and the arm of the skin test, the date, and the time it should be read (see *Description* above for readings of individual tests).

FACTORS AFFECTING DIAGNOSTIC RESULTS

Steroids and immunosuppressants given within 4 to 6 weeks can cause false negative skin test results.

A skin test performed before the body's incubation period (infectious process) can cause a false negative result.

Test results read several days after the designated time can give an inaccurate reading.

NURSING IMPLICATIONS WITH RATIONALE

Explain to the patient that the purpose of the skin test is to determine the presence of an organism. The organism and the type of skin test should be discussed.

Explain the procedure to the patient. Tell the patient that he or she will feel a pin prick as a small needle with a small amount of solution is injected under the skin.

Obtain a patient history about hypersensitivity to skin tests. Ask the patient if the skin test was performed before and, if so, whether the skin test result was positive or negative. The skin test should only be repeated if it was negative.

Note on the chart if the patient is taking steroids (e.g., Cortisone) or immunosuppressant drugs.

Inform the patient that the result of the skin test must be read during the stated time.

Record the patient's abnormal signs and symptoms. Ask the patient about his or her contact with bacterial, fungal, or parasitic organisms, if known.

Tell the patient that a positive skin test does not always indicate active infectious disease. However, the positive test does indicate that the organism is present in the body in either an active or a dormant state. If the results are positive, other studies are performed—i.e., x-rays, sputum and tissue cultures, and serum tests.

Be supportive of the patient and family and allow them time to express their concerns.

STRESS/EXERCISE TESTING, STRESS TESTING, EXERCISE ELECTROCARDIOLOGY (ECG)

NORMAL FINDING
Normal ECG (EKG) with little or no S–T segment depression with exercise.
Positive: >1 mm S–T depression.

DESCRIPTION
Stress testing is based on the theory that patients with coronary artery disease will have marked S–T segment depression on the ECG when exercising. Depression of the S–T segment and depression or inversion of the T-wave indicate myocardial ischemia. In 1928, Fiel and Siegel reported on the relationship of exercising and S–T segment depression in patients complaining of angina. Master used an exercise test (two-step) in 1929 to demonstrate ischemia but used only pulse and blood pressure to note changes. In 1931, Wood and Wolferth felt exercise was a useful tool for diagnosing coronary disease but that it could be dangerous. Later it was discovered that S–T segment depression usually occurred before the onset of pain and was still present for some time after the pain had subsided. Mild S–T segment depression after exercise can occur without coronary artery disease.

In 1956, R.A. Bruce established guidelines on performing stress testing on a treadmill. Master's Step Test (1955) was also accepted as a method for stress testing. Another method used today is the bicycle ergometer test; however, the treadmill seems to be the choice for testing cardiac status. With the treadmill stress test, the work rate is changed every 3 minutes for 15 minutes by increasing the speed slightly and the degree of incline (grade) by 3 percent each time (3 percent, 6 percent, 9 percent, etc). The body muscles do not seem to tire with the treadmill method as much as leg muscles (quadriceps) tire with the bicycle ergometer.

The uses for the stress/exercise test include: screening for coronary artery disease, evaluating the work capacity of cardiac patients, and developing a cardiac rehabilitation program.[5,7,8,14,15,21]

CLINICAL PROBLEMS
Indications: to detect coronary artery disease; to evaluate cardiac status for work capability, further diagnostic studies (e.g., cardiac catheterization), jogging or an exercise program (especially after the age of 35), cardiac rehabilitation programs.

PROCEDURE
A consent form should be signed by the patient.

The patient should not have food or liquids, especially alcoholic and caffeine-containing drinks, or smoke for 2 to 3 hours before the test. A light breakfast is indicated.

Medications should be taken, unless otherwise indicated by the physician.

Comfortable clothes should be worn—i.e., shorts or slacks with a belt and sneakers or tennis shoes with socks. Most bedroom slippers are not suitable.

The chest and/or back are shaved as needed and the skin is cleansed with alcohol. The skin sites for the chest electrodes will be sandpapered to remove the epidermis layer and excess skin oils.

Electrodes are applied to the chest according to the lead selections.

Baseline ECG, pulse rate, and blood pressure are taken and then are monitored throughout the test.

The test is stopped if the patient becomes dyspneic, suffers severe fatigue, complains of chest pain, has a rapid increase in pulse rates and/or blood pressure, or develops life-threatening arrhythmias—i.e., ventricular tachycardia, premature ventricular contractions over 10 PVC in 1 minute.

Usually the test is not stopped abruptly unless this is necessary. Vital signs and ECG tracings are recorded at the end of the testing or the recovery stage.

The test takes approximately 30 minutes, which includes up to 12 to 15 minutes of exercising.

Treadmill stress test: Usually there are five stages.

In the first stage, the speed is 2 mph at a 3 percent grade or incline for 3 minutes. In the second stage, the speed is 3.3 mph at a 6 percent grade for another 3 minutes. Normally the speed does not go beyond 3.3 mph. With each stage, the grade is increased 3 percent and the time is increased by 3 minutes, unless fatigue or adverse reactions occur. The power-driven treadmill has support rails to help the patient maintain balance but not to support his weight.

Bicycle ergometer test: The patient is instructed to pedal the bike against an increased amount of resistance. The bike handlebars are for maintaining balance and should not be gripped tightly for support.

The patient should not shower or take a hot bath for 2 hours after testing.

FACTORS AFFECTING DIAGNOSTIC TESTS

Certain drugs (e.g., digitalis preparations) can cause a false positive test result.

Leaning on support rails of the treadmill or the handlebars of the bicycle will affect the test results.

NURSING IMPLICATIONS WITH RATIONALE

Recognize when the stress/exercise test is contraindicated—i.e., with recent myocardial infarction; severe, unstable angina; uncontrolled arrhythmias; congestive heart failure; or recent pulmonary embolism.

Explain to the patient that the purpose of the test is to identify possible coronary disease *or* to determine the response of the heart to stress.

Explain the procedure to the patient in regards to having nothing by mouth (NPO); not smoking; continuing with medications; the clothing and shoes that should be worn; shaving and cleansing the chest area; electrode application; continuous monitoring of the ECG, pulse rate, and blood pressure; and not leaning on the rails of the treadmill or the handlebars of the bike.

Check that the consent form has been signed.

Inform the patient that the electrodes will not hurt. He or she may have some itching at the electrode sites.

Instruct the patient to inform the cardiologist or technician if he or she experiences chest pain, difficulty in breathing, or severe fatigue. The risk of having a myocardial infarction (heart attack) during the stress test is less than 0.2 percent.

Inform the patient that after 12 to 15 minutes of testing or when the heart rate is at a desired or an elevated rate, the test is stopped. It will be terminated immediately if there are any severe ECG changes—i.e., multiple PVC, ventricular tachycardia.

Allow the patient to ask questions. Refer questions you cannot answer to other appropriate health professionals—i.e., a cardiologist, a specialized technician, or a nurse in the stress test lab.

Instruct the patient to continue the walking exercise at the completion of the test for 3 to 5 minutes to prevent dizziness. The treadmill speed will be decreased. Tell the patient that he or she may be perspiring and may be "out of breath." Profuse diaphoresis, cold and clammy skin, severe dyspnea, and severe tachycardia are not normal.

Inform the patient that an ECG and vital signs are taken 5 to 10 minutes after the stress test (recovery stage).

Encourage the patient to participate in a cardiac/exercise rehabilitation program as advised by the physician/cardiologist. Tell the patient of the health advantages— constant heart monitoring, improved collateral circulation, increased oxygen supply to the heart, and dilating coronary resistance vessels.

Discourage the patient over 35 years old about doing strenuous exercises without having a stress/exercise test or a cardiac evaluation.

Inform the patient he or she can resume activity as indicated.

T

THERMOGRAPHY (Breast)
Mammothermography

NORMAL FINDING
No hot "white" spots; symmetric appearance of the breasts (photograph).

DESCRIPTION
Mammothermography (breast thermography), an infrared photographic test, measures and records heat energy from the skin surface of the breast. Lesions of the breast, especially cancerous ones, cause increased breast metabolism, resulting in an increased breast surface temperature and vascularity. If hot spots are recorded, then additional tests (such as low-dose mammography, ultrasonography, diaphanography, and/or biopsy) should be performed to confirm breast cancer.

Approximately 80 percent of positive thermograms are accurate for diagnosing lesions of the breast (35 percent of positive thermograms show benign breast lesions). This leaves 20 percent of the tests giving false positive results. Because one-fifth of the results are false positive, mammothermography is not commonly used, except for screening purposes. Usually it cannot detect small or deep breast cancer lesions. Mammothermography should be used in conjunction with a physical examination of the breast.[5,8]

CLINICAL PROBLEMS
Indications: to detect cancer of the breast, abscesses of the breast, fibrocystic disease of the breast; to analyze the progression of breast lesion(s).

PROCEDURE
Food and drinks are not restricted. Immediately before the test, hot or very cold drinks should be avoided.

The patient should remove jewelry and clothes from the neck to the waist. The patient is given a cloth or paper gown and the gown should be worn with the opening in the front.

Ointment or powder on the breast should be removed before the test.

The patient usually sits in a cool room (68°F) for 10 to 15 minutes before the test. This helps to equalize body temperature.

The patient is seated and will be asked to place her hands over her head or on her hips. Usually three photographs of different angles are taken of each breast. The procedure takes about 15 minutes.

The films are checked for readability before the patient removes the gown.

FACTORS AFFECTING DIAGNOSTIC RESULTS
Ointment, powder, and recent sunburn could change skin temperature and cause false positive results.

Fluctuations in room temperature could affect the test results.

Menstruation (immediately before or during) could increase vascular engorgement of the breasts.

NURSING IMPLICATIONS WITH RATIONALE

Explain to the patient that the purpose of the test is to determine if there are any tissue changes in the breast.

Explain the procedure to the patient. The respective procedures in hospitals and in private laboratories may differ slightly. Check before discussing the procedure with the patient. Tell the patient the test is not painful.

Instruct the patient not to use ointment or powder on the breast the day of the test. These could cause false positive results. Check the skin for recent exposure to sunlight.

Obtain a menstrual history. Ask the patient when she had her last menstrual period. She should not have the thermogram if she is pregnant or if she is menstruating or close to her period. The vascularity of the breasts increases at these times.

Inform the patient that the test takes about 15 minutes; however, she will be asked to wait for several minutes after the pictures are taken to be sure they are readable. Tell the patient not to be alarmed if one of the pictures needs to be repeated.

Encourage the patient to express her concerns. Answer questions, if possible, or refer questions to other appropriate health professionals.

Inform the patient that the mammothermography is generally a screening test and that if it happens to be positive, with a lesion or growth present, then other tests will be conducted to confirm the test results. Inform the patient that approximately one-third the positive results are benign lesions and one-fifth of the positive results could be false positives.

Encourage the patient to perform breast examination after each menstrual period and to keep routine medical appointments. If necessary, demonstrate breast examination technique.

U

ULTRASONOGRAPHY (Abdominal Aorta, Brain, Doppler (Arteries and Veins), Gallbladder, Heart, Kidney, Liver, Obstetrics, Pancreas, Spleen, and Thyroid)
Ultrasound, Echography (Echogram)

NORMAL FINDING
A normal pattern image of the organ.

DESCRIPTION
The terms *ultrasonography, ultrasound,* and *echography* are used interchangeably for a noninvasive diagnostic procedure used to visualize body tissue structures. A technician, the ultrasonographer, uses an ultrasound probe called a transducer held over the patient's skin surface to produce an ultrasound beam to the tissues. The reflected sound waves or echoes from the body tissues are recorded on an oscilloscope, a moving chart recorder, polaroid film, and/or videotape. The recording is referred to as an echogram or sonogram.

Ultrasound examinations frequently are used as screening tests, since they are relatively inexpensive and fast and are not known to cause any physical harm to the patient. They do not produce radiation. This noninvasive test is used to supplement other diagnostic radiologic examinations. There are limitations to this procedure such as with air-filled organs (the lung and the gastrointestinal tract with gas)—the ultrasound beam cannot penetrate air. When ultrasound studies indicate pathologic abnormalities, a more invasive procedure (i.e., computerized tomography [CT], radionuclide scanning, or radiologic studies with contrast dye) may be used to confirm the ultrasonographic results. In recent years, the accuracy of ultrasound exams has increased tremendously. In the future, they may actually replace the use of radiographic exams in some areas.

Some of the body structures which this procedure examines are the abdominal aorta, the brain, the arteries and veins (Doppler), the gallbladder, the heart, the kidney, the liver, obstetric regions (pelvic), the pancreas, the spleen, and the thyroid.

Abdominal aorta: For abdominal scanning, the umbilicus is a common reference point. "U + 7 cm" would mean 7 cm above the umbilicus. Ultrasound can detect aortic aneurysms with 98 percent accuracy. The aorta is an easy abdominal structure to examine by ultrasonic technique, from the xyphoid process to the aortic bifurication.

Brain: Ultrasound examination of the brain is usually referred to as *echoencephalography*. It is used as a quick means for checking the midline structure of the brain. Normally the third ventricle is in the midline and the echoes recorded should be at an equal distance on both sides. If the ventricle is shifted to one side, then pathologic findings (such as an intracranial lesion or an intracranial hemorrhage) could be suspected. Follow-up studies using CT and radionuclides may be indicated.

Doppler *(arteries and veins):* Doppler ultrasonography evaluates the blood flow in the major arteries and veins of the arms and legs. The Doppler transducer can detect decreased blood flow caused by partial arterial occlusion or by deep vein thrombosis. Low-frequency waves usually indicate low-velocity blood flow.

Gallbladder: Ultrasonography can evaluate the size, structure, and position of the gallbladder and can determine the presence of gallstones. The high-frequency sound waves from the transducer are directed to the upper-right quadrant of the abdomen.

Heart: The ultrasound examination of the heart is frequently called *echocardiography*.

It can determine the size, shape, and position of the heart and the movement of the heart valves and chambers. Echoes are picked up from the transducer (probe), converted to electrical impulses, and recorded on an oscilloscope, moving chart recorder, or videotape. The methods commonly used are the M-mode and the two-dimensional. The M-mode records the motion of the intracardiac structures, such as valves, and the two-dimensional records a cross-sectional view of cardiac structures. The echocardiogram is useful in detecting mitral stenosis, pericardial effusion, congenital heart disease, and enlargement of a heart chamber.

Kidney (renal): The ultrasound examination of the kidney is considered a reliable test for identifying renal masses (cyst and tumor) and can differentiate between a cyst and a tumor. The cyst is echo-free and the tumor records multiple echoes. There could be small malignant tumors surrounding a cystic mass which could be missed by the renal echogram. This test is highly recommended when the patient is hypersensitive to iodinated contrast dye used in x-ray tests—e.g., IVP.

Liver: The liver was one of the first organs examined by ultrasound, since it was large in size and difficult to x-ray. Using ultrasonography, liver masses (cyst or tumor) can be distinguished. With cysts, the echogram reflects an echo-free response, whereas with a tumor, multiple echoes are recorded. This noninvasive procedure is helpful for determining the size, structure, and position of the liver.

Obstetrics or pelvic: The obstetric or pelvic echogram is useful for determining pregnancy, the placental site, fetal growth, and/or pelvic diseases. In pregnancy, the amniotic fluid enhances reflection of sound waves from the placenta and fetus, thus identifying their size, shape, and position. Echoes from the pregnant uterus may be seen between 6 and 10 weeks and not again until 14 weeks after gestation. At that time, some of the fetal structures, such as the skull, can be identified. Ultrasonography is noninvasive and is considered a safe procedure for the mother and the unborn child (fetus). For better visualization of the uterus and its contents, a full bladder is indicated, which will displace the uterus.

Pancreas: The pancreas is a difficult organ to examine. In using ultrasound, high-frequency sound waves from the transducer are transmitted into the pancreatic region and echoes are picked up and converted to electrical impulses on the oscilloscope. Pancreatic tumors, pseudocysts, and pancreatitis can be detected by ultrasonography.

Speen: Ultrasound can be used for determining the size, structure, and position of the spleen. This procedure can identify splenic masses. In some cases it is a useful tool for evaluating a need for a splenectomy.

Thyroid: Ultrasonography of the thyroid s 85 percent accurate in determining the size and structure of the thyroid gland. This procedure can differentiate between a cyst and a tumor according to the echoes transmitted back to the transducer. It can also be used to determine the depth and dimension of thyroid nodules. Ultrasound is considered safe and does not involve radiation exposure.[5,8,15,22,23]

CLINICAL PROBLEMS

Organ Echogram	Abnormal Findings
Abdominal aorta	Aortic aneurysms
	Aortic stenosis
Brain	Intracranial hemorrhage
	Intracranial lesions (tumor, abscess)
	Hydrocephalus
Arteries and veins (Doppler)	Arterial occlusion (partial or complete)
	Deep vein thrombosis (DVT)
	Chronic venous insufficiency
	Arterial trauma

Organ Echogram	Abnormal Findings
Gallbladder	Acute cholecystitis
	Cholelithiasis (gallstones)
	Biliary obstruction
Heart	Cardiomegaly
	Mitral stenosis
	Aortic stenosis
	Pericardial effusion
	Congenital heart disease
	Atrial tumors
Kidney	Renal cysts
	Renal tumors
	Hydronephrosis
	Perirenal abscess
	Acute pyelonephritis
	Acute glomerulonephritis
Liver	Hepatic cysts and abscesses
	Hepatic tumor
	Hepatocellular disease (cirrhosis)
	Hepatic metastasis
Obstetrics and pelvic	Uterine lesions (tumor, fibroids)
	Fetal death
	Placenta previa
	Abruptio placenta
	Hydrocephalus
	Breech fetal presentation
Pancreas	Pancreatic tumors
	Pseudocysts
	Acute pancreatitis
Spleen	Splenomegaly
	Splenic cysts and abscesses
	Splenic tumors
Thyroid	Thyroid tumors (benign or malignant)
	Thyroid goiters
	Thyroid cysts

PROCEDURE

The procedures for all ultrasonography (ultrasound or echography) are very similar; however, differences and exceptions will be presented.

Food and drink restrictions will vary for abdominal aorta, brain, Doppler, heart, kidney, obstetric (pelvic), and thyroid ultrasound studies, respectively.

For the obstetrics and pelvic test, the patient should drink 3 to 4 glasses of water and not urinate until after the test.

For abdominal ultrasonography (gallbladder, liver, pancreas, and spleen), the patient should be NPO for 8 to 12 hours before the test. Patients having an ultrasound gallbladder test should eat a fat-free meal the evening before the test. These dietary preparations may vary from time to time.

Dressings at the site for the ultrasound study should be removed, if at all possible. Dressings that cannot be removed should be noted on the request slip.

The patient should lie in the supine position on the examining table. The procedure usually takes 30 minutes to 1 hour.

Mineral oil, glycerin, or a water-soluble lubricant is applied to the skin surface at the site that is to be examined. The ultrasound probe (transducer) is hand-held and moved smoothly back and forth across the oiled or lubricated skin surface. The transducer emits high-frequency sound waves. Echoes are picked up by the transducer, converted to electrical impulses on the oscilloscope, and recorded (strip recorder, photographs, or videotape).

Premedications are seldom given unless the patient is extremely apprehensive or has nausea and vomiting.

The patient should remain still during the procedure, as directed by the ultrasonographer.

FACTORS AFFECTING DIAGNOSTIC RESULTS

Dressings (bandages) and scar tissue inhibit and interfere with the transmission of ultrasound.

Residual barium sulfate in the GI tract from previous x-ray studies will interfere with ultrasound results. Ultrasonography should be performed before barium studies.

Air and gas (bowel) will not transmit the ultrasound beam.

NURSING IMPLICATIONS WITH RATIONALE

Explain to the patient the purpose of the test. Explanation could be brief, such as, "to identify the cause of the clinical problem" *or* "to determine the size and structure of the specific organ."

Explain the procedure to the patient (see *Description* and *Procedure* above). Inform the patient that food and drinks are not restricted except for abdominal ultrasonographies (gallbladder, liver, pancreas, and spleen). Tell the patient that an oil or lubricant is applied to the skin surface at the site of the organ and that a probe will move with light pressure back and forth over the area.

Inform the patient that this is a painless procedure unless there has been trauma (injury) to the area. Tell the patient that he or she will not be exposed to radiation and that the ultrasound test is considered to be safe and fast.

Instruct the patient to remain still during the procedure. Inform him or her that the test usually takes 30 minutes or less, except for a few ultrasound tests (e.g., kidney) which could take 1 hour.

Encourage the patient to ask questions and to express any concerns. Refer questions you cannot answer to the ultrasonographer or the physician.

Be supportive of the patient and the family.

V

VENOGRAPHY (Lower Limb)
Phlebography

NORMAL FINDING
Normal, patent deep leg veins.

DESCRIPTION
Lower limb venography is a fluoroscopic and/or x-ray examination of the deep leg veins after injection of a contrast dye. This test is useful for identifying venous obstruction due to a deep vein thrombosis (DVT). A thrombus formation usually occurs in the deep calf veins and at the venous junction and its valves. If DVT is not treated, it can lead to femoral and iliac venous occlusion, or the thrombus can become an embolus and cause pulmonary embolism.

This procedure is frequently done after Doppler ultrasonography to confirm a positive or questionable DVT. Almost all contrast dyes are composed of iodine, and for patients allergic to iodine products, radionuclide venography using ^{125}I fibrinogen with scintillation scanning may be done. The ^{125}I fibrinogen is given intravenously and the tagged fibrinogen collects at the site of the thrombus. It may take 6 to 72 hours for the isotope to collect at the thrombus site; thus the scanner will be used to check the leg daily for 3 days. Both venographies (contrast dye and radionuclide) will cause accumulation of radiation in the body and so these tests should not be performed for screening purposes.[5,15]

CLINICAL PROBLEMS
Indications: to detect deep vein thrombus (DVT); to identify congenital venous abnormalities, a vein for arterial bypass grafting.

PROCEDURE
A consent form should be signed by the patient or a designated family member.

The patient should be NPO for 4 hours before the test, although in some departments, clear liquids before the test will be permitted.

Anticoagulants may be temporarily discontinued.

Give a skin test and/or steroids (physician's order) to patients who have a history or allergies to iodine, seafood, or x-ray dye from other tests (e.g., IVP).

The patient lies on a tilted radiographic table at a 40° to 60° angle. There should be no weight bearing on the leg. A tourniquet is applied above the ankle, a vein is located in the dorsum of the patient's foot, a small amount of normal saline is given intravenously into the vein, and then the contrast dye is injected slowly over a period of 2 to 4 minutes. A cutdown may be necessary if a vein in the foot cannot be located or is not suitable. Fluoroscopy may be used to monitor the flow of the contrast dye, and spot films are taken.

Normal saline is used after the procedure to flush the contrast dye from the veins.

A sedative may be indicated prior to the test for patients who are extremely apprehensive and for those who have a low threshold of pain.

The test takes 30 minutes to 1 hour.

FACTORS AFFECTING DIAGNOSTIC TESTS
Weight on the leg being tested can cause a decrease in the flow of the contrast dye.

Movement of the leg being tested can interfere with the clarity of the film.

NURSING IMPLICATIONS WITH RATIONALE

Explain to the patient that the purpose of the test is to check for clots and patency of the deep veins in the legs.

Explain the procedure to the patient as regards to food and drink restrictions, the tilted table and intravenous fluids in the foot.

Inform the patient that he or she may have a slight burning sensation when the dye is injected. Inform the patient not to move the leg being tested during the injection of the dye or during x-ray filming.

Obtain a patient history of allergies to iodine, iodine substances (x-ray dye), and seafood. Antihistamines or steroids (e.g., cortisone) may be given for 2 to 3 days before the test.

Record baseline vital signs. Have the patient void before the test.

Post-test

Monitor vital signs every 15 minutes for 1 hour, every 30 minutes for the next 2 hours, and then every hour until stable or as ordered.

Check the pulse in the dorsalis pedis, popliteal, and femoral arteries for volume intensity and rate.

Observe for signs and symptoms of latent allergic reaction to the contrast dye—i.e., dyspnea, skin rash, urticaria (hives), and tachycardia.

Observe the injection site for bleeding, hematoma, and signs and symptoms of infection—i.e., redness, edema, and pain. Report abnormal changes and problems to the physician and record the observations in the patient's chart.

Elevate the affected leg as ordered. If the venogram is positive for DVT, the physician most likely will order bed rest, blood laboratory tests, heparin infusion, leg elevation, and warm, moist compresses.

Be supportive of the patient. Answer the patient's questions or refer them to the physician.

X

X-RAY (Chest; Heart; Flat Plate of Abdomen; Kidney, Ureter, Bladder; and Skull)
Roentgenography, Radiography

NORMAL FINDING
Chest: Normal bony structure and normal lung tissue.
Heart *(cardiac):* Normal size and shape of the heart and vessels.
Flat plate of abdomen: Normal abdominal structures.
Kidney, ureter, bladder *(KUB):* Normal kidney size and structure.
Skull: Normal structure.

DESCRIPTION
In November of 1895, Wilhelm Konrad Roentgen, a German physicist, discovered x-radiation for diagnosing diseases. Adequate control of the rays (roentgen rays) for the patient and the operator did not occur until 1910, and it was then when the machines and techniques were greatly improved. Today x-ray studies cause small amounts of radiation exposure due to the high quality of x-ray film and procedure.

There are four densities in the human body—air, water, fat, and bone—that will absorb varying degrees of radiation. Air has less density, causing dark images on the film, and bone has high density, causing light images. Bone contains a large amount of calcium and will absorb more radiation, thus allowing less radiation to strike the x-ray film, thus a white structure is produced.

The chest x-ray is one of the diagnostic tests most often ordered by the physician. A skull x-ray is usually ordered following head trauma. The requests for cardiac, flat plate of abdomen, and KUB x-rays have increased in the last two decades. X-ray studies are requested primarily for screening purposes and then are followed by other extensive diagnostic tests.[3,5,8,9,23]

CLINICAL PROBLEMS

Test	Abnormal Results
Chest	Atelectasis
	Pneumonias
	Tuberculosis
	Tumors (neoplasms), malignant and benign
	Lung abscess
	Pneumothorax
	Sarcoidosis
	Scoliosis/kyphosis
	Sarcoma
Heart (cardiac)	Cardiomegaly
	Aneurysms
	Anomalies of the vessels (e.g., the aorta)
Abdominal (flat plate)	Abdominal masses in the liver, stomach, pancreas, intestines
	Small bowel obstruction
	Abdominal tissue trauma
	Ascites (abnormal fluid)

Test	Abnormal Results
KUB (kidney, ureter, bladder)	Abnormal size and structure of KUB
	Renal calculi
	Kidney and bladder masses
Skull	Head trauma: intracranial pressure, skull fractures, etc.
	Congenital anomalies
	Bone defects

PROCEDURE

Chest: Food and drinks are not restricted.

A posteroanterior (PA) chest film is usually ordered with the patient standing. An AP chest film may be ordered when PA film cannot be obtained. With an AP chest film, the patient is sitting or lying down.

Clothing and jewelry should be removed from the neck to the waist and a paper or cloth gown should be worn.

The patient should take a deep breath and exhale, then take a second deep breath and hold it when told by the operator.

A lateral chest film may also be ordered.

Heart: Food and drinks are not restricted.

Posteroanterior (PA) and left-lateral chest films are usually indicated for evaluating the size and shape of the heart. The left anterior oblique (LAO) 60° rotation with the PA position may be ordered for cardiac evaluation.

Clothing and jewelry should be removed from the neck to the waist and a paper or cloth gown should be worn.

Patient instructions will include body position (usually standing) and when to take a deep breath and hold it.

Abdomen and KUB: Food and drinks are usually not restricted.

X-rays should be taken before an IVP or gastrointestinal studies.

Clothes are removed and a paper or cloth gown is worn.

The patient lies in the supine position with his or her arms away from the body on a tilted x-ray table.

The testes should be shielded as an added precaution.

Skull: Food and drinks are not restricted.

The patient should remove hair pins, glasses, and dentures before the x-ray tests.

The patient will be asked to assume various positions so that different areas of the skull can be x-rayed. X-rays may include the facial bones and sinuses.

FACTORS AFFECTING DIAGNOSTIC RESULTS

Radiopaque materials for IVP and gastrointestinal studies administered within 3 days of routine x-rays—i.e., chest, flat plate or abdomen, and KUB.

Incorrect positioning of the patient.

Obesity and ascites could affect the clarity of the x-ray film.

NURSING IMPLICATIONS WITH RATIONALE

Explain to the patient the purpose of the ordered x-ray test(s). Explanation could be brief, such as, "to determine if the chest, heart, KUB, or skull is normal" *or* "to find out if there is a clinical problem."

Describe the x-ray procedure to the patient.

Inform the patient that the x-ray test usually takes 10 to 15 minutes. Inform the patient that he or she may have to wait a half hour or so before the x-ray is taken.

Inform the patient that there may be several x-ray pictures taken—e.g., one or two chest films (PA and lateral) or five skull films. Ask the patient to remain in the waiting room for 10 to 15 minutes after the x-rays are taken to be sure the films are readable. Inform the patient that if additional x-rays are taken, this does not necessarily mean that the prior x-rays are abnormal.

Encourage the patient to ask questions or express his or her concerns to the nurse, the physician, and the technician. Also, if the patient does not understand the directions, he or she should ask to have them repeated.

Inform the patient that food and drinks are usually not restricted. Sometimes fasting for 8 hours is requested for the abdominal x-ray.

Ask the female patient if she is pregnant or if pregnancy is suspected. X-rays should be avoided during the first trimester of pregnancy. If x-ray of the chest is necessary, a lead apron should be worn by the female covering the abdomen and pelvic areas. Some dentists have women of childbearing age (12 to 48 years old) wear lead aprons.

Explain to the patient that the x-ray equipment and film today are of good quality and decrease the exposure to radiation.

REFERENCES: DIAGNOSTIC TESTS

1. Brucer, M. *What every young nurse should know about nuclear medicine.* St. Louis: Mallinckrodt, 1974.
2. Brunner, L.S., & Suddarth, D.S. *Medical–surgical nursing* (4th ed.). Philadelphia: Lippincott, 1980.
3. Brunner, L.S., & Suddarth, D.S. *The Lippincott manual of nursing practice* (2nd ed.). Philadelphia: Lippincott, 1978.
4. Cohen, S. Pulmonary function tests in patient care. *American Journal of Nursing,* 1980, *80 (6),* 1135–1161.
5. *Diagnostics.* Springhouse, Penn.: Intermed Communications, 1981.
6. Early, P. J., et al. *Textbook of nuclear medicine technology* (3rd ed.) St. Louis: Mosby, 1979.
7. Ellenstad, M. *Stress testing* (2nd ed.). Philadelphia: Davis, 1980.
8. Fischbach, F. *A manual of laboratory diagnostic tests.* Philadelphia: Lippincott, 1980.
9. French, R.M. *Guide to diagnostic procedures* (5th ed.). New York: McGraw-Hill, 1980.
10. Garb, S. *Laboratory tests in common use* (6th ed.). New York: Springer, 1976.
11. Goldberger, A.L., & Goldberger, E. *Clinical electrocardiography* (2nd ed.). St. Louis: Mosby, 1981.
12. Grossman, W. *Cardiac catheterization and angiography* (2nd ed.). Philadelphia: Lea & Febiger, 1980.
13. Haughey, C.W. CT scans. *Nursing '81,* 1981, *11 (12),* 72–77.
14. Janz, N., & Lampman, R.M. Treadmill stress test: Coaching your cardiac patient along the path to recovery. *Nursing '81,* 1981, *11 (12),* 36–41.
15. Luckmann, J., & Sorensen, K.C. *Medical–surgical nursing* (2nd ed.). Philadelphia: Saunders, 1980.
16. *Manual of radiology service.* Wilmington, Del.: Veterans Administration Center, 1978.
17. Matin, P. *Clinical nuclear medicine.* New York: Medical Examination Publishing, 1981.
18. Otto, P., & Ewe, K. *Atlas of rectoscopy and colonoscopy.* New York: Springer–Verlag, 1979.
19. Phipps, W.J., et al. *Schafer's medical–surgical nursing* (7th ed.). St. Louis: Mosby, 1980.
20. Sodee, D.B., & Early, P.J. *Technology and interpretation of nuclear medicine procedures* (2nd ed.). St. Louis: Mosby, 1975.
21. Sonnenblick, E.H., & Lesch, M. (Eds.). *Exercise and heart disease.* New York: Grune and Stratton, 1977.
22. Taylor, K. (Ed.). *Diagnostic ultrasound in gastrointestinal disease.* New York: Churchill Livingstone, 1979.
23. Thompson, T.T. *Primer of clinical radiology* (2nd ed.). Boston: Little, Brown, 1980.
24. Whaley, L.F., & Wong, D.L. *Nursing care of infants and children.* St. Louis: Mosby, 1979.
25. Whitehouse, W.M. (Ed.). *The year book of diagnostic radiology—1982.* Chicago: Year Book Medical Publishers, 1982.
26. Widmann, F.K. *Clinical interpretation of laboratory test.* (8th ed.). Philadelphia: Davis, 1980.

BIBLIOGRAPHY

BOOKS

Bio-Science directory of services. Van Nuys, Cal. Bio-Science Laboratories, 1980.

Brundage, D. *Nursing management of renal problems* (2nd ed.). St. Louis: Mosby, 1980.

Brunner, L.S., & Suddarth, D.S. *The Lippincott manual of nursing practice* (2nd ed.). Philadelphia: Lippincott, 1978.

Brunner, L.S., & Suddarth, D.S. *Medical–surgical nursing* (4th ed.). Philadelphia: Lippincott, 1980.

Byrne, C.J., et al. *Laboratory tests.* Reading, Mass.: Addison–Wesley, 1981.

Diagnostics. Horsham, Penn.: Intermed Communications, 1981.

Diseases. Horsham, Penn.: Intermed Communications, 1981.

Early, P.J., et al. *Textbook of nuclear medicine technology* (3rd ed.). St. Louis: Mosby, 1979.

Ellestad, M. *Stress Testing* (2nd ed.). Philadelphia: Davis, 1980.

Fischbach, F. *A manual of laboratory diagnostic tests.* Philadelphia: Lippincott, 1980.

French, R.M. *Guide to diagnostic procedures* (5th ed.). New York: McGraw-Hill, 1980.

Garb, S. *Laboratory tests in common use* (6th ed.). New York: Springer, 1976.

Goldberger, A.L., & Goldberger, E. *Clinical electrocardiography* (2nd ed.). St. Louis: Mosby, 1981.

Groer, M.E., et al. *Basic pathophysiology: A conceptual approach.* St. Louis: Mosby, 1979.

Grossman, W. *Cardiac catheterization and angiography* (2nd ed.). Philadelphia: Lea & Febiger, 1980.

Henry, J.B. *Todd–Sanford–Davidsohn: Clinical diagnosis and management by laboratory methods* (16th ed.). Philadelphia: Saunders, 1979.

Jones, D.A., et al. *Medical–surgical nursing.* New York: McGraw-Hill, 1978.

Kee, J.L. *Fluids and electrolytes with clinical applications* (3rd ed.). New York: John Wiley & Sons, 1982.

Krause, M.V., & Mahan, L.K. *Food, nutrition and diet therapy* (6th ed.). Philadelphia: Saunders, 1979.

Linne, J.J., & Lingsrud, K.M. *Basic techniques for the medical laboratory* (2nd ed.). New York: McGraw-Hill, 1979.

Luckmann, J., & Sorensen, K.C. *Medical–surgical nursing* (2nd ed.). Philadelphia: Saunders, 1980.

Matin, P. *Clinical nuclear medicine.* New York: Medical Examination Publishing, 1981.

Nester, E.W., et al. *Microbiology.* New York: Holt, Rinehart, and Winston, 1973.

Otto, P., & Ewe, K. *Atlas of rectoscopy and colonscopy.* New York: Springer-Verlag, 1979.

Patterson, H.R., et al. *Falconer's current drug handbook, 1980-1982.* Philadelphia: Saunders, 1980.

Phipps, W.J., et al. *Schaeffer medical–surgical nursing* (7th ed.). St. Louis: Mosby, 1980.

Ravel, R. *Clinical laboratory medicine* (3rd ed.). Chicago: Year Book Medical, 1978.

Robinson, C.H. *Normal and therapeutic nutrition* (14th ed.). New York: Macmillan, 1972.

Sodee, D.B., & Early, P.J. *Technology and interpretation of nuclear medicine procedures* (2nd ed.). St. Louis: Mosby, 1975.

Sonnenblick, E.H., & Lesch, M. (Eds.). *Exercise and heart disease.* New York: Grune & Stratton, 1977.

Strand, M.M., & Elmer, L.A. *Clinical laboratory tests* (2nd ed.). St. Louis: Mosby, 1980.

Taylor, K. (Ed.). *Diagnostic ultrasound in gastrointestinal disease.* New York: Churchill Livingstone, 1979.

Tilkian, S.M., et al. *Clinical implications of laboratory tests* (2nd ed.). St. Louis: Mosby, 1979.

Thompson, T.T. *Primer of clinical radiology* (2nd ed.). Boston: Little, Brown, 1980.

Wallach, J. *Interpretation of diagnostic tests* (3rd ed.). Boston: Little, Brown, 1978.

Whaley, L.F., & Wong, D.L. *Nursing care of infants and children.* St. Louis: Mosby, 1979.

Whitehouse, W.M. (Ed.). *The year book of diagnostic radiology—1982.* Chicago: Year Book Medical, 1982.

Widmann, F.K. *Clinical interpretation of laboratory tests* (8th ed.). Philadelphia: Davis, 1980.

PERIODICALS

Billet, E.T., & Welch, M.J. The use of clinical laboratory findings in diagnosing and managing critically ill children. *Critical Care Quarterly,* 1979, *2 (3),* 19–35.

Cohen, S. Pulmonary function tests in patient care. *American Journal of Nursing,* 1980, *80 (6),* 1135–61.

Elbaum, N. Detecting and correcting magnesium imbalance. *Nursing '77,* 1977, *7 (8),* 34–35.

Felver, L. Understanding the electrolyte maze. *American Journal of Nursing,* 1980, *80 (9),* 1591–95.

Friedman, R.B., et al. Effects of diseases on clinical laboratory tests. *Clinical Chemistry,* 1980, *26 (4),* 1–243.

Grant, M.M., & Kubo, W.M. Assessing a patient's hydration status. *American Journal of Nursing,* 1975, *75 (8),* 1306–11.

Haughey, C.W. CT scans. *Nursing '81,* 1981, *11 (12),* 72–77.

Janz, N., & Lampman, R.M. Treadmill stress test: Coaching your cardiac patient along the path to recovery. *Nursing '81,* 1981, *11 (12),* 36–41.

Kee, J.L. Clinical implications of laboratory studies in critical care. *Critical Care Quarterly,* 1979, *2 (3),* 1–17.

Lancour, J. Two hormone regulators of fluid balance. In *Nursing skillbook: Monitoring fluid and electrolytes precisely.* Horsham, Penn.: Intermed Communications, 1978.

Menzel, L.K. Clinical problems of electrolyte balance. *Nursing Clinics of North America,* 1980, *15 (3),* 559–75.

O'Dorisio, T.M. Hypercalcemic crisis. *Heart and Lung,* 1978, *7 (3),* 425–32.

Stark, J. BUN/creatinine–your keys to kidney function. *Nursing '80,* 1980, *10 (5),* 33–38.

Tiongson, J.G., & Woods, A.L. Cardiac isoenzymes: clinical implications. and limitations *Critical Care Quarterly,* 1979, *2 (3),* 47–51.

Tripp, A. Hyper and hypocalcemia. *American Journal of Nursing,* 1976, *76 (7),* 1142–45.

BOOKLETS

Brucer, M. What every young nurse should know about nuclear medicine. St. Louis: Mallinckrodt, 1974.

Manual of Radiology service. Wilmington, Del.: Veterans Administration Center, 1978.

APPENDIX A

Abbreviations of Measurements Used for Normal Values

↑	=	increased
↓	=	decreased
>	=	greater than
<	=	less than
cm^3	=	cubic centimeter
cu mm (mm^3)	=	cubic millimeter
dl	=	deciliter (100 ml)
fl	=	femtoliter
g or gm	=	gram
IU	=	International Unit
kg	=	kilogram
L	=	liter
m^2	=	square meter
mCi	=	millicuries
mcg (μg)	=	microgram
mEq	=	milliequivalent
mg	=	milligram
mg/dl	=	milligram per deciliter
mIU	=	milli-International Unit
ml	=	milliliter
mm	=	millimeter
mm^3	=	cubic millimeter
mmHg	=	millimeter of mercury
mmol	=	millimole
mOsm	=	milliosmole
mU	=	milliunit
mUU	=	mouse uterine units
mμ	=	millimicron
ng	=	nanogram
nmol	=	nanomole
pg	=	picogram
SI units	=	International system of units
U	=	unit
μ	=	micron (micrometer)
μ^3	=	cubic micron
μg	=	microgram
μIU	=	micro-International Unit
μl	=	microliter
μM	=	micromolar
μm^3	=	cubic micrometer
μmol	=	micromole
μU	=	microunit

Abbreviations for Laboratory and Diagnostic Tests

ABG	=	Arterial blood gas
ACP	=	Acid phosphatase
ACTH	=	Adrenocorticotropic hormone
AHF	=	Antihemophilic factor
ALD	=	Aldolase
ALP	=	Alkaline phosphatase
ALT	=	Alanine aminotransferase (same as SGPT)
α 1-AT	=	Alpha-1-antitrypsin
ANA	=	Antinuclear antibodies
APTT	=	Activated partial thromboplastin time
ASO	=	Antistreptolysin O
AST	=	Aspartate aminotransferase (same as SGOT)
BE	=	Base excess
BUN	=	Blood urea nitrogen
C	=	Complement—e.g., Complement C3
Ca	=	Calcium
CA	=	Cold agglutinins
CAT	=	Computerized axial tomography
CBC	=	Complete blood count
CEA	=	Carcinoembryonic antigen
CHS	=	Cholinesterase
Cl	=	Chloride
CO	=	Carbon monoxide
CO_2	=	Carbon dioxide
Cp	=	Ceruloplasmin
CPK or CK	=	Creatine phosphokinase
CPK-BB	=	Creatine phosphokinase, brain
CPK-MB	=	Creatine phosphokinase, heart
CPK-MM	=	Creatine phosphokinase, skeletal muscle
Cr	=	Creatinine
CRF	=	Corticotropin-releasing factor
CRP	=	C-reactive protein
CSF	=	Cerebrospinal fluid
CT	=	Coagulation time
CT	=	Computerized tomography
CTT	=	Computerized transaxial tomography
Cu	=	Copper
E_3	=	Estriol
ECG (EKG)	=	Electrocardiogram
EEG	=	Electroencephalogram
EMG	=	Electromyography
ESR	=	Erythrocyte sedimentation rate
FBS	=	Fasting blood sugar
FDP	=	Fibrin degradation
FSH	=	Follicle-stimulating hormone
FSP	=	Fibrin or fibrinogen split product
FTA-ABS	=	Fluorescent treponemal antibody absorption
G-6-PD	=	Glucose-6-phosphate
GGTP or GTP	=	Gamma-glutamyl (transferase) transpeptidase
GI series	=	Gastrointestinal series (upper)
HAA	=	Hepatitis-associated antigen
HAI or HI	=	Hemagglutination inhibition
Hb or Hbg	=	Hemoglobin

HBsAg	=	Hepatitis B surface antigen
HCG	=	Human chorionic gonadotropin
HCO_3	=	Bicarbonate
HCT	=	Hematocrit
HDL	=	High-density lipoprotein
5-HIAA	=	5-Hydroxyindolacetic acid
IBC	=	Iron-binding capacity (see TIBC)
Ig	=	Immunoglobulin
IVP	=	Intravenous pyelography
K	=	Potassium
17-KS	=	17-Ketosteroid
LAP	=	Leucine aminopeptidase
LDH (LD)	=	Lactic dehydrogenase
LDL	=	Low-density lipoprotein
L/S	=	Lecithin/sphingomyelin
MCH	=	Mean corpuscular hemoglobin
MCHC	=	Mean corpuscular hemoglobin concentration
MCV	=	Mean corpuscular volume
Mg	=	Magnesium
Na	=	Sodium
17-OHCS	=	17-Hydroxycorticosteroid
P	=	Phosphorus
Pco_2	=	Partial pressure of carbon dioxide
pH	=	Negative logarithm of hydrogen ion concentration
PKU	=	Phenylketonuria
Po_2	=	Partial pressure of oxygen
PPBS	=	Postprandial blood sugar (feasting blood sugar)
PT	=	Prothrombin time
PTT	=	Partial thromboplastin time
RA	=	Rheumatoid arthritis
RAI	=	Radioactive iodine uptake
RBC	=	Red blood cell
RF	=	Rheumatoid factor
RIA	=	Radioimmunoassay
RPR	=	Rapid plasma reagin
SGOT	=	Serum glutamic oxaloacetic transaminase (same as AST)
SGPT	=	Serum glutamic pyruvic transaminase (same as ALT)
So_2	=	Oxygen saturation
T_3	=	Triiodothyronine resin uptake
T_4	=	Thyroxine
TA	=	Thyroid antibodies
TIBC	=	Total iron-binding capacity (see IBC)
TSH	=	Thyroid-stimulating hormone
UA	=	Urinalysis
VCT	=	Venous clotting time
VDRL	=	Venereal disease research laboratory
VLDL	=	Very low-density lipoprotein
VMA	=	Vanilmandelic acid
WBC	=	White blood cell (leukocyte)

APPENDIX C

Laboratory Test Values for Adults and Children

The laboratory tests and their normal ranges for adults and children are listed according to the laboratory sections that analyze the specimens. The personnel from the laboratory department and nuclear medicine frequently work together in obtaining blood specimens to be tested by the radioimmunoassay (RIA) method. So that the patient does not receive several venous punctures, the laboratory personnel will collect enough blood for all lab tests, including RIA.

Arterial blood gases are analyzed in either the pulmonary function laboratory, critical care units, or the chemistry section of the laboratory. The cerebrospinal fluid tubes are distributed to the appropriate laboratory sections—i.e., Hematology, Chemistry, or Microbiology.

Hematology	Adult	Children
	Normal Range	
Bleeding time	Ivy method: 1–6 min Duke method: 1–3 min	Same as adult
Carboxyhemoglobin (CO)—see *Chemistry*		
Clot retraction	1–24 hr	Same as adult
Coagulation time (CT)	5–15 min	Same as adult

Erthrocyte sedimentation rate (ESR)	Average: 8 min
	<50 years old (Westergren)
	  Male: 0–15 mm/hr
	  Female: 0–20 mm/hr
	>50 years old (Westergren)
	  Male: 0–20 mm/hr
	  Female: 0–30 mm/hr
	Cutler method
	  Male: 0–8 mm/hr
	  Female: 0–10 mm/hr
	Wintrobe method
	  Male: 0–7 mm/hr
	  Female: 0–15 mm/hr
		Newborn:
		  0–2 mm/hr
		4–14 years old:
		  3–13 mm/hr

Factor assay		
I: Fibrinogen	200–400 mg/dl Minimum for clotting: 75–100 mg/dl	Same as adult
II: Prothrombin	Minimum hemostatic level: 10–15% concentration	
III: Thromboplastin	Variety of substances	
IV: Calcium	4.5–5.5 mEq/L or 9–11 mg/dl	
V: Proaccelerin labile factor	Minimum hemostatic level: 5–10% concentration	Same as adult
VI	Not used	
VII: Proconvertin stable factor	Minimum hemostatic level: 5–15% concentration	

VIII: Antihemophilic factor (AHF)	Minimum hemostatic level: 30–35% concentration	
IX: Plasma thromboplastin component (PTC, Christmas factor)	Minimum hemostatic level: 30% concentration	
X: Stuart factor, Prower factor	Minimum hemostatic level: 7–10% concentration	
XI: Plasma thromboplastin antecedent (PTA)	Minimum hemostatic level: 20–30% concentration	
XII: Hageman factor	0% concentration	
XIII: Fibrinase, fibrin stabilizing factor (FSF)	Minimum hemostatic level: 1% concentration	
Fibrin degradation products (FDP)	2 to 10 µg/ml	
Hematocrit (HCT)	Male: 40–54%; 0.40–0.54 SI units Female: 36–46%; 0.36–0.46 SI units	Not usually done Newborn: 42–54% 1–3 years old: 29–40% 4–10 years old: 36–38%
Hemoglobin (Hb or Hgb)	Male: 13.5–18 g/dl Female: 12–16 g/dl	Newborn: 14–24 g/dl Infant: 10–15 g/dl Child: 11–16 g/dl
Hemoglobin electrophoresis		
A_1	95–98% total Hb	
A_2	1.5–3.5%	
F	<2%	Newborn: 40–70% total Hb Infant: 2–10% total Hb Child: 1–2% total Hb
C	0%	
D	0%	
S	0%	
Osmotic fragility: erythrocyte	see table below	Same as adult
Partial thromboplastin time (PTT)	PPT: 60–70 sec APTT: 30–45 sec	

		% Hemolysis	
			Incubated at 37°C
%Saline (NaCl)		Fresh blood (3 hours)	(24 hr blood)
0.30		97–100	85–100
0.35		90–98	75–100
0.40		50–95	65–100
0.45		5–45	55–95
0.50		0–5	40–85
0.55		0	15–65
0.60		0	0–40

(continued)

Hematology	Normal Range	
	Adult	**Children**
Platelet count (thrombocytes)	150,000–400,000 mm³ (mean, 250,000 mm³) SI units: 0.15–0.4 × 10¹²/L	Premature: 100,000–300,000 mm³ Newborn: 150,000–300,000 mm³ Infant: 200,000–475,000 mm³
Prothrombin time (PT)	11–15 sec or 70–100% Anticoagulant therapy: 2–2.5 times the control in seconds or 20–30%	Same as adult
Red blood cell indices (mil/mm³)		
MCV	Male: 4.6–6.0 Female: 4.0–5.0	Newborn: 4.8–7.2 Child: 3.8–5.5
	80–98	Newborn: 96–108 Child: 82–92
MCH	27–31	Newborn: 32–34 Child: 27–31
MCHC	32–36	Newborn: 32–33 Child: 32–36
Reticulocyte count	0.5–1.5% of all RBC 25,000–75,000 mm³ (absolute count)	Newborn: 2.5–6.5% of all RBC Infant: 0.5–3.5% of all RBC Child: 0.5–2.0% of all RBC
Schilling (vitamin B12)	> 7%	
Sickle cell screening	0	0
White blood cells (WBC)	5000–10,000 mm³	Newborn: 9000–30,000 mm³ 2 years old: 6000–17,000 mm³
White blood cell Differential		
Neutrophils	50–70% of total WBC	29–47%
Segments	50–65%	
Bands	0–5%	
Eosinophils	0–3%	0–3%
Basophils	1–3%	1–3%
Lymphoctyes	25–35%	38–63%
Monocytes	2–6%	4–9%
Immunohematology (Blood Bank)		
Coombs direct	Negative	Negative
Coombs indirect	Negative	Negative
Cross-matching	Absence of agglutination (clumping)	Same as adult
Rh typing	Rh+ and Rh−	Same as adult

Chemistry

Acetone (ketone bodies)	Acetone: 0.3–2.0 mg/dl; SI units—51.6–344 µmol/L	Newborn: slightly higher than adult
	Ketones: 2–4 mg/dl	Infant and child: same as adult
Acid phosphatase (ACP)	0.1–2 U/dl (Gutman)	6.4–15.2 U/L
	0.5–2 U/dl (Bodansky)	
	0.1–5 U/dl (King–Armstrong)	
	0.1–0.8 U/dl (Bessey–Lowry)	
	0.0–0.8 U/L at 37°C (SI units)	
Alanine aminotransferase (ALT, SGPT)	5–35 U/ml (Frankel)	Same as adult
	5–25 mU/ml (Wroblewski)	
	8–50 U/ml at 30°C (Karmen)	
	4–36 U/L at 37°C (SI units)	
Alcohol	0%	
Aldolase (ALD)	3–8 U/dl (Sibley–Lehninger)	Infant: 12–24 U/dl
	22–59 mU/L at 37°C (SI units)	Child: 6–16 U/dl
Aldosterone (may be done in nuclear medicine)	1–9 ng/dl	
Alkaline phosphatase (ALP)	20–90 U/L at 30° (SI units)	Infant: 40–300 U/L
	25–97 U/L at 37°C (SI units)	Child: 60–270 U/L; 15–30 U/dl
	2–4 U/dl (Bodansky)	(King–Armstrong); 5–14 U/dl
	4–13 U/dl (King–Armstrong)	(Bodansky)
	0.8–2.3 U/dl (Bessy–Lowry)	
Alpha-1-antitrypsin	159–400 mg/dl	Newborn: slightly below level
Ammonia	1.0–1.6 g/L	Infant and child: same as adult
	3.2–4.5 g/dl	Newborn: 90–150 µg/dl
	32–45 g/L (SI units)	Child: 40–80 µg/dl
	11–35 µmol/L	
	20–120 µg/dl (diffusion)	
	40–80 µg/dl (enzymatic method)	
	12–48 µg/dl (resin method)	
Amylase	60–160 Somogyi U/dl	Not usually done
	111–296 U/L (SI units)	
Arterial blood gases (see Others)	0.6–1.6 mg/dl (plasma)	0.6–1.6 mg/dl (plasma)
Ascorbic acid (vitamin C)	34–91 µmol/L (SI units—plasma)	
	0.7–2.0 mg/dl (blood)	
	40–114 µmol (SI units—blood)	

(continued)

Chemistry	Normal Range	
	Adult	**Children**
Asparatate aminotransferase (AST, SGOT)	5–40 U/ml (Frankel) 4–36 IU/L 16–60 U/ml at 30°C 8–33 U/L at 37°C (SI units)	Newborn: four times normal level Child: Same as adult
Barbiturate	0 Therapeutic: 10–30 µg/dl	15–40 µg/dl
Bilirubin (indirect)	0.1–1.0 mg/dl 1.7–17.1 µmol/L (SI units)	
Bilirubin (total and direct)	Total: 0.1–1.2 mg/dl; 1.7–20.5 µmol/L (SI units) Direct (conjugated): 0.1–0.3 mg/dl; 1.7–5.1 µmol/L (SI units)	Newborn, total: 1–12 mg/dl Newborn, total: 17.1–205 µmol/L (SI units) Child, total: 0.2–0.8 mg/dl
Blood urea nitrogen (BUN)	8–25 mg/dl Male: 10–25 mg/dl Female: 8–20 mg/dl	Infant: 5–15 mg/dl Child: 5–20 mg/dl
Bromide	0 Therapeutic: <80 mg/dl	0
Calcium (Ca)	4.5–5.5 mEq/L 9–11 mg/dl 2.3–2.8 mmol/L (SI units)	Newborn: 3.7–7.0 mEq/L; 7.4–14 mg/dl Infant: 5.0–6.0 mEq/L; 10–12 mg/dl Child: 4.5–5.8 mEq/L; 9–11.5 mg/dl
Carbon dioxide combining power (CO_2)	22–30 mEq/L 22–30 mmol/L (SI units)	20–28 mEq/L
Carbon monoxide (CO) Carboxyhemoglobin (may be done in Hematology)	2.5% saturation of Hb 2–9% saturation of Hb (smokers)	Same as adult
Carotene	40–200 mg/dl 0.74–3.72 µmol/L (SI units)	40–130 µg/dl
Ceruloplasmin (Cp: may be done in Hematology)	23–50 mg/dl 230–500 mg/L (SI units)	Infant: <23 mg/dl or normal Child: same as adult
Chloride (Cl)	95–105 mEq/L 95–105 mmol/L (SI units)	Newborn: 94–112 mEq/L Infant: 95–110 mEq/L Child: 98–105 mEq/L
Cholesterol	150–250 mg/dl (may increase with age) 3.90–6.50 mmol/L (SI units)	Infant: 70–175 mg/dl Child: 120–240 mg/dl
Cholinesterase	0.5–1.0 units (RBC) 3–8 units/ml (plasma) 6–8 IU/L (RBC) 8–18 IU/L at 37°C (plasma)	Same as adult

Test	Values
Copper (Cu)	Male: 70–140 µg/dl; 11–22 µmol/L (SI units) Female: 80–155 µg/dl; 12.6–24.3 µmol/L (SI units)	Newborn: 20–70 µg/dl Child: 30–150 µg/dl Adolescent: 90–240 µg/dl
Corticotropin (ACTH; may be done by Nuclear Medicine)	ACTH: 8 A.M. to 10 A.M.; up to 80 pg/ml	
Cortisol	8 A.M. to 10 A.M.: 5–23 µg/dl; 138–635 nmol/L (SI units) 4 P.M. to 6 P.M.: 3–13 µg/dl; 83–359 nmol/L (SI units)	8 A.M. to 10 A.M.: 15–25 µg/dl 4 P.M. to 6 P.M.: 5–10 µg/dl
Creatine phosphokinase (CPK)	Male: 5–35 µg/ml; 15–120 IU/L 55–170 U/L at 37°C (SI units) Female: 5–25 µg/ml; 10–80 IU/L; 30–135 U/L at 37°C (SI units)	Newborn: 10–300 IU/L at 30°C Child: Male: 0–70 IU/L at 30°C Female: 0–50 IU/L at 30°C Infant to 6 years old: 0.3–0.6 mg/dl;
Creatinine (Cr)	0.6–1.2 mg/dl 53–106 µmol/L (SI units)	27–54 µmol/L (SI units) 6 years to 18 years old: 0.4–1.2 mg/dl; 36–106 µmol/L (SI units)
Fasting blood sugar (FBS)	70–110 mg/dl (serum) 60–100 mg/dl (blood)	Newborn: 30–80 mg/dl Child: 60–100 mg/dl
Feasting blood sugar (see postprandial blood sugar)		
Folate (folic acid; may be done by Nuclear Medicine)	5–20 ng/ml (bioassay) > 2.5 ng/ml (RIA; serum) > 140 ng/ml (RBC)	Same as adult
Gamma-glutamyl transpeptidase (GGTP)	Male: 10–38 IU/L Female: 5–25 IU/L; 5–40 U/L at 37°C (SI units)	
Gastrin (may be done by Nuclear Medicine)	40–200 pg/ml	
Glucose-6-phosphate dehydrogenase (G-6-PD; may be done in Hematology)	4.3–11.8 IU/g (Hb) 125–281 U/dl (packed RBC) 251–511 U/dl (cells) 1211–2111 mIU/ml (packed RBC)	Not usually done Same as adult
Glucose—fasting blood sugar (see fasting blood sugar)		

(continued)

Chemistry

Chemistry	Normal Range		
	Adult		**Children**
	Serum (mg/dl)		**Child (6 years or older)**

Glucose tolerance test (GTT)

Time	Serum (mg/dl)	Blood (mg/dl)	
Fasting	70–110	60–100	Same as adult
0.5 hr	<160	<150	
1 hr	<170	<160	
2 hr	<125	<115	
3 hr	Fasting level	Fasting level	

Immunoglobulins (see serology)

Iron — 50–150 µg/dl
- Newborn: 100–200 µg/dl
- 6 months to 2 years: 40–100 µg/dl

Iron-binding capacity (IBC, TIBC) — 250–450 µg/dl
- Newborn: 60–175 µg/dl
- Infant (6 months to 2 years): 100–350 µg/dl
- Child: same as adult

Lactic dehydrogenase (LDH or LD)
- 150–450 U/ml (Wroblewski-LaDue method)
- 60–120 U/ml (Wacker method)
- 70–200 IU/L
- Newborn: 300–1500 IU/L
- Child: 50–150 IU/L

LDH isoenzymes
- LDH_1 — 17–27%
- LDH_2 — 27–37%
- LDH_3 — 18–25%
- LDH_4 — 3–8%
- LDH_5 — 0–5%

Lead — 10–20 µg/dl
- 20–40 µg/dl (acceptable)
- 10–20 µg/dl
- 20–30 µg/dl (acceptable)

Lecithin/sphingomyelin ratio (L/S; amniotic fluid)
- 1:1 before 35 weeks of gestation
- L: 6–9 mg/dl
- S: 4–6 mg/dl
- 4:1 after 35 weeks of gestation
- L: 15–21 mg/dl
- S: 4–6 mg/dl

Leucine aminopeptidase (LAP)
- Male: 80–200 U/ml; 19.2–28 U/L (SI units)
- Female: 75–185 U/ml;
- 18–44.4 U/L (SI units)

Lipase
- 0–1.5 U/ml
- 14–280 mIU/ml
- 14–280 U/L (SI units)
- Infant: 9–105 IU/L at 37°C
- Child: 20–136 IU/L at 37°C

Lipoproteins (see cholesterol, phospholipids, and triglycerides	
Lithium	0
	Therapeutic: 0.5–1.5 mEq/L
Magnesium (Mg)	1.5–2.5 mEq/L
	Newborn: 1.4–2.9 mEq/L
	Child: 1.6–2.6 mEq/L
Osmolality	280–300 mOsm/kg/H_2O
	270–290 mOsm/kg/H_2O
Phospholipids	150–380 mg/dl
Phosphorus (P; inorganic)	1.7–2.6 mEq/L
	Newborn: 3.5–8.6 mg/dl
	2.5–4.5 mg/dl
	Infant: 4.5–6.7 mg/dl
	Child: 4.5–5.5 mg/dl
Postprandial blood sugar (feasting; PPBS)	<140 mg/dl 2 hr (plasma)
	Same as adult
	<120 mg/dl 2 hr (blood)
	Older adult: <160 mg/dl 2 hr (plasma);
	<140 mg/dl 2 hr (blood)
Potassium (K)	3.5–5.0 mEq/L
	Infant: 3.6–5.8 mEq/L
	Child: 3.5–5.5 mEq/L
Protein	6.0–8.0 g/dl
	Premature: 4.2–7.6 g/dl
	Newborn: 4.6–7.4 g/dl
	Infant: 6.0–6.7 g/dl
	Child: 6.2–8.0 g/dl
Protein electrophoresis	Albumin: 3.5–5.0 g/dl;
	52–68% of total protein
	Premature: 3.0–4.2 g/dl
	Newborn: 3.5–5.4 g/dl
	Infant: 4.4–5.4 g/dl
	Globulin: 1.5–3.5 g/dl;
	Child: 4.0–5.8 g/dl
	32–48% of total protein
Renin (may be done by Nuclear Medicine)	0.4–4.5 ng/ml/hr
Salicylate	0
	Not usually done
	Therapeutic: 15–30 mg/dl
	0
Sodium (Na)	135–145 mEq/L
	Infant: 134–150 mEq/L
	135–145 mmol/L (SI units)
	Child: 135–145 mEq/L
T_3 resin uptake (triiodothyronine; may be done by Nuclear Medicine)	110–220 ng/dl
	Not usually done
	25–35 relative % uptake
Testosterone	Male: 0.3–1.0 μg/dl; 300–1000 ng/dl
	Male adolescent: > 0.1 μg/dl
	Female: 0.03–0.1 μg/dl; 30–100 ng/dl
	Male (12–14 years old): > 100 ng/dl

(continued)

355

	Normal Range	
	Adult	**Children**
Chemistry		
Thyroxine (T₄; may be done by Nuclear Medicine)	4.5–11.5 μg/dl (T₄ by column)	Newborn: 11–23 μg/dl
	6.0–11.8 μg/dl (Murphy–Pattee)	1–4 months; 7.5–16.5 μg/dl
	5–12 μg/dl (T₄ RIA)	4–12 months: 5.5–14.5 μg/dl
	1.0–2.3 ng/dl	1–6 years old: 5.5–13.5 μg/dl
		6–10 years old: 5–12.5 μg/dl
Triglycerides	10–190 mg/dl	Infant: 5–40 mg/dl
Uric acid	0.11–2.09 mmol/L (SI units)	Child: Same as adult
	Male: 3.5–7.8 mg/dl	2.5–5.5 mg/dl
	Female: 2.8–6.8 mg/dl	
Serology		
Antinuclear antibodies (ANA)	Negative	Negative
Antistreptolysin O (ASO)	<160 U/dl (Todd units)	Newborn: similar to mother's
		Infant: <60 U/dl
		Preschool: <150 U/dl
		School age: <200 U/dl
Carcinoembryonic antigen (CEA; may be done by Nuclear Medicine)	<2.5 ng/ml	Not usually done
Cold agglutinins (CA)	1:8 antibody titer	Same as adult
Complement C3	Male: 80–180 mg/dl	Not usually done
	Female: 76–120 mg/dl	
	Blacks: 90–220 mg/dl	
Complement C4	Male: 15–60 mg/dl	Not usually done
	Female: 15–52 mg/dl	
	Blacks: 16–66 mg/dl	
C-reactive protein (CRP)	0	0
Cryoglobulins	Negative	Negative
Febrile agglutinins	Febrile group: titers	Same as adult
	Brucella: <1:20	
	Tularemia: <1:40	
	Salmonella: <1:40	
	Proteus: <1:40	
FTA–ABS (fluorescent treponemal antibody absorption)	Negative	Negative
Haptoglobin	60–270 mg/dl	Newborn: 0–10 mg/dl
	0.6–2.7 g/L (SI units)	Infant: 1–6 months: 0–30 mg/dl, then gradual increase

Test	Normal value	Children	
Hepatitis B surface antigen (HBsAg; may be done by Nuclear Medicine)	Negative	Negative	
Heterophile antibody	<1:28 titer		

Immunoglobulins (Ig)		Same as adult	
		1–3 years old	7–11 years old
Total Ig	900–2200 mg/dl		
IgG	800–1800 mg/dl	400–1500 mg/dl	700–1700 mg/dl
IgA	100–400 mg/dl	300–1400 mg/dl	600–1450 mg/dl
IgM	50–150 mg/dl	20–150 mg/dl	50–200 mg/dl
IgD	0.5–3 mg/dl	20–100 mg/dl	30–120 mg/dl

Test	Normal value	Children
Rheumatoid factor (RF)	<1:20 titer	Not usually done
RPR (rapid plasma reagin)	Negative	Negative
Rubella antibody detection (HAI or HI)	<1:8 titer susceptible	Same as adult
	1:8–1:32 titer, past rubella exposure	
	1:32–1:64 titer, immunity	
	> 1:64 titer, definite immunity	
Thyroid antibodies (TA; may be done by Nuclear Medicine)	Negative or <1:20 titer	Not usually done
VDRL (venereal disease research laboratory)	Negative	Negative

Microbiology

Test	Normal value	Children
Antibiotic susceptibility (sensitivity)	Sensitive to antibiotic	Same as adult
	Intermediate to antibiotic	
	Resistant to antibiotic	
Cultures (blood, sputum, stool, throat, wound, and urine)	No pathogen	Same as adult
Fungal organisms (mycotic infections)	No pathogen or under 8	Same as adult
Malarial smear	Negative	Negative
Occult blood (feces)	Negative	Negative
Parasites and ova (feces)	Negative	Negative

Urine Chemistry

Test	Normal value	Children
Aldosterone	6–25 µg/24 hr	Not usually done
Amylase	35–260 somogyi U/hr	Not usually done
	6.5–48.1 U/L (SI units)	
	260–950 Somogyi U/24 hr	
Ascorbic acid tolerance (4, 5, or 6 hr sample)	Oral: 10% of administered amount	Not usually done
	IV: 30–40% of administered amount	

(continued)

Urine Chemistry

Urine Chemistry	Normal Range	
	Adult	**Children**
Bence–Jones protein	Negative to trace	Same as adult
Bilirubin and bile	Negative to 0.02 mg/dl	Same as adult
Calcium (Ca)	100–250 mg/24 hr (average calcium diet) 2.50–6.25 mmol/24 hr	Same as adult
Catecholamines	<100µg/24 hr <0.59 µmol/24 hr (SI units)	Lower level than adult—weight difference
Epinephrine	0–14 µg/dl (random) <10 ng/24 hr	
Norepinephrine	<100 ng/24 hr	
Creatinine clearance	100–120 ml/min	
Creatinine	Male: 20–26 mg/kg/24 hr; 0.18–0.23 mmol/kg/24 hr (SI units) Female: 14–22 mg/kg/24 hr; 0.12–0.19 mmol/kg/24 hr (SI units)	Male: 98–150 ml/min Female: 95–123 ml/min
Estriol (E_3)	Pregnant: 10–30 mg/24 hr (30–32 weeks); 12–46 mg/24 hr (34–36 weeks); 18–60 mg/24 hr (38–40 weeks)	Not usually done
Estrogens (total)	Preovulation: 5–25 µg/24 hr Follicular phase: 24–100 µg/24 hr Luteal phase (menstruation): 12–80 µg/24 hr Postmenopause: 0–10 µg/24 hr Male: 4–25 µg/24 hr	Same as adult (postpuberty)
Follicle-stimulating hormone (FSH)	6–50 MUU/24 hr > 50 MUU/24 hr (postmenopausal)	<10 MUU/24 hr (prepubertal)
Human chorionic gonadotropin (HCG)	Positive for pregnancy: no agglutination Negative for pregnancy: agglutination	Usually not done
17-Hydroxycorticosteroids (17-OHCS)	Male: 5–15 mg/24 hr Female: 3–13 mg/24 hr	Lower than adult range
5-Hydroxyindolacetic acid (5-HIAA)	Random: negative 24 hr: 2–10 mg/24 hr	Usually not done
Ketone bodies (acetone)	Negative	Negative
17-Ketosteroids (17-KS)	Male: 8–25 mg/24 hr Female: 5–15 mg/24 hr > 65 years: 4–8 mg/24 hr	Infant: 1 mg/24 hr 1–3 years: <2 mg/24 hr 3–6 years: <3 mg/24 hr

17-Ketosteroids (17-KS) CONT.	7–10 years: <4 mg/24 hr
	10–12 years:
	  Male:<6 mg/24 hr
	  Female: <5 mg/24 hr
	Adolescent:
	  Male: <3–15 mg/24 hr
	  Female: <3–12 mg/24 hr

Osmolality	50–1200 mOsm/kg/H_2O Average: 200–800 mOsm/kg/H_2O

Phenylketonuria (PKU)	Not usually done
	Newborn: 100–600 mOsm/kg/H_2O
	Child: same as adult
	PKU: negative (positive when serum
	  phenylalanine is 12–15 mg/dl)
	Guthrie: negative (positive when serum
	  phenylalanine is 4 mg/dl)

Porphobilinogen	Random: negative 24 hr: 0–1 mg/24 hr
	Same as adult
Porphyrins Coproporphyrins	Random: 3–20 μg/dl 24 hr: 50–160 μg
Uroporphyrins	Random: negative
Potassium (K)	25–120 mEq/24 hr 25–120 mmol/24 hr (SI units)	0–80 μg/24 hr
		10–30 μg/24 hr
		Same as adult

Pregnanediol	Male: 0.1–1.5 mg/24 hr
	Female: 0.5–1.5 mg/24 hr (proliferative phase);
	  2–7 mg/24 hr (luteal phase); 0.1–1.0 mg/24 hr
	  (postmenopausal)
		0.4–1.0 mg/24 hr

Pregnanetriol	Male: 0.4–2.4 mg/24 hr Female: 0.5–2.0 mg/24 hr
Sodium (Na)	40–220 mEq/24 hr	Infant: 0–0.2 mg/24 hr Child: 0–1.0 mg/24 hr
Uric acid	251–751 mg/24 hr (low-purine diet)	Same as adult
Urinalysis		Same as adult
pH	4.5–8
Specific gravity (SG)	1.005–1.030	Newborn: 5–7 Child: 4.5–8
		Newborn: 1.001–1.020 Child: same as adult
Protein	Negative	Negative
Glucose	Negative	Negative

(continued)

	Normal Range	
	Adult	**Children**
Urine Chemistry		
Ketones	Negative	Negative
RBC	1–2/low-power field	Rare
WBC	3–4	0–4
Casts	Occasional hyaline	Rare
Urobilinogen	Random: 0.3–3.5 mg/dl	Same as adult
	0.05–2.5 mg/24 hr	
	0.5–4.0 Ehrlich units/24 hr	
	0.09–4.23 µmol/24 hr (SI units)	
Vanilmandelic acid (VMA)	1.5–7.5 mg/24 hr	Same as adult
	7.6–37.9 µmol/24 hr (SI units)	
Others		
Arterial blood gases (ABGs)		
pH:	7.35–7.45	7.36–7.44
PCO_2	35–45 mmHg	Same as adult
PO_2	75–100 mmHg	Same as adult
HCO_3	24–28 mEq/L	Same as adult
BE	+2 to −2 (± 2 mEq/L)	Same as adult
Cerebrospinal fluid (CSF)		
Pressure	75–175 mmH$_2$O	50–100 mmH$_2$O
Cell count	0–8 mm^3	0–8 mm^3
Protein	15–45 mg/dl	15–45 mg/dl
Chloride	118–132 mEq/L	120–128 mEq/L
Glucose	40–80 mg/dl	35–75 mg/dl
Culture	No organism	No organism
Chloride (sweat)	<60 mEq/L	<50 mEq/L
	60–150 mil/ml	Not usually done
Semen examination	Volume: 1.5–5.0 ml	
	Morphology: > 75% mature spermatozoa	
	Motility: > 60% actively mobile spermatozoa	

Index